Physical Activity Across the Lifespan

Issues in Children's and Families' Lives

Series Editors:

Thomas P. Gullotta, *Child and Family Agency of Southeastern Connecticut,*
New London, Connecticut
Herbert J. Walberg, *University of Illinois at Chicago, Chicago, Illinois*
Roger P. Weissberg, *University of Illinois at Chicago, Chicago, Illinois*

For other titles published in this series, go to
http://www.springer.com/series/6110

A Continuation Order Plan is available for this series. A continuation order will bring
delivery of each new volume immediately upon publication. Volumes are billed only
upon actual shipment. For further information please contact the publisher.

Aleta L. Meyer · Thomas P. Gullotta
Editors

Jessica M. Ramos
Research Assistant

Physical Activity Across the Lifespan

Prevention and Treatment for Health and Well-Being

A Sponsored Publication of the Child & Family Agency of Southeastern Connecticut

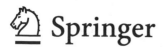 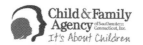 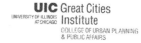

Editors
Aleta L. Meyer
Office of Planning, Research,
  and Evaluation
Administration for Children and Families
Washington, DC, USA

Thomas P. Gullotta
Child and Family Agency of Southeastern
  Connecticut
New London, CT 06320, USA

ISSN 1572-1981
ISBN 978-1-4614-3605-8   ISBN 978-1-4614-3606-5 (eBook)
DOI 10.1007/978-1-4614-3606-5
Springer New York Heidelberg Dordrecht London

Library of Congress Control Number: 2012939063

Printed on acid-free paper

Springer is part of Springer Science+Business Media (www.springer.com)

This volume is dedicated to Elizabeth Ann Fries, whose scientific efforts to seek ways to address multiple health outcomes together continue to inspire.

Preface

Putting the Volume in Context

This book was written during the Obama administration, an administration with a focus on universal health care. While the bulk of this policy discussion centers on strategies for containing costs and making affordable treatment available, there is a small undercurrent taking into consideration such questions as "What can be done to prevent the chronic diseases that drive most health care costs?" and "How can we best prepare for unpredictable adversities that pose challenges to physical and mental health, such as new strains of influenza, natural disasters, and war?" Responses to these questions often focus on lifestyle behaviors that promote physical and mental health, increase immune function, and protect against injury. From both a treatment and prevention standpoint, primary among the lifestyle behaviors that could have the biggest impact on health care costs are avoiding tobacco, eating nutritious foods, and being physically active (National Center for Chronic Disease and Health Promotion, 2009). This book focuses on the last of these—physical activity—and the role it might play in treatment and prevention across multiple areas of health, from chronic disease to mental health.

Social commentary on how the United States has gotten itself into such a conundrum regarding the health of its citizens often includes reflection on how human beings have had the same biology for thousands of years, yet the way that Americans use their bodies has changed significantly in the past 50 years. While our bodies, well suited to the hunter-gatherer lifestyle, have not changed, our lifestyles have. In an examination of recent secular changes in physical activity in Australia, researchers used triaxial accelerometers to compare the activity levels of actors who were paid to live like early Australian settlers to a group of present-day sedentary office workers (Egger, Vogels, & Westerperp, 2001). They found a difference in daily activity levels equivalent to walking 6–18 km (e.g., 5–10 miles) per day between previous and modern times (Egger et al., 2001). Given the likelihood that this shift toward a sedentary lifestyle was not an intentional goal in and of itself, but rather a product of larger changes in the culture toward expediency and convenience, some public health experts have noted that it will take much more than the motivation of individuals to produce enduring changes that promote health (Farley & Cohen, 2005; Orleans, Gruman, Ulmer, Emont, & Hollendonner, 1999). In other words, increasing physical activity is much easier said than done.

While substantial evidence has established that a sedentary lifestyle combined with an unhealthy diet contributes to premature deaths (e.g., McGinnis & Foege, 1993), the amount of evidence indicating that physical activity can function as treatment and/or prevention varies greatly across and within health outcomes (National Center for Chronic Disease and Health Promotion, 2009). The recent physical activity guidelines weigh the evidence across many health outcomes, including all-cause mortality, cardiorespiratory health, metabolic health, energy balance, musculoskeletal health, functional health, cancer, and mental health. For example, studies of the impact of increased physical activity for individuals with Type I or Type II diabetes indicate reduced macrovascular complications for those with Type II (e.g., Hu et al., 2004), yet any exercise prescription in Type I diabetes must address the issue of avoiding exercise-induced hypoglycemia (Durak, Jovanovic-Peterson, & Peterson, 1990). In the area of cardiorespiratory health, exercise training has been found to be an effective secondary preventive measure for those with established peripheral arterial disease (e.g., Killewich, Macko, Montgomery, Wiley, & Gardner, 2004; Tsai et al., 2002). In terms of primary prevention, lifestyle interventions that increase physical activity and promote modest weight loss have been shown to prevent coronary heart disease in men (e.g., Chiuve, McCullough, Sacks, & Rimm, 2006) and in women (Stampfer, Hu, Manson, Rimm, & Willet, 2000) and to prevent Type II diabetes in those at heightened risk, substantially outperforming medications used for that purpose (e.g., Tuomilehto et al., 2001). In contrast, little is known about the role of physical activity in drug use and it is not included as a primary health outcome of interest in the recent physical activity guidelines (Physical Activity Guidelines Advisory Committee, 2008).

Given the dearth of scientific information regarding physical activity and drug use, in June of 2008, the National Institute on Drug Abuse (NIDA) held a science meeting to explore the potential role of physical activity in preventing drug use and addiction. The meeting was designed to build on existing knowledge regarding physical activity and health; many of the presentations drew from physical activity research on depression and obesity, disorders that can co-occur and/or have shared etiologies with substance use and addiction. After the meeting, it was clear that while some of the knowledge gaps identified during this meeting should be tackled through new scientific inquiry, other gaps could be attended to through methodical and innovative application of existing data and wisdom. Subsequent to the meeting, to deal with gaps in the science base regarding the interaction between physical activity and drug use, NIDA issued a funding opportunity announcement to promote a full range of new science, from clinical neuroscience and epidemiology to treatment and prevention. As a parallel activity, we proposed this volume to establish a benchmark of what is known and what avenues to explore toward using physical activity to promote health and to prevent disease, particularly as it relates to depression, obesity, and drug use.

Broadly speaking, three ways to think about physical activity as a strategy for prevention and treatment include: (1) physical activity as an end in itself (e.g., Physical Activity Guidelines Advisory Committee, 2008), (2) physical activity as an experiential approach to learning (e.g., Dewey, 1938) and/or intervention theory (e.g., Kellam, Koretz, & Moscicki, 1999), and (3) physical activity as a fundamental component of key social activities that promote human development, such as work and play (e.g., Vgotsky, 1978). In the first approach where physical activity is viewed as an end in itself, prevention and treatment strategies focus on the physiological and mechanical enhancements that occur to tissue and organ function within the body as a result of physical activity. This focus emphasizes aspects of physical activity such as duration, intensity, and strength building. The aforementioned research studies focused on Type I and Type II diabetes are an example of this way of thinking about physical activity.

A second way of thinking about physical activity as an intervention strategy is to consider its potential as an experiential approach to doing the "work" of an intervention. Whereas most interventions are comprised didactic educational approaches aimed at building knowledge and skills, an experiential approach uses intentional experiences to provide concrete opportunities for behavioral enactment and rehearsal, immediate feedback, and reinforcement. More importantly, experiential approaches can evoke strong emotions that help facilitate engagement and recollection of learned skills in new environments. Sports programs that provide training to coaches to plan ahead for "teachable moments" in conflict resolution skills and emotion regulation are an example of thinking about physical activity as an experiential approach to intervention design.

A third way to think about physical activity as treatment or prevention is to consider the primary role of physical activity in endeavors such as work and play. While conveniences and technology have reduced the amount of physical effort that needs to go into a daily routine such as preparing a meal (e.g., instead of needing to gather and prepare food, going to the freezer and pulling out a prepared meal for the microwave), it is important to take into account the additional benefits one received when preparing a meal, above and beyond the nutritional content of the food. Included in the benefits of preparing a meal for others are the development of competencies such as the fine motor skills necessary for using knives and utensils properly, the physical strength and judgment needed to build and maintain a fire, the time-management skills needed to make sure things are ready at the same time, and the ability to recall and utilize memories of having observed another person make what you are preparing. Taking such an approach, one could argue that conveniences deprive humans of "old-fashioned" hard work and play, thus contributing to high levels of chronic disease and mental health problems as seen in modern culture. Moreover, when competencies such as time management and physical strength are taught as stand-alones, without a context such as play or work, this viewpoint argues their potency as intervention is diluted. Intervention approaches that emphasize the reinstatement of physical activity into daily activity, such as gardening and walking to work, are examples of viewing physical activity's therapeutic and preventive aspects as embedded within normative contexts such as play and work.

Overview of Chapters

Our hope for this volume is that students, practitioners, and researchers who read these chapters will move beyond contemplating physical activity as a potent tool for promoting health and preventing disease to acting on that potential through their professional efforts. To facilitate this, we have organized the volume in three sections: Setting the Stage (Chaps. 1–4); Physical Activity as Treatment and Prevention (Chaps. 5–10); and Real-World Applications (Chaps. 11 and 12). To set the stage, the first section provides in-depth explorations into the topic of physical activity. In Chap. 1, Augusto Diana articulates the varied ways in which physical activity is defined and knowledge gaps related to those various ways of defining physical activity. In Chap. 2, Jaak Panksepp and Eric Scott offer their reflections on the implications of society changing away from natural ways of living toward highly structured ways of living, with a focus on the central role of rough and tumble play for social development in early childhood, including considerations of the ways rough and tumble play might address attention-deficit hyperactivity disorders (ADHD). In the third chapter, Darla Castelli and Charles Hillman provide a detailed description, from neurons to neighborhoods, of the ways that physical activity affects school performance through its influence on cognition. In Chap. 4, Fuzhong Li takes a look at physical activity later in the lifespan by examining the roles of social and built environments on physical activity in middle-aged and older adults.

The second section is organized around the simple yet complex task of delving into the ways that physical activity could function as part of treatment and prevention for three health areas: depression, obesity, and substance use. For each of these chapters, we asked the authors to consider theoretical and empirical support for physical activity as intervention in that area, to describe existing research on the effectiveness of such approaches, to provide suggestions for practitioners, and to identify areas for future research. Lynette Craft starts off this section with Chap. 5 by providing an examination of theory and research that support physical activity as treatment for depression. In Chap. 6, coauthors Bethany Kwan, Kyle Davis, and Andrea Dunn discuss how physical activity might be used to prevent depression. With Chap. 7, Elissa Jelalian and Amy Sato continue this endeavor by describing physical activity as treatment for obesity. In Chap. 8, Nicole Zarrett and Dawn Wilson illustrate the opportunities for physical activity as obesity prevention. In Chap. 9, coauthors Dori Pekmezi, Lucas Carr, Brook Barbera, and Bess Marcus explain the role that physical activity can play in the treatment of substance use disorders. In closing to this section, coauthors Aleta Meyer, Augusto Diana, and Elizabeth Robertson present research and theory in support of the potential of physical activity for drug abuse prevention, with a focus on its potential for promoting self-regulation in early childhood and adolescence.

In the final chapters, specific applications for increasing levels of physical activity and sustaining that change over time are provided. In Chap. 11, coauthors Kyle Davis, Samuel Hubley, and Jenn Leiferman provide specific guidance on behavior change strategies that can promote physical activity for individuals. In Chap. 12, coauthors John Ratey and Jacob Sattelmair present a mandate for movement through explicating the specific ways that schools can serve as agents of change to promote health at a population level. In the Epilogue, Thomas Gullotta and Aleta Meyer offer their reflections on next steps for applying what is known about physical activity as treatment, prevention, and a way of living, as well as for building the knowledge base about physical activity.

Momentarily, the reader's journey through this book will begin. Encouragingly, active living is a positive health promotion activity with significant demonstrable results for those with obesity. The benefits appear helpful and awaiting more evidence may be significant in preventing depression or its reoccurrence. Tantalizing threads of evidence gleaned from animal studies and case reports suggest that active living may be a positive intervention assisting in a child's proper brain development and in the treatment and relapse prevention of substance abusers. Across all of these health outcomes, it appears that physical activity could provide an effective booster for enacting the active ingredients of an intervention. For the professionals and graduate students in psychology, education, social work, and allied health fields who will read this book, we urge you to grab those interventions proven to work and use them. More importantly, though, is to actively investigate and push forward programmatically promising approaches for the treatment and prevention of obesity, depression, drug abuse, and ADHD. Real progress in the field of treatment and prevention awaits your findings. For policy makers and government officials, this book should be taken seriously. It offers the possibility of significantly less-expensive interventions, including changes to the built and social environment, that may prove to be as effective as and more sustainable than programs currently in use. Supporting the implementation and research to determine the effectiveness of this programming and environmental change is money well spent.

Washington, DC, USA
New London, CT, USA

Aleta L. Meyer
Thomas P. Gullotta

References

Chiuve, S. E., McCullough, M. L., Sacks, F. M., & Rimm, E. B. (2006). Healthy lifestyle factors in the primary prevention of coronary heart disease among men. *Circulation, 114*(2), 160–167.

Dewey, J. (1938). *Experience and education.* New York: Collier.

Durak, E. P., Jovanovic-Peterson, L., & Peterson, C. M. (1990). Randomized crossover study of effect of resistance training on glycemic control, muscular strength, and cholesterol in type I diabetic men. *Diabetes Care,* October 13, (10), 1039–1043.

Egger, G., Vogels, N., & Westerperp, K. (2001). Estimating historical changes in physical activity levels. *Medical Journal of Australia, 175,* 635–636.

Farley, T., & Cohen, D. (2005). *Prescription for a healthy nation: A new approach to improving our lives by fixing our everyday world.* Boston, MA: Beacon.

Hu, G., Eriksson, J., Barengo, N. C., Lakka, T. A., Valle, T. T., Nissinen, A., et al. (2004). Occupational, commuting, and leisure-time physical activity in relation to total and cardiovascular mortality among Finnish subjects with type 2 diabetes. *Circulation,* August 10, 110(6), 666–673.

Kellam, S., Koretz, D., & Moscicki, E. (1999). Core elements of developmental epidemiologically based prevention research. *American Journal of Community Psychology,* 27(4), 463–482.

Killewich, L. A., Macko, R. F., Montgomery, P. S., Wiley, L. A., & Gardner, A. W. (2004). Exercise training enhances endogenous fibrinolysis in peripheral arterial disease. *Journal of Vascular Surgery.* October, 40(4), 741–745.

McGinnis, J., & Foege, W. (1993). Actual causes of death in the U.S. *Journal of the American Medical Association,* 270, 2207–2212.

National Center for Chronic Disease and Health Promotion. (2009). *Chronic diseases: The power to prevent, the call to control. At a glance 2009.* Washington, DC: U.S. Department of Health and Human Services. Retrieved November 11, 2011, from http://cdc.gov/nccdphp/publications/AAG/chronic.htm.

Orleans, C., Gruman, J., Ulmer, C., Emont, S., & Hollendonner, J. (1999). Rating our progress in population health promotion: Report card on six behaviors. *American Journal of Health Promotion,* 14, 75–82.

Physical Activity Guidelines Advisory Committee. (2008). *Physical activity guidelines advisory committee report.* Washington, DC: U.S. Department of Health and Human Services. Retrieved November 11, 2011, from http://www.health.gov/paguidelines/committeereport.aspx.

Stampfer, M. J., Hu, F. B., Manson, J. E., Rimm, E. B., & Willet, W. C. (2000). Primary prevention of coronary heart disease in women through diet and lifestyle. *New England Journal of Medicine,* 343(3), 16–22.

Tsai, J. C., Chan, P., Wang, C. H., Jeng, C., Hsieh, M. H., Kao, P. F., et al. (2002). The effects of exercise training on walking function and perception of health status in elderly patients with peripheral arterial occlusive disease. *Journal of Internal Medicine,* November, 252(5), 448–455.

Tuomilehto, J., Lindstrom, J., Eriksson, J. G., Valle, T., Hamalainen, H., Ilanne-Parikka, P. et al. (2001). Prevention of type 2 diabetes mellitus by changes in lifestyle among subjects with impaired glucose tolerance. *The New England Journal of Medicine,* 344, 1343–1350.

Vgotsky, L. (1978). *Mind in Society.* Cambridge, MA: Harvard University Press.

Contents

WITHDRAWN

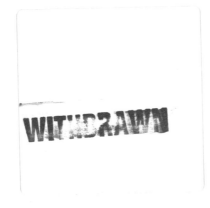

About the Editors

Aleta L. Meyer, Ph.D., is President of Prevention Opportunities, LLC, and is a senior social science research analyst at the Administration for Children and Families, in the Office of Planning, Research and Evaluation, in the Division of Child and Family Development. From 2007 to 2010, she was a health scientist administrator in the Prevention Research Branch at the National Institute on Drug Abuse (NIDA). Prior to joining NIDA, she was an Associate Professor of Psychology in the Clark-Hill Institute for Positive Youth Development at Virginia Commonwealth University. From 1994 to 1996, she was a Gimbel Child and Family Scholar. She completed her doctoral work in Human Development and Family Studies at The Pennsylvania State University. The focus of her research has been to translate theory and empirical research across multiple health outcomes into effective and feasible health promotion and prevention programs for early adolescents.

Thomas P. Gullotta, M.A., M.S.W., L.C.S.W., is the C.E.O. of Child and Family Agency and a member of the psychology and education departments at Eastern Connecticut State University. His scholarship encompasses coauthorship of two college textbooks, the founding editorship of *The Journal of Primary Prevention* (Kluwer/Academic 1980–2000), coeditor of *Advances in Adolescent Development: An Annual Book Series* (Sage 1985–2000), editor of *Prevention in Practice Library: A Monograph Series* (Plenum, 1996–2001), and senior editor of *Issues in Childrens' and Families' Lives: A Book Series* (Springer 1990–present). In addition to authoring nearly 100 chapters, papers, or reviews, he has coedited or authored over 30 volumes devoted to illness prevention/promotion of health or the treatment of children, adolescents, and families. Tom was the senior editor for the first edition of the Encyclopedia of Primary Prevention and Health Promotion (Kluwer/Academic, 2003) and has returned to that same role for the anticipated four volume second edition of that reference work (Springer, in progress). His most recent edited volume with Bob Hampton, *Handbook of African American Health* (Guilford, 2010), was recently recognized by the *American Journal of Nursing* as the most valuable text of 2010 in the category Community Public Health.

About the Authors

Brooke Barbera, Ph.D., is a postdoctoral fellow at The NeuroMedical Center in Baton Rouge, Louisiana. Her degree is in Clinical Psychology with an emphasis on behavioral medicine. Dr. Barbera's research focuses on obesity and pain, the impact of surgical treatment for obesity, and physical activity promotion. Her current clinical emphases include the assessment and treatment of psychopathology among patients with various neurodegenerative disorders.

Dr. Lucas J. Carr, Ph.D., is an Assistant Professor in the Department of Kinesiology at East Carolina University in Greenville, NC. Dr. Carr received a master's degree in Exercise Physiology and doctoral degree in Physiology from the University of Wyoming. He also completed a postdoctoral fellowship in Cardiovascular Behavioral Medicine at The Miriam Hospital and Brown University in Providence, RI. Dr. Carr's current research focuses on both the physiological and psychosocial health benefits of reducing sedentary behaviors and increasing physical activity behavior.

Darla M. Castelli, Ph.D., has been working with school-age youth in physical activity settings for over 20 years. Since 2002, she has been investigating the effects of physical activity and fitness on motor competency and cognitive health in children. Recently Darla was asked to present her work at a US Congressional and Senate Briefings in Washington, DC as a means of supporting the Fit Kids Act. For her role in this research, Darla was named a 2006 Young Scholar by the International Association of Physical Education in Higher Education (AIESEP), 2007 Illinois Association for Health, Physical Education, Recreation, and Dance (IAHPERD) Past-Presidents' Scholar, and a Fellow in the AAHPERD Research Consortium. Her research has been funded by the National Institutes of Health and US Department of Education. She enjoys spending time with her two children, Brian and Abby, as well as participating in a variety of physical activities.

Dr. Lynette L. Craft, Ph.D., is an Assistant Professor in the Department of Preventive Medicine, Feinberg School of Medicine, at Northwestern University. Dr. Craft completed her Ph.D. in Kinesiology from Michigan State University and a postdoctoral fellowship in Health Psychology from Boston University School of Medicine.

Dr. Craft's area of specialization is Exercise Psychology, with a secondary focus on Exercise Physiology and Epidemiology. Her research expertise is in the use of exercise as an adjunct to traditional treatments for clinical depression and the mechanisms underlying the exercise–depression relationship. This has included studies examining psychosocial factors predictive of exercise participation among depressed women, the use of home and facility based exercise interventions to alleviate depressive symptoms, and studies examining psychological factors that moderate the exercise–depression relationship. In addition, Dr. Craft studies the effect of exercise on cancer-related symptoms and quality of life in breast cancer survivors.

Kyle J. Davis, M.A., a fourth year Clinical Psychology graduate student at the University of Colorado, is at the beginning of a research career focusing on the relationship between physical activity and mood. Specific interests include the relationship between physical activity and self-efficacy in the treatment of depression as well as the relationship between physical activity and mood in underrepresented populations. Kyle enjoys rock climbing, snowboarding, cycling, and hiking to help regulate his own mood.

Dr. Augusto Diana, Ph.D., began as a Health Scientist Administrator in the Prevention Research Branch (PRB) in April, 2006. At NIDA, Augie is overseeing Small Business Innovation Research/Small Business Technology Transfer grants, which focus primarily on the use of technology in developing products to enhance access and widespread use of effective prevention strategies. In addition, Augie has been working to build a portfolio of research focused on physical activity's potential as a prevention intervention. Prior to joining NIDA, Augie worked as a Senior Public Health Analyst at the Center for Substance Abuse Prevention (CSAP) within the Substance Abuse and Mental Health Services Administration (SAMHSA) where he oversaw CSAP's national cross-site evaluation of the Strategic Prevention Framework State Incentive Grant (SPF SIG) project, and CSAP's major data/technology initiative, the Data Coordination and Consolidation Center (DCCC). Dr. Diana received his Ph.D. in Sociology from Northeastern University and his undergraduate degree from Fordham University.

Dr. Andrea L. Dunn, Ph.D., is a Senior Scientist at Klein Buendel, Inc. Her research focuses on behavioral interventions for physical activity for children and adults and on exercise as an alternative treatment for mild-to-moderate major depressive disorder. She is the author or coauthor of over 100 published peer-reviewed articles, book chapters, and abstracts. Dr. Dunn formerly served as Director, Behavioral Science Research Group at The Cooper Institute. She has an M.S. in psychology from Virginia Polytechnic Institute and a Ph.D. in Exercise Science from the University of Georgia and was a postdoctoral fellow in the Department of Psychiatry at the University of Colorado Health Sciences Center. Dr. Dunn is a Fellow and former member of the Board of Trustees of The American College of Sports Medicine, a Fellow of the Society for Behavioral Medicine and a member of the American Academy of Health Behavior.

Charles H. Hillman, Ph.D., received his bachelor's degree in psychology from the University of Miami in 1994 before earning his master's degree in Exercise and

Sport Sciences from the University of Florida in 1997. He continued his education in the Department of Kinesiology at the University of Maryland, College Park, where he received his doctorate in Cognitive Motor Behavior in 2000. Currently, he is an associate professor in the Departments of Kinesiology & Community Health, Psychology, Internal Medicine, and an affiliate of the Illinois Neuroscience Program, the Division of Nutritional Sciences, and the Beckman Institute for Advanced Science and Technology. He directs the Neurocognitive Kinesiology Laboratory at the University of Illinois at Urbana-Champaign, and his research focuses on the relationship between physical activity–exercise and neurocognitive function across the human lifespan.

Samuel Hubley, M.A., grew up in the Finger Lakes region of upstate New York, earned his bachelor's degree from Cornell University and is now a third year doctoral student in clinical psychology at the University of Colorado at Boulder. Along with Dr. Sona Dimidjian, he is working to identify mechanisms of change in behavioral activation therapy for depression and develop training paradigms for new and experienced therapists. In his spare time, Sam enjoys playing soccer, teaching kids how to ski, and trying to emulate his Food Network idols.

Dr. Elissa Jelalian, Ph.D., is an Associate Professor of Psychiatry and Human Behavior at the Alpert Medical School of Brown University and staff psychologist at The Miriam Hospital Weight Control and Diabetes Research Center and Bradley Hasbro Children's Research Center. Her research program focuses on development and implementation of weight control interventions for children and adolescents, as well as evaluation of policy to promote healthier school nutrition and physical activity environments. She is the recipient of several NIH grants evaluating weight control interventions for overweight adolescents, with a focus on peer-based physical activity and parent involvement. Dr. Jelalian has published in the areas of pediatric weight control, risk-taking and injury in adolescents, and nutrition and illness in children with chronic medical conditions.

Bethany M. Kwan, M.A., M.S.P.H., is a fifth year doctoral student in social psychology in the Department of Psychology and Neuroscience at the University of Colorado at Boulder. Her work to date includes investigations into the effectiveness of theory-based exercise interventions, adherence to antidepressant treatment, and the application of theories of judgment and decision making to health behaviors. Her current research concerns the relationship between emotions and self-regulation of exercise behavior, with an additional focus on the effects of depression on exercise behavior change.

Jenn Leiferman, Ph.D., is an Assistant Professor in the Colorado School of Public Health, Department of Behavioral and Community Health. She received a B.S. in Psychology; a M.S. in Kinesiology; and a Ph.D. in Health Education and Health Promotion. She also completed NIH NRSA postdoctoral training in population studies and epidemiology. Her research interests lie in the area of maternal and child health, focusing on parental mental health and how it affects parenting practices and child health outcomes. She is currently working at designing ways to improve the prevention, detection, and treatment of maternal depression. She has published several articles related to parental depression, parenting and health behaviors, and health services research.

Fuzhong Li, Ph.D., is a Senior Scientist at the Oregon Research Institute (ORI). He received his Ph.D. from the Oregon State University in Exercise Science and joined ORI in 1996. His research areas include falls prevention for the elderly, exercise training on balance for people with Parkinson's disease, community health promotion and research dissemination, and built environment influences on obesity and physical activity. He has published a series of papers on randomized controlled trials evaluating the effectiveness of alternative-based exercise interventions on a range of psychosocial and biomedical outcomes, and falls in older adults, as well as papers that deal with social and built environment influences on physical activity and obesity.

Bess H. Marcus, Ph.D., is a Professor of Community Health and Psychiatry and Human Behavior at the Alpert Medical School of Brown University and Director of The Centers for Behavioral and Preventive Medicine at The Miriam Hospital. She is a clinical health psychologist who has spent 20 years conducting research on physical activity behavior and has published over 175 papers and book chapters as well as four books. She developed a series of assessment instruments to measure psychosocial mediators of physical activity behavior and has also developed low-cost interventions to promote physical activity behavior in community, workplace, and primary care settings. Dr. Marcus has participated in American Heart Association, American College of Sports Medicine, Centers for Disease Control and Prevention, and National Institutes of Health panels that have created recommendations regarding the quantity and intensity of physical activity necessary for health benefits. Dr. Marcus is currently Principal Investigator or Co-investigator on 12 National Institutes of Health grants.

Jaak Panksepp, Ph.D., is a Professor and Bailey Endowed Chair of Animal Well-Being Science, College of Veterinary Medicine, Washington State University, Head of Affective Neuroscience Research at the Falk Center for Molecular Therapeutics at Northwestern University, and research codirector for the new nonprofit Hope for Depression Research Foundation. His scientific contributions include more than 400 papers devoted to the study of basic emotional and motivational processes of the mammalian brain. His recent work has focused primarily on the subcortical brain mechanisms of sadness (separation distress) and joy (play and animal laughter), work that has implications for the treatment of autism and ADHD. His work is informed by exploring the consequences of basic knowledge about emotional endophenotypes for better understanding of human mental health. His monograph Affective Neuroscience (Oxford, 1998) outlined ways to understand brain affective processes mechanistically, and his edited Textbook of Biological Psychiatry (Wiley, 2004) relates this knowledge to psychiatric issues.

Dori W. Pekmezi, Ph.D., is a postdoctoral fellow at the Centers for Behavioral and Preventive Medicine at The Miriam Hospital and the Alpert Medical School of Brown University. Her degree is in Clinical Psychology with an emphasis on behavioral medicine. Dr. Pekmezi's research focuses on physical activity promotion, primarily among underserved populations. She is currently involved in the Commit to Quit-YMCA program, which tests the efficacy of providing cognitive behavioral group treatment for smoking cessation with either a physical activity or wellness component to sedentary female smokers in a YMCA setting.

Jessica M. Ramos, B.A., received her B.A. in Psychology from Eastern Connecticut State University. She is a Research Assistant at Child and Family Agency of Southeastern Connecticut. Jessica has assisted in the editorial process of books on primary prevention, prevention and treatment of behavioral problems in childhood and adolescents, Asperger Syndrome, promotion of prosocial behavior, and interpersonal violence in the African American community. She is involved in agency research and reviews cases for Quality Assurance.

John J. Ratey, M.D., is an Associate Clinical Professor of Psychiatry at Harvard Medical School, and has a private practice in Cambridge, Massachusetts. He has lectured and published many articles on the topic of Aggression, Autism, ADHD, and other issues in neuropsychiatry. Dr. Ratey has most recently Authored "Spark: The Revolutionary New Science of Exercise and the Brain" published by Little Brown. As well, he authored "A User's Guide to the Brain" (2000). He has coauthored "Shadow Syndromes" (1997) with Catherine Johnson, Ph.D., and also coauthored "Driven to Distraction" (1994), "Answers to Distraction" (1995), and Delivered from Distraction (2005) with Edward Hallowell, M.D., all published by Pantheon Press/Random House. Additionally, he has edited several books including "The Neuropsychiatry of Personality Disorders" (1994), published by Blackwell Scientific.

Elizabeth Robertson, Ph.D., came to National Institute on Drug Abuse (NIDA) in 1995; she has served as Chief of the Prevention Research Branch (PRB) and Senior Advisor for Prevention. As Chief of PRB, Liz broadened the mission of preventing drug use initiation and progression to include a developmental focus from early childhood through adulthood and an expansive contextual focus to include contexts such as the family, the criminal justice system, social welfare systems, clinical settings, recreation, the media, and governmental and nongovernmental organizations. Over time she advanced the development of portfolios on drug-related HIV infection and the dissemination and implementation of evidence-based practices. Her published articles and book chapters on drug abuse prevention include topics such as: inhibitory control, the effects of parental incarceration children, and the contributions of social support and economic stress to family/adolescent dysfunction. She has received awards from the Society for Prevention Research, the Department of Health and Human Services, and the National Institutes for Health.

Dr. Amy Sato, Ph.D., is a T32 postdoctoral fellow at the Bradley Hasbro Children's Research Center affiliated with Alpert Medical School of Brown University and Rhode Island Hospital. She has conducted research in the area of children's and parent's psychological adjustment to chronic pediatric medical conditions. Her research interests focus on the role of parent and family factors in implementation of pediatric obesity interventions and the intersection of pediatric chronic pain and obesity. Dr. Sato has published in the areas of school absenteeism and pain, and the application of cognitive behavioral therapy via telehealth to youth with functional abdominal pain, as well as the role of social support in adjustment to Type I diabetes.

Jacob Sattelmair, B.A., M.Sc., D.Sc., is a Doctoral Candidate in Epidemiology at the Harvard School of Public Health, where he researches the impact of exercise on cardiovascular and cognitive health. He has a master's degree from the University of Oxford in the "Science and Medicine of Athletic Performance." Jacob is an avid proponent for the necessity of movement and exercise to prevent chronic disease and promote optimal physical and mental health and performance. In particular, Jacob focuses on schools, workplaces, and the use of technology as opportunities to encourage physical activity.

Eric L. Scott, Ph.D., is an Assistant Professor of Clinical Psychology in Clinical Psychiatry and the Director of the Riley Pain Center. The Center is housed within Riley Hospital for Children and affiliated with the Indiana University School of Medicine. He uses cognitive behavioral therapy, hypnosis, and biofeedback for the treatment of psychological disorders and chronic pain. Dr. Scott is also a member of the Indiana University Health Riley Pain Council involved in helping guide institutional policy regarding pain treatment and management within inpatient units and outpatient clinics. Dr. Scott also works within the Child and Adolescent Psychiatry Clinic at Riley Hospital where he specializes in Cognitive Behavioral Therapy for anxious youth. Formerly, he was a Clinical Director of the Pediatric Psychiatry Consultation-Liaison Service at Riley Hospital for Children. He received his masters' degree in Psychology from Loyola University in Chicago and then his Ph.D. in clinical psychology from Bowling Green State University.

Dr. Dawn K. Wilson, Ph.D., is a Professor of Psychology at the University of South Carolina. She completed her Ph.D. in Psychology at Vanderbilt University and a postdoctoral fellowship in Public Health at University of California, Berkeley. She is a fellow of the American Psychological Association, and the Society of Behavioral Medicine, and is a member of the Academy of Behavioral Medicine. Her expertise is in the areas of dietary modification, diabetes management, hypertension prevention, and blood pressure regulatory mechanisms in minority populations. Her NIH-funded research program is currently evaluating theoretically based community interventions for promoting physical activity and healthy lifestyles in minority populations.

Dr. Nicole Zarrett, Ph.D., is an Assistant Professor of Psychology at the University of South Carolina. She completed her Ph.D. in Developmental Psychology at the University of Michigan and a postdoctoral fellowship at the Institute for Applied Research in Youth Development at Tufts University. Her area of expertise is in developmental theories of youth motivation and choice, with a primary focus on understanding the contextual, social, and intrapersonal predictors of children's healthy developmental pathways. This research has included understanding the role of out-of-school activities, as well as community, family, peers, and intrapersonal factors for promoting youth physical activity and other indicators of adolescents' short- and long-term positive physical, psychosocial, and achievement-related functioning.

Contributors

Brooke Barbera, Ph.D. Centers for Behavioral and Preventive Medicine, The Miriam Hospital and Alpert Medical School of Brown University, Providence, RI, USA

Lucas J. Carr, Ph.D. Department of Health and Human Physiology, University of Iowa, Iowa City, IA, USA

Centers for Behavioral and Preventive Medicine, The Miriam Hospital and Alpert Medical School of Brown University, Providence, RI, USA

Darla M. Castelli, Ph.D. Department of Kinesiology and Health Education Physical Education Teacher Education, The University of Texas at Austin, Austin, TX, USA

Lynette L. Craft, Ph.D. Department of Preventive Medicine, Feinberg School of Medicine, Northwestern University, Chicago, IL, USA

Kyle J. Davis, M.A. Department of Psychology, University of Colorado, Boulder, Boulder, CO, USA

Augusto Diana, Ph.D. Division of Epidemiology, Services and Prevention Research, Prevention Research Branch, National Institute on Drug Abuse (NIDA), Bethesda, MD, USA

Andrea L. Dunn, Ph.D. Klein Buendel, Inc., Golden, CO, USA

Thomas P. Gullotta, M.A., M.S.W., L.C.S.W. Child and Family Agency of Southeastern Connecticut, New London, CT, USA

Charles H. Hillman, Ph.D. Departments of Kinesiology and Community Health, Psychology, and Internal Medicine, University of Illinois at Urbana-Champaign, Urbana, IL, USA

The Beckman Institute for Advanced Science and Technology, University of Illinois at Urbana-Champaign, Urbana, IL, USA

Division of Neuroscience, University of Illinois at Urbana-Champaign, Urbana, IL, USA

Samuel Hubley, M.A. Department of Psychology, University of Colorado, Boulder, CO, USA

Elissa Jelalian, Ph.D. Psychiatry and Human Behavior, Brown Medical School, Providence, RI, USA

Bethany M. Kwan, M.A., M.S.P.H. Colorado Health Outcomes Program, Aurora, Boulder, CO, USA

Jenn Leiferman, Ph.D. Department of Community and Behavioral Health, Colorado School of Public Health, Aurora, CO, USA

Fuzhong Li, Ph.D. Oregon Research Institute, Eugene, OR, USA

Bess H. Marcus, Ph.D. Centers for Behavioral and Preventive Medicine, The Miriam Hospital and Alpert Medical School of Brown University, Providence, RI, USA

Aleta L. Meyer, Ph.D. Office of Planning, Research, and Evaluation, Administration for Children and Families, Washington, DC, USA

Jaak Panksepp, Ph.D. Department of Veterinary Comparative Anatomy, Pharmacology and Physiology (VCAPP), Washington State University, Pullman, WA, USA

Department of Psychology, Bowling Green State University, Bowling Green, OH, USA

Dori W. Pekmezi, Ph.D. Department of Health Behavior, School of Public Health, University of Alabama at Birmingham, Birmingham, AL, USA

John J. Ratey, M.D. Harvard Medical School, Cambridge, MA, USA

Elizabeth Robertson, Ph.D. Division of Epidemiology, Services, and Prevention Research, National Institute on Drug Abuse, Bethesda, MD, USA

Amy Sato, Ph.D. Department of Psychology, Kent State University, Kent, OH, USA

Jacob Sattelmair, B.A., M.Sc., D.Sc. Department of Epidemiology, Harvard School of Public Health, Boston, MA, USA

Eric L. Scott, Ph.D. Department of Psychiatry, Indiana University Medical School, Indianapolis, IN, USA

Dawn K. Wilson, Ph.D. Department of Psychology, Barnwell College, University of South Carolina, Barnwell College, Columbia, SC, USA

Nicole Zarrett, Ph.D. Department of Psychology, Barnwell College, University of South Carolina, Columbia, SC, USA

Chapter 1
Physical Activity: Definitional Issues and Knowledge Gaps

Augusto Diana

Introduction

This chapter presents issues associated with the definition of physical activity, and potential ways these definitional issues can help fill gaps in our knowledge about physical activity as an intervention strategy to address public health problems. Why does this matter? Physical activity, including exercise, sport, recreation, play, and its many other manifestations, is generally thought to be a positive thing. This is true in popular culture and also in much scientific literature. It is rare, however, for experts to clarify what types of activity bring the most benefit. This chapter explores the current base of knowledge and suggests ways that future scientific studies can help clarify these uncertainties.

The chapter is organized into four areas: (1) examples of the wide range of definitions of physical activity, including the wide variety of disciplines from which these definitions derive; (2) the way these definitions and related disciplines matter in considering how to develop, implement, and study public health interventions that incorporate physical activity; (3) measurement considerations; and (4) knowledge gaps on physical activity and where to go from here.

A. Diana (✉)
Division of Epidemiology, Services and Prevention Research, Prevention Research Branch,
National Institute on Drug Abuse (NIDA), 6001 Executive Blvd., Room 5163,
MSC 9589, Bethesda, MD 20892-9589, USA
e-mail: dianaa@nida.nih.gov

A.L. Meyer and T.P. Gullotta (eds.), *Physical Activity Across the Lifespan*,
Issues in Children's and Families' Lives 12, DOI 10.1007/978-1-4614-3606-5_1,
© Springer Science+Business Media New York 2012

The Range of Definitions of Physical Activity

To show the range in definitions, it would be easy to fill an entire chapter with quotes of diverse definitions of physical activity. These definitions run the gamut—from simple statements about movement to complex sets of categories and concepts. The two examples provided below provide a nice summation of this variety.

> Physical activity is bodily movement produced by skeletal muscles that results in varying amounts and rates of energy expenditure that are positively related to physical fitness depending on the stimulus features of physical activity such as type, intensity, regularity, and timing of the activity. Physical activity can occur in short bursts of low to high intensity or, long, sustained periods of lower intensity … Exercise is a specific form of physical activity that is structured and repetitive, with the goal of improving or maintaining physical fitness, function, or health (Dishman, 2006, p. 350).

> 'Physical activity,' 'exercise,' and 'physical fitness' are terms that describe different concepts. However, they are often confused with one another, and the terms are sometimes used interchangeably. Physical activity in daily life can be categorized into occupational, sports, conditioning, household, or other activities. Exercise is a subset of physical activity that is planned, structured, and repetitive and has a final or an intermediate objective, the improvement or maintenance of physical fitness. Physical fitness is a set of attributes that are either health- or skill-related. The degree to which people have these attributes can be measured with specific tests (Caspersen, Powell, & Christenson, 1985; Gabriel, Pettee, & Morrow, 2010).

Youth activity involvement has been operationalized and analyzed using a wide range of approaches. Some have studied the effects of involvement vs. noninvolvement, while others have focused on the intensity of involvement in particular activities. Research has also addressed the "multiple unique effects" of individual activities, as compared with the individual's breadth, or diversity, of activity participation (for some, "dosage") (Bohnert, Martin, & Garber, 2007; Busseri & Rose-Krasnor, 2010; Feister, Simpkins, & Bouffard, 2005).

Some researchers and policy makers have differentiated physical activity from non-activity, and "purposeful" activity. Physical activity is seen as behavior that drives "human movement"; human movement, in turn, results in change in physiological attributes such as greater "energy expenditure" and improved "physical fitness." Sedentary behavior, meanwhile, produces little or no human movement resulting in minimal physiological gain. Health-enhancing physical activity is movement that, when added to normal daily (usually light intensity) activities, produces health benefits (Hagstromer & Bowles, 2010).

To help the public make good decisions about their participation in physical activity, and to integrate scientific conceptualizations, Health and Human Services Secretary, Mike Leavitt, formed a scientific advisory committee, comprised primarily of physical activity researchers was formed to discuss appropriate participation in physical activity. This committee work culminated in a set of guidelines regarding physical activity. The guidelines are organized around a number of dimensions: type of activity (e.g., aerobic, anaerobic); frequency of participation; intensity of participation; duration of participation; appropriate participation across age groups; and by other targeted groupings (e.g., pregnant women) (Physical Activity Guidelines Advisory Committee, 2008). The Physical Activity Guidelines consider the way to maximize health benefits from activity participation (Physical Activity Guidelines Advisory Committee, 2008).

These recommendations echo those of an earlier federal advisory committee formed around a similar purpose: "(1) aerobic exercise a minimum of 3 to 5 times per week for a duration of approximately 30 minutes per session at moderate (noticeably increased breathing and heart rate) to vigorous intensity (substantial increases in breathing and heart rate); (2) a strength/resistance program 2 to 3 times per week with 1 to 3 sets of 8 to 15 repetitions of the major muscle groups; and (3) a flexibility or stretching program of the major muscle groups 2 to 3 times per week" (American College of Sports Medicine, 1998).

Though prescriptive in identifying the amount of activity, the guidelines do not make explicit the kinds of activities that might best satisfy activity needs and goals across the life span. Are particular types of aerobic activity more or less desirable, and does this depend on the subgroup? The scientific literature tends to focus on activities that can occur in both natural and controlled settings. For instance, running and cycling can be done in a fitness center, an outdoor track, on public streets, or in public parks. Most studies, such as those measuring physiological characteristics of participants, have been done in a controlled environment. Because activities like running and cycling can occur in natural environments and the nature of the participation is likely to be fairly similar, the learnings from controlled environment studies should enhance our understanding of the impact of physical activity participation.

At the same time, a number of other dimensions of people's participation in physical activity are typically left out of scientific analyses. These include the potential importance of the context (where the physical activity takes place). For instance, are there differences between indoor and outdoor participation? Does it matter if the participation occurs on a marked field or arena (as in team sports), or in an open space, such as a park setting? Does it matter if the environment is housed in an urban, suburban, or rural setting? What if the activity is associated with a workplace or school context? Does it make a difference if the activity occurs in a dangerous vs. a safe location?

Beyond the geographical context of the activity, a number of other contextual factors may affect activity participation. For instance, does it matter if the activity is individual or team-oriented? What if the activity is part of a formal vs. an informal structure (e.g., formal league play, intramural league play, casual or pickup activity)? Are the physiological or social-psychological effects different if the activity is cooperative or competitive? Most important to this discussion, does it matter if the activity is designed to build skills, if it is more or less structured, if there are defined roles and responsibilities? Are there greater benefits of individual activities, such as running, nature walks, and cycling, when they are done in conjunction with someone else or multiple others? What if the walk, run, or ride is part of a charitable event?

Though these contextual issues are too numerous to address in this chapter, we can provide an illustration using one subfield of physical activity study, sport sociology. This example points to the need to consider activity type in determining potential health benefits.

Sport sociologists focus on the 'deeper game' associated with sports, the game through which sports become part of the social and cultural worlds in which we live. … [C]an we say that two groups of children playing a sandlot game of baseball in a Kansas town and a pickup game of soccer on a Mexican beach are engaged in sports? Their activities are quite different from what occurs in connection with Major League Baseball games and World Cup soccer matches. … what [about] hunting? weight lifting? jumping rope and jogging? darts? automobile racing? scuba diving? professional wrestling? skateboarding? X games? paintball? a piano competition? These differences become significant when parents ask if playing sports is good for their children, when community leaders ask if they should use tax money to pay for sports, or when school officials ask if sports contribute to the educational missions of their schools (Coakley, 2007, pp. 4–6).

The Many Subdisciplines Addressing Physical Activity

Knowing the possible definitions of physical activity belies another critical dimension of physical activity's possible relationship to health: the diversity of fields, disciplines, and perspectives that researchers and others bring to bear in explaining or studying physical activity. Among the many fields that directly address the health benefits of physical activity are Health and Exercise Sciences, Leisure Studies, Physical Education and Kinesiology, Urban Planning and Landscape Architecture, Nutrition Counseling, Parks and Recreation and Play Associations, and the General Social Sciences, especially Sociology and Psychology (with subdisciplines dedicated to Sport Sociology and Sport Psychology) (Coakley, 2007; Ottoson et al., 2009; Sallis et al., 2009; Trost, Owen, Bauman, Sallis, & Brown, 2002).

One place where physical activity as a lifestyle choice has received particular attention derives from the field of outdoor recreation and has been called Active Living. Active Living has been defined as a way of life that integrates physical activity into everyday routines encompassing both leisure-time physical activity and walking and biking for transportation purposes (Orleans, Kraft, Marx, & McGinnis, 2003).

In an analysis of the Active Living initiative funded by the William T. Grant Foundation, researchers found that grantee investigators represented the variety of disciplines described above. These authors provide an activity classification scheme:

> **physical environment-related** (architecture, environmental science, geography, landscape architecture, transportation, and urban planning); **health-related** (epidemiology, medicine, nursing, public health, and statistics); **social science-related** (anthropology, behavioral science, education, and psychology); **recreation- and leisure-related** (physical activity/exercise science and recreation/leisure science); and **policy science-related** (business, economics, and policy studies.) (Gutman, Barker, Samples-Smart, & Morley, 2009, p. S27).

The Active Living researchers closely parallel the work of researchers in many other fields. For instance, Lloyd Johnston discussed healthy physical activity as it links to school, work, and other social environments (Safron, Schulenberg, & Bachman, 2001). In Johnston's categorization, school-related sports participation was associated with work intensity, though curricular and extracurricular activities were not.

Similarly, Coakley (2007, p. 13) differentiated the approaches taken by psychologists and sociologists to sport participation. Sports sociologists focus on formal sports and consider three dimensions of sport: the physical nature of the activity, the competitive nature of the activity, and the activity's institutionalization. Institutionalization, for sociologists, refers to the patterns of social actions and relationships, over time and across situations. Most importantly, activities that have become institutionalized have formal rules and organizational structures that guide people's actions (Coakley, 2007, p. 6). A key feature of sport from the sociological perspective is that it produces both intrinsic and extrinsic rewards. Here, the crossover with sport psychology becomes evident. Sport psychologists focus on motivation, perception, cognition, self-esteem, self-confidence, attitudes, and personality, as well as interpersonal dynamics, including communication, leadership, and social influence, specifically as these exist inside individuals. While both fields incorporate intrinsic or internal rewards into their work, historically this has been a primary domain of psychology.

Still another field of study with physical activity as a primary focus is that of play. "Play is an expressive activity done for its own sake. It may be spontaneous or guided by informal norms. An example of play is three four-year-olds who, during a recess period at preschool, spontaneously run around a playground, yelling joyfully while throwing playground balls in whatever directions they feel like throwing them" (Coakley, 2007, p. 7). According to cultural historian Howard Chudacoff, "… when we talk about play today, the first thing that comes to mind are toys, … when I would think of play in the nineteenth century, I would think of *activity* rather than an object … for most of human history, what children did when they played was roam in packs large and small, more or less unsupervised, and engage in freewheeling imaginative play. They were pirates and princesses, aristocrats and action heroes … They improvised their own play; they regulated their play; they made up their own rules" (in Spiegel, 2008).

Why Definitional Issues Matter for Assessing the Public Health Benefits of Physical Activity

The information presented thus far has focused generically on the types of definitions utilized in a variety of fields of study. For our purposes, what matters more is whether, and if so, how, these definitions might help determine the potential health benefits of participation in physical activity. This area is especially important when considering how to incorporate physical activity into prevention and treatment interventions.

Among the ways definitions of physical activity have been explored in relation to health benefits are: the relationship of differential access and responsiveness to activity opportunities; diversity of settings in which activity occurs; type and intensity of activity; and skills-building potential of physical activity (can include physiological, cognitive, social-emotional, and general social skills, such as social interaction, role playing, and development of respect for rules and team processes). Some of these areas are briefly explored below.

Physical Activity Viewed as Health-Enhancing or Therapeutic

"Health-enhancing" physical activity has been defined as any form of activity that can benefit health and fitness, without producing undue harm or risk (European Union Public Health and Information Knowledge System, 2009). Importantly, not all physical activity is seen as beneficial to health. To have health benefits, in line with federal guidelines, activity should be vigorous or moderate. Moderate-intensity physical activity raises the heart beat, leaves the individual feeling slightly out of breath, increases the body's metabolism, and can include activities like brisk walking. Vigorous physical activity leads to sweating, becoming out of breath, and raising the body's metabolism to at least six times its resting level; this type of activity usually involves sports or exercise, including running and cycling (Gabriel et al., 2010).

An illustration of the overlay of definitions and health outcomes is provided by the field of leisure studies. This field, and a parallel area called wilderness therapy or outdoor behavioral health care, focuses on what about the activity is "therapeutic" for participants (Marchand, Russell, & Cross, 2009). As Caldwell (2005, p. 8) notes, there are two primary academic traditions in the USA that focus on leisure.

> Leisure studies or sciences (including the professional field of recreation and parks management) focuses on understanding what and why people do what they do with their free time, the impact of their participation (e.g. economic, community development, and health benefits) and how to manage environments where leisure occurs. The field of therapeutic recreation (or recreational therapy) was initially established to assist people who had trouble in their leisure, caused by illness, disability, or some other condition (e.g. poverty).

What makes recreation therapeutic? First, the leisure has to promote problem prevention, coping, and transcending negative life events. Second, the leisure activity can benefit either physical well-being, such as "a positive body feeling" and the amelioration of disease indications, or psychological well-being, including happiness and general life satisfaction. Merging these benefits, the activity promotes a greater sense of meaningfulness (Bengel, Strittmayer, & Willmann, 1999; Caldwell, 2005).

This body of literature is replete with studies that demonstrate positive health benefits (Caldwell, 2005). Though the evidence base is not as strong, the research on non-physically active leisure, such as music appreciation, viewing aesthetic scenery, and humor gained through leisure, shows that these are "functionally equivalent" in improving mood and decreasing anxiety (Snowball & Szabo, 1990; Szabo et al., 1998). Meanwhile, uninvolving leisure (e.g., watching television) has been regularly associated with negative mental health outcomes (Passmore & French, 2000). Several unique protective factors help to understand why leisure contributes to health (Caldwell, 2005, p. 17; Bengel et al., 1999). These include competence, self-efficacy, experience of challenge, absorption, self-determination/self-control over leisure time, relaxation/disengaging from stress, distraction from negative life events, life continuity after disability, social support, friendships, and social acceptance.

Research in the field of leisure studies have introduced dimensions of activity type, such as dance and "creative" exercise, as well as form, including "long-duration" vs. "steady-state" exercise, "progressive cycling," and others (Gondola, 1987). Others have focused on the importance of contact with nature in creative play and the safe and healthy development of youth (Louv, 2005; Sallis et al., 2009). Children are less active when they are inside; they are less healthy when they are inactive. Exposure to nature is seen to have restorative power. Activity for nature advocates is not always vigorous—wildlife viewing, photography and nature journaling, and "wildcrafting" (hunting and gathering of plants for food, herbal medicine, or crafts) are examples (Louv, 2005). In the adventure field, it is common to conceptualize healthy activity as "natural risk" (Erickson, 2004).

Physical Activity Viewed as Enhancing Cognitive Function

Most studies of cognitive function have shown positive results from participation in physical activity. Studies comparing both experienced and inexperienced, and high-skill/low-skill, soccer players showed significant increases in response speed and decision making (Marriott, Reilly, & Miles, 1993). Tennenbaum, Yuval, Elbaz, Bar-Eli, and Weinberg (1993) found that team handball players walking or running on a treadmill improved their decision-making abilities, regardless of handball playing experience. Improvements were significantly better during high exercise levels than during low exercise levels. Other studies have suggested that exercise influences peoples' response speeds on decision-making processes as well.

In a review by Tomporowski (2003), more than two-thirds of studies evaluated indicated that multiple cognitive processes were enhanced when "submaximal aerobic exercise" was performed between 20 and 60 min. These cognitive processes are critical to optimal performance and adaptive behavior, suggesting that aerobic exercise better prepares people to engage in action, concentrate, and solve complex problems. Another line of studies reviewed by Tomporowski (2003) showed improvements in participants' cognitive performance with moderate-intensity aerobic exercise. It was less clear if more intense, anaerobic exercise resulted in improvements but this activity did not impair cognitive function. There are so many other ways that researchers and activity proponents have utilized definitional/descriptive language to put forth "best practice" recommendations.

Researchers have also discussed the "activation of … systemic changes in physiological functions (e.g. cardiorespiration, endocrine function, body temperature change)," particularly in terms of the "acute effects" on cognitive performance (while in the midst of exercising or shortly thereafter) (Tomporowski, 2003, p. 298). A consistent theme in these studies is that high-performance athletes (among the fittest humans), of widely varying activity types, perform better cognitively with more intense exercise. Meanwhile, less fit people, including athletes, also do better with exercise, but only in moderation. This line of research appears to suggest a continuum of fitness and cognitive benefit. Those who benefit the most are the fittest who engage in the most intensive activity, usually very well-conditioned athletes. For less fit athletes and the rest of the population, less intense activity may be recommended and provide cognitive benefit. These findings suggest that there are important differences in what people do and how they do it.

Physical Activity Viewed as Addressing Social Problems

A number of theorists have discussed the benefits of physical activity as a means of mitigating social problems. In his seminal work that introduced Social Control theory, Travis Hirschi (1969, p. 187) argued that youth need engagement because, relative to adults, they have a lot of leisure time: "[t]he child playing ping-pong, swimming in he community pool, or doing his homework is not committing delinquent acts."

Hirschi alerted us to the need to differentiate types of activity. He noted that some activities, like watching TV, are not protective: "[we] must consider ... *what* the child is doing, and assiduously avoid the idea that doing 'something'—anything—is ... inhibitive of the commission of delinquent acts" (Hirschi, 1969, p. 190). Other researchers have studied the relationship between varying types of activity and other problem areas as well. For instance, club and group, but not individual, sports participation has been identified as a protective factor against drinking and cigarette smoking and other illicit drug use (Barnes, Hoffman, Welte, Farrel, & Dintcheff, 2006). However, it appears that as the vigorousness of the activity increases, this distinction disappears (Vilhjalmsson & Thorlindsson, 1992). Yusko, Buckman, White, and Pandina (2008a) found that male athletes are less likely to use cigarettes in season than out of season. Rutten and Lantz (2004) tried controlling for the "sporting context" (i.e., how it is structured) and it appeared to have an influence on athletes' antisocial and prosocial behavior choices. Correia, Carey, Simons, and Borsari (2003) found low levels of involvement in substance-free activities, such as hiking and arts projects, among heavy drinkers.

Physical Activity Viewed as Building Community, and Group Identity

Other areas extensively studied in regard to physical activity's potential benefits involve skills-building, and community and social support. Dating back to at least the Progressive Era in American history (post Civil War to the turn of the twentieth century), theorists have been extolling the virtues of activity in promoting "positive American values" and enabling immigrant cultures to assimilate more easily (Coakley, 2007). While political and social systems at the time were driven by a desire to minimize difference, this approach was certainly more humane than the extermination practices exercised against American Indians and the vitriolic racial practices in the American south in the nineteenth and twentieth centuries.

During the Progressive Era, people were encouraged to invent or adapt activities for use with immigrant populations. Generally, these activities were thought to be functional if they could take place in groups, and in publically available spaces such as parks. Often, Parks and Recreation Departments sponsored these activities. The birth and diffusion of volleyball and basketball took hold at this time (Coakley, 2007).

Extending into the early twentieth century, the value of athletics in relation to education played out on college campuses across the USA. One analysis of this period describes football coach Alonzo Stagg at the University of Chicago, both of which sought to align sport values to education. Stagg identified core values of sport, including hard work, achievement, efficiency, and competitiveness/winning (Lester, 1999).

Some who praise the social benefits of activity participation talk about the potential to create or sustain community and even national political identity. While the health benefits of an outcome like this are less clear, often the activity is described as having transcendent qualities.

> In sport, community often manifests itself in celebration of team unity and sacrifice. If a group (or team) can come together leaving individual desires and characteristics behind, the team as a unified and harmonious group is more likely to accomplish its goals (Helstein, 2005, p. 1).

Physical Activity Viewed as Skills-Building and Positive Youth Development

There is now a considerable literature base suggesting that adolescent patterns of leisure activity may have important developmental implications. Some studies have found benefits of adult-guided and supervised leisure activities and prosocial identity development, emotion regulation, and academic achievement (Eccles, Barber, Stone, & Hunt, 2003; Mahoney, Harris, & Eccles, 2006). High-quality leisure activity appears to be especially protective for youth at risk of academic failure (Mahoney et al., 2006; Mahoney & Cairns, 1997). While involvement in organized activities provides a context for healthy adolescent development (Mahoney et al., 2006), unstructured, unsupervised leisure activities, such as youth centers, are associated with greater risk of substance use, delinquency, and sexual activity, perhaps due to a lack of adult supervision and/or exposure to delinquent peers (e.g., Bartko & Eccles, 2003; Caldwell, Baldwin, Walls, & Smith, 2004; Linville & Huebner, 2005). Other research has shown that youth involved in unstructured out-of-school activities may engage in greater delinquency. One study of school-based physical education programs, extracurricular physical activity, and in-school, intraschool, or intramural sport found that an additional hour of curricular time devoted to physical activity/physical education seems to improve GPA in elementary school students, and increases seem to correspond to improvements in teacher performance (Trudeau & Shephard, 2008, p. 1). The authors argue that this improvement may be related to simultaneous improvements in concentration, memory, and classroom behavior.

With regard to social support and social relationships, leisure may afford individuals the opportunity to form and maintain social networks (Warner-Smith, 2003) and to provide "palliative coping, mood enhancement, leisure companionship" (Iwasaki & Mannell, 2000). Social relationships formed in leisure have also been identified with the overall well-being for the disabled. One group used leisure to adjust to living with a spinal cord injury (Kleiber, Brock, Dattilo, Lee, & Caldwell,

1995) and the Toronto Front Runners used running as "therapeutic landscapes of social relations" for sexual minorities (van Ingen, 2004).

From a positive youth development perspective (Damon, 2004; Lerner, Almerigi, Theokas, & Lerner, 2005), structured activities have been seen as supportive contexts within which youth have growth-related experiences that promote personal and interpersonal development (Larson, Hansen, & Moneta, 2006). Related to youth development, other research on leisure activities suggests that motivation for participation and feelings about activities may also influence outcomes (Caldwell, 2005). Busseri and Rose-Krasnor (2009, 2010) have emphasized that it is the diversity of involvements (a broader range of activities) that is critical to skills development for youth, and allows them to build stronger support networks and prosocial bonds. Outward Bound programming utilizes an approach called "Scaffolding" in which skills built in an activity are built upon for the next activity or learning experience. Outdoor leaders and their relationships with participants are also seen as critical to the learning outcomes of youth participants (Ewert & Sibthorp, 2009; Shooter, Paisley, & Sibthorp, 2009).

Physically Active as Play

Current-day thinkers have not abandoned much of the rhetoric of the Progressive Era, described above in the section "Physical Activity Viewed as Building Community, and Group Identity." For example, cultural historian Howard Chudacoff (in Spiegel, 2008) has argued that as parents became increasingly concerned about safety, they sought to create secure play environments protected from outside threats. The highly organized types of activity this has led parents to encourage for their children—Karate classes, gymnastics, summer camps—are seen to enhance this sense of safety and also to enrich children's minds.

Children's play has also been tied to nutrition. Focusing on the timing of recess, some schools are encouraging young children (second graders in one study) to "move" before eating lunch, usually in the form of playground activity and freeform running. One study discovered that the timing of recess combined with the freeform play led to a 40% drop in nurse visits, and the children had fewer headaches and stomachaches. Concerns about the likely effectiveness in urban or cold winter settings make clear why the nature and context of the activity matter (Parker-Pope, 2010).

Those studying the world of play also pay attention to how certain types of activity may foster enhanced executive function (self-regulation) in children. For instance, "make-believe" is seen to enhance the development of "private speech," which in turn helps children build self-discipline. When engaged in make-believe play, children talk to themselves about what they are going to do and how they are going to do it (Parker-Pope, 2010). These authors highlight the distinction between free play and more structured activity. They suggest that in the modern world of extensive and highly structured activity, including "soccer moms and dads" who run their kids from event to event, younger children have less opportunity to develop certain cognitive skills.

Physical Activity Involving Athletes

Some researchers have explored the effects of activity participation for scholastic and professional athletes. One study found that elite sports participation often was associated with greater substance use, especially binge drinking; drinking is seen as a response to stress, the added pressure of higher status college athletics, and the higher time constraints for athletes (Yusko, Buckman, White, & Pandina, 2008b). More well documented is the relationship between athletic performance and performance-enhancing drugs (National Institute on Drug Abuse, 2006). Perhaps most troubling about the pattern of use among elite and lower level athletes in activities as diverse as cycling and football is that many athletes use the substances for both athletic and nonathletic purposes. For instance, one study (Elliot & Goldberg, 2000) found that retired athletes reported injecting themselves with vegetable oil and Armor All upholstery protectant, among other substances, believing the fluids to have "steroid-like" qualities. While athletes seek increases in speed and strength, nonathletes seek increases in muscularity to sustain their "athletic" appearance and for greater physical appeal (Denham, 2009). "Recent studies also suggest that adolescents who use [steroids] may be more likely to continue using the drugs" (Denham, 2009, p. 277).

Even within sports, criticism centers around the grouping of athletes into one category. Is it methodologically sound to combine all kinds of sports together, considering the differences in physical, socioeconomic, psychological, and disciplinary demands of the various sports? (Bovard, 2008). For example, female soccer players were significantly more likely to report binge drinking, marijuana use, and other illicit drug use than females in other sports, and to have more school problem behaviors (Ford, 2007; Sokol-Katz, Kelley, Basinger-Fleischman, & Braddock, 2006)—Could this be because soccer is one of the sports where women have a publically defined and even "elite" status?

When Duration and Intensity of Physical Activity Are the Focus?

Dimensions of activity that have most often been associated with health benefits are duration and intensity of participation. One study explored in great depth the importance of each of these dimensions (Mahoney et al., 2006). The authors confirmed the importance of minimum number of hours and minimum degree of intensity of activity participation (as expressed in the Physical Activity Guidelines). However, the authors found that intensity of activity participation, or the general distinction between involvement and noninvolvement, may have less positive developmental significance than the "breadth of involvement" in the adolescent period (Lerner, Freund, De Stefanis, & Habermas, 2001). Breadth represents both the amount and the variety of activities in which youth are involved. The authors offer an important interpretation of this finding:

it may be premature to conclude that all youth should be encouraged to participate in as many activities as possible, irrespective of the intensity of involvement. Some indicators of development, including the development of mastery and expertise within a particular domain (e.g., fine arts) could be predicted best through more intense involvement. ... a certain level of intensity of involvement may be necessary before the benefits of involvement begin to accrue (Busseri & Rose-Krasnor, 2010, pp. 607–608).

Measurement Questions

One of the most critical factors in determining which definition(s) of physical activity we want to prioritize is how we can most efficiently and effectively collect data in the area we choose. In many ways the literature on physical activity measurement parallels the discussion of definitional issues presented thus far.

> Decisions concerning measurement and analysis of youth activity involvement have important implications both for the interpretation of a given set of results and integration across studies. ... Often, however, no rationale is provided in published reports, nor is substantive discussion provided concerning the implications of such choices (Busseri & Rose-Krasnor, 2010, p. 583).

This section briefly discusses some of the tools and related issues in the measurement of physical activity.

Tools to Measure Activity

Tools available for the measurement of physical activity include survey instruments, technological devices, tracking tools, and qualitative assessments. Many standard survey instruments include items assessing physical activity participation. The national Monitoring the Future study asks youth about any and vigorous activity, as well as participation in specific types such as athletic teams (Johnston, 2008). Others, such as the Behavioral Risk Factor Surveillance System (BRFSS), Neighborhood Selection Questionnaire, NEXT Generation Health Survey, NHANES, and Healthy People 2010 studies and guidelines focus on measures of moderate and vigorous aerobic activity, including walking (and environment walkability), as well as sedentary lifestyles and muscular strengthening, flexibility (stretching), and balance and coordination activity. Most of these survey tools also allow for correlational analysis of activity and substance use and other health concerns. Self-report tools can also include guided checklists and journals (Sternfeld & Rosas, 2010).

Self-report tools have many advantages including cost, access to greater numbers, familiarity to participants, and others. But they suffer from problems of inaccurate recall, dangers of overreporting, and the difficulty of assessing the accuracy of responses (Atienza, 2008). In one case, participants were asked if they had ever exercised regularly for 6 months or more and then stopped for 3 months or more

(Chambliss et al., 2006). In general, surveys vary greatly on the amount and type of participant recall expected (e.g., 24-h, 3-day, or 7-day recall) (Atienza, 2008).

Numerous researchers have assessed the physiological impact of activity thru the use of "wearable monitors," including pedometers, accelerometers, mobile phones, doubly labeled water, oxygen sensors, the *Fitnessgram*, and GIS devices (Castelli & Hillman, 2012; Freedson, 2008; Intille, 2008; Masse, 2010; Patrick, 2008). Technological tools have the advantage of being directly, physiologically objective and they can allow for cross-validation with self-report data. However, most of the devices are not readily available for general public use due to cost, and most also require more of a controlled setting for their implementation, given the need to monitor the participant's activity (Atienza, 2008). It can also be hard to know whether the body would respond in identical ways in a more "natural" environment.

The Variety in Physical Activity Measurement and the Implications for Analysis

The detail provided in activity measurement can be overwhelming. Approaches to the measurement of physical activity participation must consider the types of question areas and response categories needed for a useful and accurate assessment. As noted above, surveys can vary greatly on the amount and type of participant recall expected (from as recent as the current day to a several month period of time). Surveys also distinguish among dichotomous scoring (involved or not), ordinal measures of "more" or "less" activity (e.g., Zajacova & Burgard, 2010), counts of the number of activities, and indices of frequency or intensity of participation or time spent in the activity (Feister et al., 2005). Sometimes the counts and indices address a wide variety of activities, including performing arts, housework, and gardening, and other times only more traditional team or individual sports are queried (Chambliss et al., 2006; Fredricks & Eccles, 2006).

Other measurement areas may have implications both type and analytic opportunities. For instance, whether the participation is seen as voluntary or nondiscretionary (taking a leisurely walk in a park on weekends vs. walking to work) may feel quite different both subjectively and objectively. The nature of the built or natural environment should be considered as part of the measurement discussion in producing walkability indices (Sallis et al., 2009). In the case of the NIfETy study, multiple raters, traveling in pairs, assess neighborhood conditions, safety, and physical activity (including biking and walking, and daytime vs. nighttime patterns) thru observational and data recording strategies (Furr-Holden et al., 2008). And whether surveys, travel diaries, or technological tools such as GIS are used will have great bearing on the types of analysis possible, and the types of conclusions one can draw from the data.

As was extensively discussed in a workshop organized by NIH (Hagstromer & Bowles, 2010) on the measurement of active and sedentary behaviors, our goals must be to simultaneously maximize the quality of our measurement of activity and to minimize the error in our reporting. Reducing specification error (question or measurement method does not match the target concept), measurement error related to data collection, and processing errors in the manipulation or analysis of raw data (Nusser, 2010) all need to be carefully attended to while maintaining sensitivity to change (Masse, 2010).

How the Context Affects Measurement

Just as built and natural environments affect measurement opportunities, other systems will affect what we can measure, how we measure it, and what we are able to conclude from data derived from the measurement. The Active Living Research project (Sallis et al., 2009) laid out several measurement areas for considering physical activity and its social context. For instance, city and state transportation departments, and metropolitan transportation improvement programs, might consider planning walk lights at traffic signals, bridge walkways, bicycle and other nonmotorized projects, etc. Other policy-making organizations such as forest and park services, mayor's and county councils, and planning boards can discuss open-space planning, including parks, activity guidelines for residents to reduce obesity risk, and smart-growth planning related to pedestrian safety and exercise paths.

In discussing their typology, the Active Living researchers include components of each of the categories as well. For example, transportation includes roads, sidewalks, and street-crossing aids; public recreation includes parks and trails; and private recreation includes gyms and health clubs, etc. (Sallis et al., 2009). Policies might have to do with physical education requirements, space for free or leisure activity and play, and disabled access. Worksites increasingly are addressing these issues as well.

The type of research study for which physical activity data are collected is another contextual dimension in measurement approaches (Masse, 2010). Epidemiological studies use more static data to assess relations between physical activity and health. Surveillance studies monitor levels of physical activity and patterns of change at population levels. Intervention studies, which are needed to detect change in participant outcomes related to their physical activity participation, have been conducted across a wide range of outcomes, including physical health, mental health, and academic, work, and other areas (Castelli & Hillman, 2012; Dishman, 2006; Marcus, 2008).

Finally, as with any good-quality research endeavor, measurement must take into consideration factors outside the immediate dimension under study. For example, pre-intervention or pre-study activity levels, as well as some common confounding variables—precursors, and concomitant and situational factors—are likely to affect not only the outcomes detected but also the interpretability of the data. Among the factors researchers have recommended for consideration are pre-experience anxiety, motivations and expectations, group characteristics (e.g., group personality, cohesion, maturity), weather, and trainer/instructor roles (Gass, 2005; Henderson, 2004).

There is no shortage of measurement devices to get at this physical activity stuff. The National Cancer Institute has identified 33 different self-report measures and 5 different accelerometers in its funded grants alone (Bowles, 2010). Most important is how we can use this information in a manageable way to address future priorities.

Conclusions: Knowledge Gaps on Physical Activity and Where to Go from Here

While definitional issues do not hold the same central place as designing and implementing physical activity interventions that help make healthier people, they do represent an important undercurrent to our understanding of what works. As identified in the Physical Activity Guidelines Advisory Committee (2008), there are still major unresolved issues in regard to how much of what type of activity we need to engage in to improve health. Similar calls have been put out by others:

> we need to know how the impact of exercise is influenced by the type of exercise, whether or not it is voluntary, its intensity, the timing and duration of a single session, and the number and frequency of sessions (Dishman, 2006, p. 351).

Given this overriding need, how can we capitalize on the existing knowledge to further build the field?

For starters, researchers can be more explicit in identifying the type, nature, and context of the activity they study that matter in producing outcomes. Most physical activity researchers delineate what their research participants do, and carefully measure their activity participation. However, seldom is attention given to whether it matters that this activity was chosen, where the activity took place, whether the activity had a structured or social dimension, and many other things. It seems that more attention could be given to these issues without undue burden to the research. For example, studies in a fitness center could assess whether having two people running side by side on a treadmill and interacting with one another would change the nature of the observed outcomes. Those studying team sports or extracurricular activities could assign participants to different types to compare and contrast the participation experience and observed outcomes.

Exploring Unexplored Areas

There are many areas that could benefit from additional research. There is a need for better, more culturally sensitive measures. Does physical activity occur and is it experienced in similar ways across gender, race/ethnic, and other population groups? People of color and low income have high rates of obesity and other problems, and more limited access to physical activity. Creating "cultural equivalence, relevance and sensitivity" in programming and measurement is needed to understand whether even the widely broadcast activity guidelines can be expected to work equally across subgroups of the population (Arredondo, 2010; Physical Activity Guidelines Advisory Committee, 2008). Linguistic relevance is only part of the cultural landscape. Exploring physical activity as a means of managing physical disability, optimizing mind-body functioning, and creating greater "inclusion" for those with disabilities are examples of ways studies can incorporate a wider range of definitional and measurement issues into research (Guthrie & Castelnuevo, 2001; Promis, Erevelles, & Matthews, 2001).

Another area where the definition and experience of physical activity are likely to be quite different is Internet and video-gaming. Internet and TV-based fitness and activity, such as Wii and WiiFit, are increasingly available and seen as health-promoting resources. Early research in this area suggests significant relationships between Internet video-game cues and the anterior cingulate area of the brain (Han, Kim, Lee, Min, & Renshaw, 2010). Better understanding of the physiological and social participation in and reactions to these vicarious forms of physical activity can benefit the physical activity measurement and assessment knowledge base. For instance, tools like the Videogame Experience Questionnaire (VEQ) assess participants' experience of games (are they realistic?), the importance of their aggressive and violent features, how playing helps or interferes with other areas of their lives, and whether the video-gamers playing alone or with others affects perceptions (Dauphin & Heller, 2010).

Policy Implications

Other future research areas might include indirect barometers of the physical activity experience. A small set of studies have explored the meaning and benefit of "assistance" in the physical activity experience. Assistance can be in the form of personal trainers, physical activity counseling, monitoring, and reinforcement of participation, all of which appear to improve attendance (Jeffry, Wing, Thorson, & Burton, 1998). "Non-active" incentives, such as pedaling to power TV or video games and offering points to purchase toys and games, have led children to spend more time and intensity pedaling a stationary bicycle and to reduce body fat (DeLuca & Holborn, 1992; Faith, Berman, & Heo, 2001).

Some have been more explicit in recommending policy approaches to increase physical activity, and these policy approaches can enhance definition and measurement needs. The Active Living research group (Sallis et al., 2009), for instance, suggested the need for the following measures of policy for obesity, diet, and physical activity:

1. Better measurement tools of physical activity and its correlates for target populations, particularly those at high risk for obesity
2. Better health impact assessment techniques and data-collection systems
3. Better measures to support surveillance of food- and activity-related policies (Sallis et al., 2009, pp. S74–S76)

The policy group also urged use of multiple methodological approaches (quantitative and qualitative methods, case studies, ethnography), an accessible compendium of metrics/indicators to draw from, ways to relate measurement to community values, and variability in policies, their implementation, and enforcement.

An additional area to enhance our understanding of the nature and measurement of physical activity concerns best ways to sustain activity involvement. Researchers have debated whether it is more important to help people initiate or maintain their exercise regimens. The 50% dropout rate among exercise program participants suggests that maintenance is where attention is needed (Dishman, 1994; Wing, 2000). Complicating this issue is that starting physical activity generally incurs costs (e.g., related to time, clothing, shoes, and equipment), compared with smoking cessation, for instance, which saves money. Additional research on financial incentives and the social-emotional costs and benefits of physical activity could help to understand how to increase initiation and maintenance participation (Buchner & Schmid, 2009).

CDC and RWJF have begun some of this financial work. Marcus (2008) has suggested that, similar to tobacco control, changing social norms about physical activity is crucial to success. In California, coalitions have been engaged to address barriers to physical activity such as deteriorating playgrounds or unsafe parks, with some promising policy successes (Blackwell, 2009). Urban planning and community design, including land-use mix, street connectivity, and greater availability of public transit, are additional policy approaches associated with greater physical activity that may help to promote initiation and maintenance of activity (Frank, Saelens, Powell, & Chapman, 2007; Morandi, 2009).

Though much remains to be done, the physical activity literature benefits from a very wide diversity of approaches to its issues. The fact that so many different disciplines include activity and its potential for addressing social problems, and these disciplines have offered such a wide range of ways to consider activity's definition, measurement, implementation, and outcomes, provides a unique and worthwhile base of knowledge for ongoing analysis. It is our hope that future work will incorporate more careful delineations of what we mean by physical activity when we study it.

References

American College of Sports Medicine. (1998). American college of sports medicine, position stand: the recommended quantity and quality of exercise for developing and maintaining cardiorespiratory and muscular fitness in health adults. *Medical Science Sports Exercise, 30,* 975–991.

Arredondo, E. (2010). *Language translation & cultural adaptation of self-report instruments.* Presented at Measurement of Active and Sedentary Behaviors: Closing the Gaps in Self-Report Methods, National Institutes of Health Workshop, July 21, Bethesda, MD.

Atienza, A. (2008). Technological tools for assessing physical activity—product demonstrations. Presented at NIDA Workshop, Can Physical Activity and Exercise Prevent Drug Abuse?: Promoting a Full Range of Science to Inform Prevention, June 5–6, Bethesda, MD.

Barnes, G. M., Hoffman, J. H., Welte, J. W., Farrel, P., & Dintcheff, B. A. (2006). Adolescents' time use: effects on substance use, delinquency, and sexual activity. *Journal of Youth and Adolescence, 36*, 697–710.

Bartko, W. T., & Eccles, J. S. (2003). Adolescent participation in structured and unstructured activities: a person-oriented analysis. *Journal of Youth and Adolescence, 32*, 233–241.

Bengel, J.R., Strittmayer, R., & Willmann, H. (1999). What keeps people healthy? The current state of discussion and the relevance of Antonovsky's salutogenic model of health. *Research and Practice of Health Promotion* (Vol. 4). Cologne, Germany: Federal Centre for Health Education.

Blackwell, A. G. (2009). Active living research and the movement for healthy communities. *American Journal of Preventive Medicine, 36*(2s), S50–S52.

Bohnert, A. M., Martin, N. C., & Garber, J. (2007). Predicting adolescents' organized activity involvement: the role of maternal depression history, family relationship quality, and adolescent cognitions. *Journal of Research on Adolescence, 32*, 233–241.

Bovard, R. S. (2008). Risk behaviors in high school and college sport. *Current Sports Medicine Reports, 7*(6), 359–366.

Bowles, H. (2010). Think tank overview and objectives. Measurement of Active and Sedentary Behaviors: Closing the Gaps in Self-Report Methods, July 21. National Institutes of Health, Bethesda, MD.

Buchner, D. M., & Schmid, T. L. (2009). Active living research and public health: natural partners in a new field. *American Journal of Preventive Medicine, 36*(2s), S44–S46.

Busseri, M., & Rose-Krasnor, L. (2009). Breadth and intensity: salient, separable, and developmentally significant dimensions of structured youth activity involvement. *British Journal of Developmental Psychology, 27*, 907–933.

Busseri, M., & Rose-Krasnor, L. (2010). Addressing three common issues in research on youth activities: an integrative approach for operationalizing and analyzing involvement. *Journal of Research on Adolescence, 2*(3), 583–615.

Caldwell, L. (2005). Leisure and health: why is leisure therapeutic? *British Journal of Guidance and Counseling, 33*(1), 7–26.

Caldwell, L. L., Baldwin, C. K., Walls, T., & Smith, E. A. (2004). Preliminary effects of a leisure education program to promote healthy use of free time among middle school adolescents. *Journal of Leisure Research, 36*, 310–335.

Caspersen, C. J., Powell, K. E., & Christenson, G. M. (1985). Physical activity, exercise, and physical fitness: definitions and distinctions for health-related research. *Public Health Reports, 100*, 126–131.

Castelli, D., & Hillman, D. (2012). Physical activity, cognition, and school performance: from neurons to neighborhoods, In A. L. Meyer & T. P. Gullotta (eds), *Physical Activity as Intervention: Promoting Health and Preventing Disease*. (pp. TBD). NY: Springer.

Chambliss, H.O., Greer, T.L., Grannemann, B.D., Jordan, A.N., Glaper, D.I., & Church, T.S. (2006). Baseline physical activity characteristics of individuals seeking exercise as an adjuvant treatment for depression. Presented at the American College of Sports Medicine Annual Meeting, May 31–June 3, Denver, CO.

Coakley, J. (2007). *Sports in society: issues and controversies* (9th ed.). Boston, MA: McGraw Hill.

Correia, C. J., Carey, K. B., Simons, J., & Borsari, B. E. (2003). Relationship between binge drinking and substance-free reinforcement in a sample of college students: a preliminary investigation. *Addiction Behavior, 2003*(28), 361–368.

Damon, W. (2004). What is positive youth development? *Annals of the American Academy of Political and Social Sciences, 591*, 13–24.

Dauphin, B., & Heller, G. (2010). Going to other worlds: the relationships between videogaming, psychological absorption, and daydreaming styles. *CyberPsychology, Behavior, and Social Networking, 13*(2), 169–172.

DeLuca, R., & Holborn, S. (1992). Effects of a variable-ratio reinforcement schedule with changing criteria on exercise in obese and non-obese boys. *Journal of Applied Behavioral Analysis, 25*, 671–679.

Denham, B. E. (2009). Determinants of anabolic-androgenic steroid risk perceptions in youth populations. *Journal of Health and Social Behavior, 50*(3), 277–292.

Dishman, R. K. (1994). *Advances in exercise adherence*. Champaign, IL: Human Kinetics.

Dishman, R. (2006). Neurobiology of exercise. *Obesity, 14*(3), 345–356.

Eccles, J. S., Barber, B. L., Stone, M., & Hunt, J. (2003). Extracurricular activities and adolescent development. *Journal of Social Issues, 59*, 865–889.

Elliot, D. L., & Goldberg, L. (2000). Women and anabolic steroids. In C. E. Yesalis (Ed.), *Anabolic steroids in sports and exercise*. Champaign, IL: Human Kinetics.

Erickson, B. (2004). Style matters: explorations of bodies, whiteness and identity in rock climbing. *Sport Sociology Journal, 21*(2), 373–396.

European Union Public Health Information and Knowledge System. (2009). EU Public Health Information and Knowledge System (EUPHIX), Version 1.11, December 17.

Ewert, A., & Sibthorp, J. (2009). Creating outcomes through experiential education: the challenge of confounding variables. *Journal of Experiential Education, 31*(3), 376–389.

Faith, M. S., Berman, N., & Heo, M. (2001). Effects of contingent television on physical activity and television viewing in obese children. *Pediatrics, 107*, 1043–1048.

Feister, L. M., Simpkins, S. D., & Bouffard, S. M. (2005). Present and accounted for: measuring attendance in out-of-school time programs. *New Directions for Youth Development, 105*, 91–107.

Ford, J. (2007). Alcohol use among college students: a comparison of athletes and nonathletes. *Substance Use and Misuse, 42*(9), 1367–1377.

Frank, L. D., Saelens, B. E., Powell, K. E., & Chapman, J. E. (2007). Stepping toward causation: do built environments or neighborhood and travel preferences explain physical activity, driving and obesity? *Social Science and Medicine, 65*, 1898–1914.

Fredricks, J. A., & Eccles, J. (2006). Extracurricular involvement and adjustment: impact of duration, number of activities, and breadth of participation. *Applied Developmental Science, 10*(3), 132–146.

Freedson, P. S. (2008). Assessment of physical activity using wearable monitors: novel analytic techniques and multiple sensor devices. Presented at NIDA Workshop, Can Physical Activity and Exercise Prevent Drug Abuse?: Promoting a Full Range of Science to Inform Prevention, June 5–6, Bethesda, MD.

Furr-Holden, C. D. M., Smart, M. J., Pokorni, J. L., Ialongo, N. S., Leaf, P. J., & Holder, H.D. (2008). The NIfETy method for environmental assessment of neighborhood-level indicators of violence, alcohol, and other drug exposure. *Prevention Science, 9*, 245–255.

Gabriel, K., Pettee, K., & Morrow, J.R. (2010). A framework for physical activity as a complex and multidimensional behavior. Presented at Measurement of Active and Sedentary Behaviors: Closing the Gaps in Self-Report Methods, National Institutes of Health Workshop, July 21, Bethesda, MD.

Gass, M. (2005). Comprehending the value structures influencing significance and power behind experiential education research. *Journal of Experiential Education, 27*(3), 286–296.

Gondola, J. C. (1987). The effects of a single bout of aerobic dancing on selected tests of creativity. *Journal of Social Behavior and Personality, 2*, 275–278.

Guthrie, S., & Castelnuevo, S. (2001). Disability management among women with physical impairments: the contribution of physical activity. *Sociology of Sport Journal, 18*(1), 5–20.

Gutman, M., Barker, D., Samples-Smart, F., & Morley, C. (2009). Evaluation of active living research: progress and lessons in building a new field. *American Journal of Preventive Medicine, 36*(2S), S22–S33.

Hagstromer, M., & Bowles, H. (2010). A checklist for evaluating the validity and suitability of existing physical activity and sedentary behavior instruments. Presented at Measurement of Active and Sedentary Behaviors: Closing the Gaps in Self-Report Methods, National Institutes of Health Workshop, July 21, Bethesda, MD.

Han, D. H., Kim, Y. S., Lee, Y. S., Min, K. J., & Renshaw, P. F. (2010). Changes in cue-induced, prefrontal cortex activity with video-game play. *Cyberpsychology, Behavior, and Social Networking, 13*(6), 655–661.

Helstein, M. T. (2005). Rethinking community: introducing the 'whatever' female athlete. *Sociology of Sport Journal, 22*(1), 1–18.

Henderson, K. A. (2004). Got research in experiential education? theory and evidence. *Journal of Experiential Education, 26*(3), 184–189.

Hirschi, T. (1969). *The causes of delinquency*. Berkeley, CA: University of California Press.

Intille, S.S. (2008). Towards real-time recognition of type, duration, intensity, and location of physical activity on mobile phones. Presented at NIDA Workshop, Can Physical Activity and Exercise Prevent Drug Abuse?: Promoting a Full Range of Science to Inform Prevention, June 5–6, Bethesda, MD.

Iwasaki, Y., & Mannell, R. C. (2000). Hierarchical dimensions of leisure stress-coping. *Leisure Sciences, 22*, 163–181.

Jeffry, R. R., Wing, R. R., Thorson, C., & Burton, L. (1998). Use of personal trainers and financial incentives to increase exercise in a behavioral weight loss program. *Journal of Consulting Clinical Psychology, 66*, 777–783.

Johnston, L.D. (2008). The association of exercise and sports participation with various forms of substance use in adolescence: findings from monitoring the future. Presented at NIDA Workshop, Can Physical Activity and Exercise Prevent Drug Abuse?: Promoting a Full Range of Science to Inform Prevention, June 5–6, Bethesda, MD.

Kleiber, D. A., Brock, S. C., Dattilo, J., Lee, Y., & Caldwell, L. (1995). The relevance of leisure in an illness experience: realities of spinal cord injury. *Journal of Leisure Research, 27*, 283–299.

Larson, R., Hansen, D. M., & Moneta, G. (2006). Differing profiles of developmental experiences across types of organized youth activities. *Developmental Psychology, 42*, 849–863.

Lerner, R. M., Almerigi, J. B., Theokas, C., & Lerner, J. V. (2005). Positive youth development: a view of the issues. *Journal of Early Adolescence, 25*, 10–16.

Lerner, R. M., Freund, A. M., De Stefanis, I., & Habermas, T. H. (2001). Understanding developmental regulation in adolescence: the use of the selection, optimization, and compensation model. *Human Development, 44*, 29–50.

Lester, R. (1999). *Stagg's University: the rise, decline, and fall of big-time football at Chicago.* Champaign, IL: University of Illinois Press.

Linville, D. C., & Huebner, A. J. (2005). The analysis of extracurricular activities and their relationship to youth violence. *Journal of Youth and Adolescence, 34*, 483–494.

Louv, R. (2005). *Last child in the woods: saving our children from nature deficit disorder*. Chapel Hill, NC: Algonquin Books.

Mahoney, J. L., & Cairns, R. B. (1997). Do extracurricular activities protect against school dropout? *Developmental Psychology, 33*, 241–253.

Mahoney, J. L., Harris, A. L., & Eccles, J. S. (2006). Organized activity participation, positive youth development, and the over-scheduling hypothesis. *Social Policy Report, 20*, 3–30.

Marchand, G., Russell, K. C., & Cross, R. (2009). An empirical examination of outdoor behavioral healthcare field instructor job-related stress and retention. *Journal of Experiential Education, 31*(3), 359–375.

Marcus, B. (2008). Physical activity interventions for smoking cessation among women. Presented to NIDA Workshop, Can Physical Activity and Exercise Prevent Drug Abuse?: Promoting a Full Range of Science to Inform Prevention, June 5–6, Bethesda, MD.

Marriott, T., Reilly, T., & Miles, T. (1993). The effect of physiological stress on cognitive performance in a simulation of soccer. In T. Reilly, J. Clarys, & A. Stibbe (Eds.), *Science and football II* (pp. 261–264). London, UK: E and FN Spon.

Masse, L. (2010). Assessing PA with self-report: a methodological overview. Presented at Measurement of Active and Sedentary Behaviors: Closing the Gaps in Self-Report Methods, National Institutes of Health Workshop, July 21, Bethesda, MD.

Morandi, L. (2009). Essential nexus: how to use research to inform and evaluate public policy. *American Journal of Preventive Medicine, 36*(2s), S53–S54.

National Institute on Drug Abuse. (2006). Anabolic steroid abuse. http://drugabuse.gov/PDF/RRSteroids.pdf. Accessed 11 Nov 2011.

Nusser, S. (2010). Modeling errors in physical activity data. Presented at Measurement of Active and Sedentary Behaviors: Closing the Gaps in Self-Report Methods, National Institutes of Health Workshop, July 21, Bethesda, MD.

Orleans, C. T., Kraft, M. K., Marx, J. F., & McGinnis, J. M. (2003). Why are some neighborhoods active and others not? charting a new course for research on the policy and environmental determinants of physical activity. *Annual Behavioral Medicine, 25*, 77–79.

Ottoson, J. M., Green, L. W., Beery, W. L., Senter, S. K., Cahill, C. L., Pearson, D. C., et al. (2009). Policy-contribution assessment and field-building analysis of the Robert Wood Johnson Foundation's active living research program. *American Journal of Preventive Medicine, 36*(2S), S34–S43.

Parker-Pope, T. (2010.) Play, then eat: Shift brings gains at school. http://www.nytimes.com/2010/01/26/health/26well.html. Accessed 11 Nov 2011.

Passmore, A., & French, D. (2000). A model of leisure and mental health in Australian adolescents. *Behavior Change, 17*, 208–221.

Patrick, K. (2008). Physical activity location measurement system (PALMS). Presented at NIDA Workshop, Can Physical Activity and Exercise Prevent Drug Abuse?: Promoting a Full Range of Science to Inform Prevention, June 5–6, Bethesda, MD.

Physical Activity Guidelines Advisory Committee. (2008). Physical activity guidelines for Americans. http://odphp.osophs.dhhs.gov/pubs/pubslist.pdf. Accessed 11 Nov 2011.

Promis, D., Erevelles, N., & Matthews, J. (2001). Reconceptualizing inclusion: the politics of university sports and recreation programs for students with minority impairments. *Journal of Sport Sociology, 18*(1), 37–50.

Rutten, D., & Lantz, C. (2004). Violent, delinquent, and aggressive behaviors of rural high school athletes and non-athletes. *Physical Education, 61*(4), 170–176.

Safron, D. J., Schulenberg, J. E., & Bachman, J. G. (2001). Part-time work and hurried adolescence: the links among work intensity, social activities, health behaviors, and substance use. *Journal of Health and Social Behavior, 42*, 425–449.

Sallis, J. F., Kraft, K., Cutter, C. L., Kerr, J., Weitzel, J., & Wilson, A. (2009). The active living research program. *American Journal of Preventive Medicine, 36*(2s), S10–S21.

Shooter, W., Paisley, K., & Sibthorp, J. (2009). The effect of leader attributes, situational context, and participant optimism on trust in outdoor leaders. *Journal of Experiential Education, 31*(3), 395–399.

Snowball, J., & Szabo, A. (1990). Anxiety, affect, and exercise: preliminary evidence lends support to the distraction hypothesis. *Journal of Sport Science, 17*, 67–68.

Sokol-Katz, J., Kelley, M., Basinger-Fleischman, L., & Braddock, J. (2006). Re-examining the relationship between interscholastic sport participation and delinquency: type of sport matters. *Sociological Focus, 39*(3), 173–192.

Spiegel, A. (2008). Old-fashioned play builds serious skills. http://www.npr.org/templates/story/story.php?storyId=19212514. Accessed 11 Nov 2011.

Sternfeld, B., & Rosas, L.G. (2010). Typology for linking self-report methods to study design and data modeling strategies. Presented at Measurement of Active and Sedentary Behaviors: Closing the Gaps in Self-Report Methods, National Institutes of Health Workshop, July 21, Bethesda, MD.

Szabo, A., Mesko, A., Caputo, A., & Gill, E. (1998). Examination of exercise induced feeling states in four modes of exercise. *International Journal of Sport Psychology, 29*, 376–390.

Tennenbaum, G., Yuval, R., Elbaz, M., Bar-Eli, M., & Weinberg, R. (1993). The relationship between cognitive characteristics and decision making. *Canadian Journal of Applied Physiology, 18*, 48–62.

Tomporowski, P. D. (2003). Effects of acute bouts of exercise on cognition. *Acta Psychologica, 112*, 297–324.

Trost, S. G., Owen, N., Bauman, A. E., Sallis, J. F., & Brown, W. (2002). Correlates of adults' participation in physical activity: review and update. *Medical Science Sports Exercise, 34*, 1996–2001.

Trudeau, F., & Shephard, R. J. (2008). Physical education, school physical activity, school sports and academic performance. *International Journal of Behavioral Nutrition and Physical Activity, 5*, 1–12.

van Ingen, C. (2004). Therapeutic landscapes and the regulated body in the Toronto front runners. *Sociology of Sport Journal, 21*(3), 253–269.

Vilhjalmsson, R., & Thorlindsson, T. (1992). The integrative and physiological effects of sport participation: a study of adolescents. *The Sociological Quarterly, 33*(4), 637–647.

Warner-Smith, P. (2003). Women's health Australia longitudinal study: leisure valued for well-being, http://www.abc.net.au/rural/ruralhealth2003/stories/s797687.htm. Accessed 11 Nov 2011.

Wing, R. R. (2000). Cross-cutting themes in maintenance of behavior change. *Health Psychology, 19S*, 84–88.

Yusko, D., Buckman, J., White, H., & Pandina, R. (2008a). Alcohol, tobacco, illicit drugs, and performance enhancers: a comparison of use by college student athletes and nonathletes. *Journal of American College Health, 57*(3), 281–289.

Yusko, D., Buckman, J., White, H., & Pandina, R. (2008b). Risk for excessive alcohol use and drinking-related problems in college student athletes. *Addictive Behaviors, 33*, 1546–1556.

Zajacova, A., & Burgard, S. A. (2010). Body weight and health from early to mid-adulthood: a longitudinal analysis. *Journal of Health and Social Behavior, 51*(1), 92–107.

Chapter 2
Reflections on Rough and Tumble Play, Social Development, and Attention-Deficit Hyperactivity Disorders

Jaak Panksepp and Eric L. Scott

Introduction

The urge for physical play in mammals, including humans, is built into the nervous system (Panksepp, 2008). This has been rigorously demonstrated in laboratory animals (Ikemoto & Panksepp, 1992). Although the precise functions of physical play remain unspecified, it is likely essential for optimal childhood development, both body and mind, with many demonstrated benefits (Burgdorf, Kroes, Beinfeld, Panksepp, & Moskal, 2010; Panksepp, 1993, 2010). We propose that play forms the backbone of young children's daily life through spontaneous social learning that enhances social interactions, promotes learning, and provides positive affect that may increase psychological resilience. In fact, we now know that play provides considerable benefits in young animals, where the necessary detailed behavioral work can be done (as summarized in Burgdorf et al., 2010; Burgdorf, Panksepp, & Moskal, 2011; Gordon, Burke, Akil, Watson, & Panksepp, 2003; Panksepp, Siviy, & Normansell, 1984; Pellis & Pellis, 2009; Vanderschuren, 2010).

As society has moved away from natural ways of living, where children were allowed abundant free time to spend as they wished, toward more structured educational demands on their time and energy, we may be having an inadvertent and unsystematic societal experiment underway on the consequences of taking natural

J. Panksepp (✉)
Program in Neuroscience, Department Veterinary Comparative Anatomy,
Pharmacology and Physiology, College of Vet. Med., Washington State University,
Pullman, WA 99164, USA

Department of Psychology, Bowling Green State University, Bowling Green, OH, USA
e-mail: jpanksepp@vetmed.wsu.edu

E.L. Scott
Department of Psychiatry, Indiana University Medical School,
705 Ridley Hospital Drive, Indianapolis, IN 46202, USA

A.L. Meyer and T.P. Gullotta (eds.), *Physical Activity Across the Lifespan*,
Issues in Children's and Families' Lives 12, DOI 10.1007/978-1-4614-3606-5_2,
© Springer Science+Business Media New York 2012

play away from many of our children. The consequences are bound to be multifold (Panksepp, 2007a, 2010).

The possibility has been proposed that the dramatically increased prevalence of attention-deficit hyperactivity disorders (ADHD) in our children during the past few decades may be partly due to the failure of increasing numbers of children to have adequate physical play which promotes maturation of higher brain abilities, especially executive functions in medial frontal regions of the brain (Panksepp, 1998a, 1998b, 2007a) that mediate joy (Burgdorf, Wood, Kroes, Moskal, & Panksepp, 2007; Panksepp, 2007b). It is widely believed that ADHD is typically characterized by deficient frontal cortical executive functions, and one of the biophysical characteristics of ADHD is increased electroencephalographic slow-wave-activity in frontal regions of the brain (Barkley, 1997). Interestingly, preliminary preclinical work, using a juvenile rat model, has shown that impulsivity, hyperactivity symptoms and attention deficits may be diminished with abundant physical play in young animals surgically prepared with hyperactivity-promoting frontal cortical lesions, which offer a potential etiologically coherent model system for the study of ADHD (Panksepp, Burgdorf, & Gordon, 2003). While it is important to be cautious when translating information from preclinical work to humans, we think it is compelling to consider play as an important form of physical activity for children. In this chapter, we offer our reflections on the value of rough and tumble play and positive role it can play in social development in childhood.

The Value of Play

The lament over the inadequate provision of playtime has been growing steadily in the past decade. It is no longer news that in recent years the amount and frequency of unstructured playtime (e.g., recess) has declined (Sumpner & Blatchford, 1998). In stark contrast to this trend, there have been many writers, both past and present, that have declared physical play as one of the more important activities of youngsters whose brains are still in the most active phase of maturation. Consider Plato's declaration: "Our children from their earliest years must take part in all the more lawful forms of play, for if they are not surrounded with such an atmosphere they can never grow up to be well conducted and virtuous citizens" (The Laws [VII, 794]). Indeed, there have been many in the modern age who have pointed to an increasing volume of evidence for the value of play (Erikson, 1950; Frost, Wortham, & Reifel, 2001; Piaget, 1962). Richard Louv (2008) in *Last Child in the Woods*, has extolled the need for children to freely engage with the natural world, and a key part of that world is the freedom to play. Of course, now it is a dictum of neuroscience that everything we do modifies the brain circuits that create mentality.

Pellegrini and Smith (1998) summarize abundant research on the natural play of young children, especially the type of play called Rough and Tumble (R&T). They emphasized that R&T is a normal part of children's everyday activity play pattern and even though it is highly energized, often with abundant assertive gestures, it is quite distinct from aggression. But even as discussion of the benefits of R&T play has continued (Blurton-Jones, 1976; Boulton & Smith, 1992; Panksepp, 1998b; Pellegrini & Smith, 1998), school districts have been removing recess from the curriculum, increasing the likelihood that children will be deprived of R&T play. While the consequences of this for normal human child development are hard to document, examining studies of preclinical animal models offer disturbing evidence of the harm that occurs when play is limited or removed from the developmental process. Juvenile rats that have been deprived of play, exhibit various symptoms including increased aggression (Potegal & Einon, 1989) and diminished quality of other social interactions (van den Berg et al., 1999).

Research on Play

Much has been written about children's desire for engaging in joyous and exciting activities (e.g., Bekoff & Byers, 1998; Groos, 1898; Power, 2000; Sutton-Smith & Kelly-Byrne, 1984). There has been a recent upsurge in high quality neurobiological work on this research topic (for summary, see Siviy & Panksepp, 2011). This trend has been highlighted by the inauguration of the *American Journal of Play* [please note that the whole Winter issue of the journal (Vol. 2(3))] was devoted to readable articles on the neurobiology of play, and also contains an in-depth interview with the lead author of this chapter that provides a personal perspective on the field (Panksepp, 2010).

Still a generally accepted definition of play does not exist. However, many modern scholars have tried to identify the most salient aspects of what children do when they play including the following descriptions captured by Bernard Gilmore (1971) citing previously published work:

> "**Spencer**: Activity performed for the immediate gratification derived, without regard for ulterior benefits. **Lazarus**: Play is activity, which is in itself free, aimless, amusing or diverting. **Seashore**: Free self-expression for the pleasure of expression. **Dewey**: Activities not consciously performed for the sake of any result beyond themselves. **Stern**: Play is voluntary, self-sufficient activity. **Patrick**: Those human activities which are free and spontaneous and which are pursued for their own sake alone, interest in them is self-sustaining, and they are continued under any internal or external compulsion. **Allin**: Play refers to those activities, which are accompanied by a state of comparative pleasure, exhilaration, power, and the feeling of self-initiative. **Curti**: Highly motivated activity which, as free from conflicts is usually, though not always, pleasurable" (pp. 86–87, bold highlighting added).

Many writers have tried to capture a dynamic sequence of behaviors through verbal descriptions, which has proved to be a difficult endeavor (Sutton-Smith & Kelly-Byrne, 1984). Indeed, even famous development clinician Eric Erikson, found it difficult to define play, saying: "play is a borderline phenomena…and, in its own playful way, it tries to elude definition." (Erikson, 1950, p. 185).

Setting aside definitions of what play is, scholars from a variety of fields have tried to explain why children engage in playful behavior (Sutton-Smith & Kelly-Byrne, 1984). Most have relied on a functional definition outlining purposes for ludic activities (Byers & Walker, 1995; Pellegrini & Smith, 1998). Classical views such as the "surplus energy" theory discussed by Gilmore (1971) argued that animals released excess reserves of energy through play. This theory had difficulty explaining why play diminished across the life cycle. To explain such an enigma, Karl Groos (1898) postulated that play is mostly necessary for young animals to practice instinctual behaviors critical for survival.

More recent models of play behavior come from psychoanalytic theorists, behavioral theorists, cognitive theorists and social learning theorists (Gilmore, 1971). The supposed benefits include cognitive development and the ability to turn actual behavior into internal mental schemas as well as other developmental skills (Piaget, 1962). Some have theorized that play helps develop increased cardiovascular endurance, stronger muscles, and better motor coordination in both the young animal and child (Byers & Walker, 1995; Fagen, 1981). As outlined below, Pellegrini and Smith (1998) argued that play hones children's social skills. Finally, recent neurobiological perspectives suggest that Rough and Tumble (R&T) play may promote normal development of the areas of the brain responsible for behavioral inhibition (Panksepp, 1998a, 1998b; Panksepp et al., 2003). It is this theory that underscores the current study.

Rough and Tumble Play in Young Animals and Humans

One of the most commonly observed behaviors in young animals is their playfulness, specifically pouncing, chasing, wrestling and play biting. This activity, known as Rough & Tumble play (R&T), has received relatively detailed behavioral descriptions within the animal literature in comparison to human studies (Aldis, 1975; Boulton & Smith, 1992; Burghardt, 2005; Fagen, 1981; Gandelman, 1992; Groos, 1898; Panksepp, 1998a; Panksepp, Siviy, & Normansell, 1984).

Much of what is known about R&T play was learned by observing animals and establishing taxonomies of their behavior (Aldis, 1975; Burghardt, 2005; Fagen, 1981; Gandelman, 1992; Groos, 1898). Gandelman (1992) included the following categories when he reported work others had done to describe the play of Colombian ground squirrels: wrestling, pounce, side jump, box, pushes away, and chase. Bertrand (1976) noticed similar behaviors when observing Stumptail monkeys including lunge, play wrestling, pull, pinch, chase, and tag. Others have described it as having a joyous and energetic quality where organisms "rapidly begin to exhibit vigorous fighting: animals chase and pounce on each other, sometimes unilaterally, sometimes mutually with rapid role reversals" (Panksepp et al., 1984, p. 466). Many play scholars have noted that during play chase sequences there were significant role reversals. For example, the chased animal changed directions and begins to pursue the animal that has been chasing. Other characteristics included self-handicapping on the part of larger animals, thus letting smaller ones pin or chase them.

R&T in humans is presumably the most fundamental form of play because it is shared with so many other mammalian species ranging from rats (Panksepp, 1980; Panksepp & Beatty, 1980) to monkeys (Aldis, 1975; Gandelman, 1992) but, despite many similarities, it has received relatively little attention in the human empirical literature (Pellegrini & Smith, 1998). One similarity is the developmental time course play follows. In the rat, it reaches its peak between 32 and 40 days of age, and begins to decrease in frequency shortly thereafter (Panksepp, 1980). This corresponds to results found by Humphreys and Smith (1984) who found that R&T is most prevalent in children between the ages of 7 and 9 but then declines. As they grow older, human children begin to incorporate other skills like linguistics, fantasy, and sociodramatics into their play patterns. The categorical dimensions of human R&T play are examined next.

Categories Established for R&T Play

There is considerable consensus within the field as to which behaviors should be included in the broad category of R&T play (Pellegrini & Smith, 1998). Blurton-Jones (1972) has written extensively on the categories of behavior that should be included in descriptions of R&T play and as one of the first researchers to apply the term R&T play to humans, Jones included many of the same categories used by animal researchers such as: laugh, run, jump, open hand beat, wrestle, chase and flee. To determine which behaviors were emitted most commonly, he made extensive ethological observations of nursery school-aged children.

Using continuous recording techniques, Blurton-Jones recorded each child for fifteen 5-min periods during the course of the 2-month study. During each recording period frequency, counts of each of 22 social behaviors were coded. Then using temporal sequencing analysis (a variant of factor analysis) Blurton-Jones determined which of the 22 behaviors co-occurred. The results indicated that three factors could be rotated out of the analysis. The first factor included such behaviors as laugh, run, jumps, hit and wrestles. The second factor formed another category labeled aggression, and included behaviors like frown, hit, push, and take-tug-grab. The third and final factor was labeled "social" because it contained behaviors like give, receive, talk and smile. Blurton-Jones argued that the separation of the behaviors on the first and second factor indicated that the two sets of behaviors were conceptually distinct. He therefore only considered the first factor as the essential description of R&T play.

Humphreys and Smith (1984) listed similar behaviors under the category of R&T play but tried to distinguish reliably between it and a variety of other activity categories. Most importantly the R&T play category included tease/taunt, hit/kick, poke/maul, pounce, sneak up, carry child, pile on, play fight (study) and play-fight (lie), chase, hold/grab, push, and be chased or hit. These categories were considered distinct from rule games, such as skipping, marbles, football, hopscotch, and jump rope. "Locomotion" and "non-locomotor-active" were two other categories that resembled R&T play. Representative behaviors falling under these categories included walk, run, and skip/hop (for "locomotion") and ball play, climb, roll/spin, piggyback, dance and gymnastic moves (for non-locomotor-active play).

The reason Humphreys and Smith gave for distinguishing the many behaviors exhibited was to distinguish objectively the percentage of time spent in various playground activities. This kind of analysis (quantifying time spent in types of play) had not been done in previous research with school-aged children, and thereby provided important information regarding the relative frequency of children's playground behaviors. R&T play averaged about 10% of overall playground activities.

Pellegrini (1984, 1988a, 1988b, 1992, 1993) used behavioral categories similar to those of Humphreys and Smith (1984) to describe children's playground behavior. In addition to recording R&T play, he coded the affect of participants during the various activities (Pellegrini, 1992). The presence of a smile or play face was necessary in order to discriminate between R&T play and aggression. Further distinctions included the presence of role reversals, for example, if one child dominated another, yet lost the next bout. Blurton-Jones (1972) first described this necessary element. Indeed, the play literature now generally affirms that role reversals are essential for the establishment of playful mood and positive social interactions (Fry, 1987; Pellegrini, 1992).

Gender Differences in R&T Play

Humphreys and Smith (1987) have shown that there is a significant difference in the amount of R&T play a child participates in based upon the child's gender. When examining a cross section of children from one particular school in England, Humphreys and Smith noted that boys participated in significantly more R&T play than girls do at ages 7 and 11 but not at age 9. This finding is consistent with others reported by Pellegrini (1987, 1989a, 1989b) in which boys engage in more R&T play than girls in kindergarten, second and fourth grades. DiPietro (1981) has cited gender as differentially affecting the amount of R&T play in children. In a fixed interval sampling procedure of triadic groups of children, males' triadic groups were involved in more R&T play than female triadic groups.

What could account for the discrepancies in conclusions regarding gender? Humphreys and Smith (1984) argue that parents' may reinforce boys R&T but discourage it in their daughters leading to an argument that adult presence directly influences children's play behavior. Consequently, children, especially girls, may be more sensitive to the presence of the observer and may engage in less rough and tumble behavior. In any event, gender effects can be due to the methods used in a study, and we have found this to be the case in studies of rats. If one uses our "paired-encounter" (Panksepp, 1980) procedure where all play bouts from early development are studied there are no major gender effects, but if one uses the alternative "focal-observation" procedure, where socially housed family groups are periodically inspected for play behaviors, sex difference are evident (Meaney & Stewart, 1981). Indeed, when we allow 5 min of mixed gender play, the females begin exhibiting less play than the males, suggesting a rapid social-learning effect (Panksepp, unpublished observations in 1985).

Individual Difference in R&T Play

Few studies have examined personality variables that influence R&T play. Pellegrini (1992) examined R&T play and its relation to social problem solving flexibility. Children demonstrated this ability by resolving hypothetical problems presented to them by a researcher. In addition, Pellegrini used a paper and pencil measure of flexibility from the Dimensions of Temperament Survey. The results indicated that flexibility was not related to any dimension of R&T play. However, R&T play was related to social problem solving. Those children involved in more R&T play showed greater ability to solve problems in a flexible and adaptive way, relying less on aggression, and relying more on cooperation than those not engaging in R&T play. This is not necessarily a causative factor, but it is certainly worth pursuing.

Earlier work done by Pellegrini (1988a, 1988b) suggests that other child characteristics, such as popularity, may also play a role in the amount of R&T play a child engages in and the interpretation he or she makes about the interaction. For example, children nominated as popular in their class were more likely to engage in R&T play than those nominated and labeled "rejected." Indeed, Pellegrini (1988a, 1988b) has demonstrated that popular children moved readily into social games and other positive social interactions after engaging in R&T play, possibly making it more likely children choose them more frequently as play partners. On the other hand, aggressive and socially rejected children's R&T play often culminated in aggression, which could make it less likely that the child will be chosen again as a playmate. In addition, teacher's ratings of antisocial behavior for socially rejected children positively correlated with their R&T play, indicating that vigorous play may mean something different to these kids. Determining which came first, the aggression or the rejection was not addressed in the Pellegrini work, but it could be that popular children possess more social resources and skills than rejected kids and therefore can engage in more physically vigorous play without it turning aggressive. Thus, it comes as no surprise that individuals within play bouts are likely to be friends, even best friends, (Boulton, 1991b; Humphreys & Smith, 1987; and Smith & Boulton, 1990) while children that are antisocial have fewer friends resulting in less chance to participate in R&T play. Longer developmental studies are necessary to determine if the rejection preceded the aggression or if being aggressive with one's peers precludes later friendships.

Another important variable to consider is how temperament may influence a child's play. There are few studies where children's temperamental factors other than aggression and social dominance have been taken into account when studying play. Work by Kagan, Reznick and Snidman (1987) has shown that social inhibition or shyness is an important variable to consider when examining play behavior in children. Unfortunately, no studies have yet examined if children labeled as shy engage in less R&T behavior.

Additional Variables that Influence R&T Play

There are a number of variables that influence the amount and intensity of R&T in children that are relevant to the discussion of an intervention using vigorous play. Most important are gender, age, dimensions of play areas, type of play surfaces, and composition of the groups.

There is debate within the developmental literature regarding gender differences in play (Maccoby, 1997). Many researchers have concluded that boys' preferences of play partners (Maccoby & Jacklin, 1987), objects and activities are different from girls', especially in mixed gender social settings (Maccoby, 1997). Most researchers used playgrounds and other naturalistic settings where groups of boys and girls were together. Based on such studies, certain investigators have concluded that robust gender differences exist in the R&T play of boys and girls, with boys' playing more roughly than girls (Humphreys & Smith, 1987; Pellegrini, 1989a; Pellegrini & Smith, 1998). However, others have found only modest gender differences (Blurton-Jones, 1972; Boulton, 1996; DiPietro, 1981; Maccoby & Jacklin, 1987). As noted earlier, animal studies using mixed gender groups in complex social situations yield large gender effects (Meaney & Stewart, 1981), while "paired-encounters" procedures generally do not (Panksepp & Beatty, 1980). This is an observation that has been replicated in formal ethological studies of (Scott & Panksepp, 2003).

In one study of young (4–7 year olds) same-gender, same-age play pairs, Scott and Panksepp (2003) reported only a few modest differences between boys' and girls' R&T play behaviors. This is in contrast to previous work with older children where gender differences have commonly been evident (DiPietro, 1981; Humphreys & Smith, 1984, 1987; Pellegrini, 1989a). Scott & Panksepp, 2003 found that boys showed only modest increases in physical play solicitations like taps on the chest, but no difference in wrestling type behavior. Female pairs demonstrated more gross motor activities like rolling, walking and gymnastics. Pellegrini and Smith (1998), in a review of the literature, noted a slightly higher rate of play solicitations between boys compared with girls. Elsewhere, Pellegrini (1989a) noted that boys were more likely to engage in contact that is more physical during play bouts than girls, and concluded that boys are generally rougher than girls.

Another variable that influences amount of R&T play is age. Humphreys and Smith (1984, 1987) report a developmental curve in which 13% of 7 year olds' time is spent in R&T play, but declines to 9% and 5% respectively, in 9 and 11 year olds (Humphreys & Smith, 1987). However, Boulton (1996) found no differences in the relative percentage of time spent in R&T when he tested 8–11 year old children. (Scott & Panksepp, 2003) studied the free play of 3–6 year old children and performed separate analyses for two age groups (children 36–52 months of age and 52–72 months of age) and found no reliable and systematic differences in frequency of R&T play in these two age groups. These observations, combined with those of Humphreys and Smith (1987) suggest that R&T play remains constant until age 7 when it starts to decline in frequency.

Another factor influencing R&T play is the size and characteristics of the play space. Outdoor areas with few toys or playground equipment and that are soft, grassy, open and have high densities of children generally increase the likelihood of

R&T play (Humphreys & Smith, 1987; Pellegrini, 1989a, 1989b). Spacious indoor rooms allow more freedom of movement and generally increase R&T play (Smith & Connolly, 1980). However, when the area is below 25 square feet per child social interaction decreases and aggression increases (Smith & Connolly, 1980).

Probably more important than mere space, is the issue of group composition. Children are most likely to engage in R&T play in groups of three or more (McGrew, 1972; Pellegrini, 1984; Smith & Connolly, 1980). Larger groups greatly increase the number of potential play partners and in natural environments increases the likelihood that friends or groups of friends are present to facilitate play.

Another element influencing R&T play is the time that has elapsed since their last play bout. Animal researchers have demonstrated that animals deprived of play for periods of time will engage in more play after reintroduction to a playful situation (Panksepp & Beatty, 1980). Smith and Hagan (1980) compared the amount of R&T play children participated in based upon time spent in classroom activities. They found that the group of children that spent an additional 1.5 h in class played more vigorously when allowed to play on the playground at recess time (Smith & Hagan, 1980) than those held inside for only one hour. In the only study to date to test the relative developmental course of human R&T play bouts, Scott and Panksepp (2003) found that most play behaviors declined over the course of a one half-hour play period. This is consistent with past animal work (Panksepp et al., 1984), showing R&T behaviors systematically diminished during the course of the play sessions. Those behaviors that were the most physically demanding showed the most dramatic reductions, e.g., running, chasing, and other play behaviors.

Distinction of R&T Play from Aggression

When some parents and educators hear the descriptions of R&T, they sometimes confuse it with fighting or violence. Indeed, some of the action sequences in R&T play mimic aggression, but there are subtle differences. The next section contains a clear distinction between R&T play and aggression and why it is safe to encourage children to engage in R&T play.

Though R&T play and aggression appear similar on the surface, observations of R&T bouts yield clear distinctions between play and aggression (Blurton-Jones, 1972; Boulton, 1991a; Pellegrini, 1987; Scott & Panksepp, 2003). Aggression has a low occurrence rate in children's R&T play. In addition, both children and adults can reliably distinguish the two sets of behaviors (Smith & Boulton, 1990).

Usually, friendly verbal or physical solicitations or invitations (Smith & Boulton, 1990) initiate the beginning of the play bout and can be accepted or totally ignored with few negative consequences. In contrast, fights often begin when one child makes either verbal or physical threats against another, and to avoid humiliation, the threatened child retaliates with corresponding verbal jabs or physical violence (Smith & Boulton, 1990). Another difference is that fights often start when one child desires another's toy or play object (Blurton-Jones, 1972), whereas R&T play bouts are usually preceded by the participants playing together (Boulton, 1991b).

The specific interactions in R&T play fighting and aggression are very different. Physical aggression involves hitting with fists, pushing, and frowning, while R&T encompasses wrestling, jumping, hitting at and laughing (Blurton-Jones, 1976). Verbally, the interactions are very different. During physically aggressive interactions, the use of demeaning language, insulting, harassing, crying, and grimacing are common, whereas laughter and smiling characterize R&T play bouts (Blurton-Jones, 1976). Children's reports are positive after participating or watching R&T play on video clips (Boulton, 1993). However, when viewing an aggressive interaction they correctly characterize it as negative and aversive (Smith & Boulton, 1990).

An additional behavioral difference that occurs is that during play bouts, the larger or stronger participant engages in self-handicapping behaviors so the weaker partner has a chance to dominate periodically (Boulton, 1991a). This is done apparently in order to prolong the fun (Fry, 1987). In contrast, the dominant participant in an aggressive interaction will maintain superiority over the submissive partner (Blurton-Jones, 1976).

The consequences of aggressive interactions and friendly play also differ. Directly following R&T the children continue playing together either in more roughhousing or in other social games, such as tag, hopscotch, marbles or jump roping, but they move away from one another after aggression with little likelihood of a friendship developing (Blurton-Jones, 1972; Humphreys & Smith, 1987; Pellegrini, 1989a, 1989b). Play bouts rarely draw crowds of observers on a playground whereas aggressive interactions draw other children's attention (Smith & Boulton, 1990).

In addition to the behavioral and affective differences between R&T play and aggression, when studied carefully, children and adults can reliably distinguish between them about 80–90% of the time (Boulton, 1993; Smith & Boulton, 1990; Smith & Lewis, 1985). When asked, children name specific behaviors and accompanying affect as the features separating aggression from play. They are able to identify that participants are having fun, because they are smiling, laughing and the blows inflicted are either missing the other child or seem to be much less serious than in fighting (Blurton-Jones, 1976; Smith & Boulton, 1990).

Play as a Strategy to Address ADHD

A great deal of the literature has dealt with the description of play, namely that it is a common childhood phenomenon which can be observed, measured and facilitated under controlled and semi-controlled settings. Only a few have speculated about potential benefits or functions it can have in the life of a child, causing others to call for further work to demonstrate potential benefits human children may derive from regular vigorous R&T play (Panksepp, 1998a, 1998b; Pellegrini, 1988a, 1988b; Scott & Panksepp, 2003). The next section will detail one promising possibility—the provision of extra play opportunities—that may benefit children diagnosed with ADHD.

ADHD and Play

While there is a growing school of thought that ADHD is primarily a brain disorder, there are those in the scientific community who view it as a set of behaviors at the extreme end of the normal developmental continuum. For example, Panksepp (1998a) has argued that the symptoms diagnosed as ADHD are an overactive playfulness based on the similarity between behavioral descriptions of R&T play and the symptoms of ADHD outlined in the DSM-IV (American Psychiatric Association, 1994). Additionally, drugs given to reduce impulsiveness also reduce R&T play dramatically in both animals and children (Talmadge & Barkley, 1983; Siviy & Panksepp, 2011). As seen above, those with ADHD have hypoarousal of the frontal cortex, which may make it difficult to inhibit playful urges. By giving these children extra time to play, and become play satiated, this may lead to reduced hyperactivity later in the classroom. Further, a sustained increase in the availability of R&T play may lead to better maturation of higher behavior regulatory regions of the brain such as the frontal lobes.

Such possibilities seem especially pertinent since the potential benefit of allowing extra natural play to reduce inattentive and disruptive behavior in the classroom has not been evaluated. As noted earlier, R&T play and the urge to roughhouse makes up nearly 10% of all play that children engage in between the ages of 7 and 11. Additional aspects of R&T play that make it particularly conducive for this intervention are that it is a normal part of children's behavioral repertoire, kids find it enjoyable, and it is safe (Humphreys & Smith, 1987; Scott & Panksepp, 2003). R&T play is often found in larger groups of children (Humphreys & Smith, 1984), and is more likely to occur after a long period of deprivation (Panksepp & Beatty, 1980; Smith & Hagan, 1980). Since R&T play is a regulated brain function (Panksepp, 1980), children who are not allowed to play regularly may find other ways of exhibiting these urges. Thus, efforts to increase R&T play could provide a treatment that side steps safety concerns associated with medications (e.g., decreased appetite, weight loss, retarded growth, drug tolerance, an increased risk for future substance abuse) specifically avoiding the specter of sensitization, while providing ample time for children to engage in developmentally appropriate behaviors.

It is not the intent of this paper to argue that R&T should be the only form of play in which young children are engaged. However, we believe providing this form of play could bestow clear benefits for children and expand the types of play to which children are exposed. Bornstein, Haynes, Pascual, Painter, and Galperin (1999) advocates for a balance in the amount and variety of forms of play when he highlighted the importance of exploratory and symbolic play, not viewing one form as superior to another. Each form of play is a building block for additional skills. For example, younger children typically engage in more exploratory play (e.g., moving toys about the room, stacking blocks) and later move to more symbolic play (e.g., placing telephone to ear, creating a tea party with friends) (Bornstein et al., 1999). Without exploring, symbolic representations of the world could not take place. Howes and Matheson (1992) described the increasing frequency of the use of social and pretend play (similar to symbolic play of Bornstein), as children grow older. In a recent study they indicated that cooperative social pretend play (e.g., one child is the customer the other the storekeeper) and complex social pretend play (e.g., children decide on and agree to take roles and talk about it together) reach their peaks in children between the ages of 35 and 60 months of age (Howes & Matheson, 1992). This was precisely the age of children in a preliminary study we conducted (Scott, 2001), as noted below.

Yet, another perspective is provided by Piaget's formulation of psychosocial stages. Children in this study would fall into the sensorimotor and preoperational stages. According to Piaget, 2-year-old children begin the capacity to use symbols to represent reality, which happens at the end of the sensorimotor stage and extends to the preoperational stage. Using this skill, the slightly older 3-year-old (now in the preoperational stage) engaging in R&T symbolically hits and swings, without connecting or at less than full strength. In response, his or her play partner will dramatically fall to the floor feigning pain. This example illustrates both the symbolic nature of R&T (sensorimotor stage) and the dramatic nature of more advanced play (preoperational stage). It should be no surprise then that many of the investigators examining R&T play in naturalistic settings also observed older children moving directly to games with rules immediately following R&T play (concrete operational stage) (Humphreys & Smith, 1984). In many ways the roles that children often take in the R&T play bout are analogous to the symbolic play of Bornstein, the complex social pretend play described by Howes and Matheson (1992) and the preoperational child described by Piaget. Allowing children to play in this manner enhances their development. Frost, Wortham, and Reifel (2001) indicate that children within the preschool years engage in exercise, gross motor play, make believe and dramatic play beginning around age two and continue through the school age years. These are important skills for academic and social success. Pellegrini and Smith (1998) reviewed the literature regarding the benefits of R&T play, which include increased problem-solving behavior, increased cardiovascular endurance, strength training, and enhanced cognitive performance.

Suggestions for Practitioners

We believe that play is likely a safer treatment for children with attention problems than psychostimulant medication. As outlined in the introduction section, the reduction in playfulness noted after the use of psychostimulant medication, the potential for addiction, and the possibility of brain sensitization all make looking for other forms of treatment desirable.

Play circuitry of the brain and its neurochemical controls, which regrettably has been only highlighted in experimental animals such as laboratory rats (Siviy & Panksepp, 2011) is perhaps the major functional tool, provided by our ancestral genetic heritage, to allow fully social brains to mature, nourished by powerful neurotrophic functions of play (Burgdorf et al., 2010, 2011; Gordon et al., 2003).

The prime vocal indicator of playfulness in humans, namely laughter (Scott & Panksepp, 2003), has now been modeled in animals (Panksepp, 2007b). We postulate that sustained satisfaction of the primal urge for physical play in all mammals, throughout early life, should facilitate brain maturation through the release of growth factors such as Brain Derived Neurotrophic Factor (Gordon et al., 2003) and Insulin Like Growth Factor-1 (Burgdorf et al., 2010), and thereby perhaps promote prosocial regulatory functions of the frontal lobes which are deficient in ADHD, and thereby reduce impulse control disorders as children grow up. We have been pleasantly surprised by the numbers of genes that are activated by physical brain within the neocortex (Burgdorf et al., 2011), brain tissue that is not necessary for the expression of play (Panksepp, Normansell, Cox, & Siviy, 1994).

In our informal clinical experience, we have also found that fathers of single-child families who are trained to regularly indulge in vigorous physical play for about half an hour before the child is sent to sleep, typically have fewer of the all too common going-to-sleep difficulties children experience when they sleep alone. Furthermore, parents of single-child families who have come to us for advice on how to rear their child, who seem to be on the ADHD track, have been given the uniform instruction to have at least two rough-and-tumble play periods with their children, one in the morning after breakfast and one before bed-time. We have only received positive reports of such informal interventions. This has made us convinced that it is very important to evaluate such variables in formal outcome studies, but we have found that funding for such research is not available.

We are currently evaluating the potential of play for alleviating depression in animal models. The results have been clear. If animals are given various stressors that seem to produce depressive states, play or tickling given soon after the stressors diminishes the long-term impact of those vicissitudes. Thus, another beneficial effect of abundant childhood play is that it may promote a resilience prone nervous system, and potentially thereby reduce incidence of childhood and adult depression. It is well recognized that childhood depression is devastating for playfulness (Mol Lous, de Wit, De Bruyn, & Riksen-Walraven, 2002). We should also not forget that long-term administration of psychostimulants to animals and humans, as is so common in the treatment of ADHD can promote depressive rebounds after the medications are removed. In short, clinicians specializing in the treatment of troubled children, many of whom use various forms of play therapies, should keep in mind the potentially vast benefits of physical play for both brain and mind development. Indeed, we have identified potential new antidepressant medications by analyzing the effects of play on gene expression patterns in animal brains (Burgdorf et al., 2011).

Of course, most clinicians are not comfortable getting physically playful with the children they are trying to help, but they would be wise to consider the benefits. When a child psychoanalyst friend of the senior author, Mark Smaller of Chicago, recognized the potential importance of such ludic activities, he decided that the games he had long been using in his practice might be less effective than direct physically playful engagements with young children. Indeed, as he chose to be physically playful with his young clients, the children more easily opened up to him as a valuable person in their lives, making the therapeutic enterprise move along much more rapidly, probably because of the sheer joy involved. By helping restore their primal nature to them, Mark found the therapeutic enterprise moved along much more rapidly, and since then he had less and less use for the toys and games he had used before.

Future Directions for Research on Rough and Tumble Play

We are at the very beginning of formal studies of the benefits of play in human children. Indeed, the first formal ethologically oriented experimental analysis of play in our species happened a little over a decade ago (Scott & Panksepp, 2003). Once we begin to realize that the playful urge is built into the brains of our children, and that it is a fundamental social experience-expectant function of their minds that helps them learn about the social nuances of their species, we may begin to return play to its rightful, most-prominent place in young children's development—a process that can only be fully expressed in the safety of stable social-bonds, a secure base that is essential for the full and spontaneous expression of play. Chronic separation anxiety depletes the capacity of children to have the full benefits of play.

Play allows children a safe place to develop the social skills they will need for the rest of their lives—the capacity to engage other's positively, and to understand what may be going on in other minds. Through play they learn to be productive and happy individuals in their social groups. Their playful mock battles also prepare them for skills needed in social competition, but in our experience, if ongoing play is supervised by sensitive adults, it will not lead to bullying and marginalization of others, which is always a distinct possibility in unsupervised play.

Ever increasingly in modern societies, more and more young children have few rough-and-tumble play opportunities. The activities they are offered by adult all too commonly pale in comparison to the games children themselves devise. In our estimation, it is long past time for someone to fund the concept of "play sanctuaries" where young children can be taken to have free play each day among others of their age. We instituted such a societal project in Bowling Green, Ohio in the late 1990s, and it served as the junior authors dissertation project (Scott, 2001). We found that when preschool children were allowed free play for half an hour before classes, that they largely enjoyed the activities, and that we could easily diminish naughty behaviors by allowing a prompt return to play as the reward for agreeing not to act in ways that had been clearly emotionally disturbing to other children. We could see the hard to document benefits of play in front of our eyes, even though significantly improved behavior was hard to demonstrate in formal classroom observations, perhaps because of low base-rates for bad behaviors in our group of children. We would be glad to send copies of the dissertation to anyone who is interested in pursuing the details.

In sum we suspect that children who have a meager diet of joyous physical play in their childhood are likely to become more socially dysfunctional in adulthood. They will be less able to handle the social complexities of adult life, to develop strong positive relationships with others, and to provide the blessing of secure social-bonds down to their own children. We think adequate amounts of early play will allow children to "thrive by five" (the optimistic early-learning slogan in the State of Washington)—to become ever better prepared to cope with the complexities that will confront them as they grow up (Panksepp, 2010). But the really good science that needs to be done on this issue has yet to materialize (in our experience, largely for lack of funding). Let the research begin.

References

Aldis, O. (1975). *Play fighting*. New York: Academic.

American Psychiatric Association. (1994). *Diagnostic and statistical manual of mental disorders* (4th ed.). Washington, D.C.: American Psychiatric Association.

Barkley, R. A. (1997). *ADHD and the nature of self-control*. New York: Guilford.

Bekoff, M., & Byers, J. A. (1998). *Animal Play: evolutionary, comparative, and ecological perspectives*. New York: Cambridge University Press.

Bertrand, M. (1976). Rough-and-tumble play in stumptails. In J. S. Bruner, A. Jolly, & K. Sylva (Eds.), *Play—its role in development and evolution* (pp. 320–327). New York: Basic.

Blurton-Jones, N. (1972). Categories of child-child interaction. In N. Blurton- Jones (Ed.), *Ethological studies of child behavior* (pp. 97–129). New York: Cambridge University Press.

Blurton-Jones, N. (1976). Rough-and-tumble play among nursery school children. In J. S. Bruner, A. Jolly, & K. Sylva (Eds.), *Play—its role in development and evolution* (pp. 352–363). New York: Basic.

Bornstein, M. H., Haynes, O. M., Pascual, L., Painter, K. M., & Galperin, C. (1999). Play in two societies: pervasiveness of process, specificity of structure. *Child Development, 70*, 317–331.

Boulton, M. J. (1991a). A comparison of structural and contextual features of middle school children's playful and aggressive fighting. *Ethology and Sociobiology, 12*, 119–145.

Boulton, M. J. (1991b). Partner preferences in middle school children's playful fighting and chasing. *Ethology and Sociobiology, 12*, 177–193.

Boulton, M. J. (1993). Children's abilities to distinguish between playful and aggressive fighting: a developmental perspective. *British Journal of Developmental Psychology, 11*, 249–263.

Boulton, M. J. (1996). A comparison of 8- and 11-year-old girls' and boys' participation in specific types of rough-and-tumble play and aggressive fighting: Implications for functional hypothesis. *Aggressive Behavior, 22*, 271–287.

Boulton, M. J., & Smith, P. K. (1992). The social nature of play fighting and play chasing: mechanisms and strategies underlying cooperation and compromise. In J. H. Barkow, L. Cosmides, & J. Tooby (Eds.), *The adapted mind: evolutionary psychology and the generation of culture* (pp. 429–449). New York: Oxford University Press.

Burgdorf, J., Kroes, R. A., Beinfeld, M. C., Panksepp, J., & Moskal, J. R. (2010). Uncovering the molecular basis of positive affect using rough-and-tumble play in rats: a role for insulin-like growth factor I. *Neuroscience, 168*, 769–777.

Burgdorf, J., Panksepp, J., & Moskal, J. R. (2011). Frequency-modulated 50 kHz ultrasonic vocalizations: a tool for uncovering the molecular substrates of positive affect. *Neuroscience & Biobehavioral Reviews, 35*, 1831–1836.

Burgdorf, J., Wood, P. L., Kroes, R. A., Moskal, J. R., & Panksepp, J. (2007). Neurobiology of 50-kHz ultrasonic vocalizations in rats: electrode mapping, lesion, and pharmacology studies. *Behavioral Brain Research, 182*, 274–283.

Burghardt, G. M. (2005). *The genesis of animal play*. Cambridge, MA: MIT.

Byers, J. A., & Walker, C. (1995). Refining the motor training hypothesis for the evolution of play. *American Naturalist, 146*, 25–40.

DiPietro, J. A. (1981). Rough and tumble play: a function of gender. *Developmental Psychology,* *17*, 50–58.

Erikson, E. H. (1950). *Childhood and society.* New York: W.W. Norton.

Fagen, R. (1981). *Animal play behavior.* New York: Oxford.

Frost, J. L., Wortham, S., & Reifel, S. (2001). *Play and child development.* Upper Saddle River, NJ: Merrill Prentice Hall.

Fry, D. P. (1987). Difference between play fighting and serious fighting among zapotec children. *Ethology and Sociobiology, 8,* 285–306.

Gandelman, R. (1992). Play: *The psychobiology of behavioral development.* (Monogragh) New York: Oxford University Press.

Gilmore, J. B. (1971). Play: a special behavior. In R. E. Herron & B. Sutton-Smith (Eds.), *Child's play* (pp. 311–325). New York: Wiley.

Gordon, N. S., Burke, S., Akil, H., Watson, J., & Panksepp, J. (2003). Socially induced brain fertilization: play promotes brain derived neurotrophic factor expression. *Neuroscience Letters, 341,* 17–20.

Groos, K. (1898). *The play of animals.* New York: D. Appleton.

Howes, C., & Matheson, C. (1992). Sequence in the development of competent play with peers: social and pretend play. *Developmental Psychology, 28,* 961–974.

Humphreys, A., & Smith, P. (1984). Rough-and-tumble in preschool and playground. In P. K. Smith (Ed.), *Play in animals and humans* (pp. 241–270). London, UK: Blackwell.

Humphreys, A., & Smith, P. (1987). Rough-and-tumble, friendship, and dominance in school children: Evidence for continuity and change with age. *Child Development, 58,* 201–212.

Ikemoto, S., & Panksepp, J. (1992). The effects of early social isolation on the motivation for social play in juvenile rats. *Developmental Psychobiology, 25,* 261–274.

Kagan, J., Reznick, J. S., & Snidman, N. (1987). The physiology and psychology of behavioral inhibition in children. *Child Development, 58,* 1459–1473.

Louv, R. (2008). *Last child in the woods: saving our children from nature-deficit disorder.* Chapel Hill, NC: Algonquin Books of Chapel Hill.

Maccoby, E. E. (1997). Gender and relationships: a developmental account. *American Psychologist, 45,* 513–520.

Maccoby, E. E., & Jacklin, C. N. (1987). Gender segregation in childhood. In H. W. Reese (Ed.), *Advances in child development and behavior* (Vol. 20, pp. 239–288). New York: Academic.

McGrew, W. C. (1972). *An ecological study of children's behaviour.* London, UK: Academic.

Meaney, M. J., & Stewart, J. (1981). Neonatal androgens influence the social play of prepubescent rats. *Hormones and Behavior, 15,* 197–213.

Mol Lous, A., de Wit, C. A., De Bruyn, E. E., & Riksen-Walraven, J. M. (2002). Depression markers in young children's play: a comparison between depressed and nondepressed 3- to 6-year-olds in various play situations. *Journal of Child Psychology and Psychiatry, 43,* 1029–1038.

Panksepp, J. (1980). The ontogeny of play in rats. *Developmental Psychobiology, 14,* 327–332.

Panksepp, J. (1993). Rough and tumble play: a fundamental brain process. In K. McDonald (Ed.), *Parent-child play: description and implications* (SUNY series, Children's Play in Society, pp. 147–184). Albany, New York: State University of New York Press.

Panksepp, J. (1998a). *Affective neuroscience.* New York: Oxford University Press.

Panksepp, J. (1998b). The quest for long-term health and happiness: to play or not to play, that is the question. *Psychological Inquiry, 9,* 56–66.

Panksepp, J. (2007a). Can PLAY diminish ADHD and facilitate the construction of the social brain. *Journal of the Canadian Academy of Child and Adolescent Psychiatry, 10,* 57–66.

Panksepp, J. (2007b). Neuroevolutionary sources of laughter and social joy: modeling primal human laughter in laboratory rats. *Behavioral Brain Research, 182*(2), 231–244.

Panksepp, J. (2008). PLAY, ADHD and the construction of the social brain: Should the first class each day be recess? *American Journal of Play, 1,* 55–79.

Panksepp, J. (2010). Science of the brain as a gateway to understanding play: An interview with Jaak Panksepp. *American Journal of Play, 2,* 145–277.

Panksepp, J., & Beatty, W. W. (1980). Social deprivation and play in rats. *Behavior and Neural biology, 30*, 197–206.

Panksepp, J., Burgdorf, J., & Gordon, N. (2003). Modeling ADHD-type arousal with unilateral frontal cortex damage in rats and beneficial effects of play therapy. *Brain and Cognition, 52*, 97–105.

Panksepp, J., Normansell, L., Cox, J. F., & Siviy, S. M. (1994). Effects of neonatal decortication on the social play of juvenile rats. *Physiology & Behavior, 56*, 429–443.

Panksepp, J., Siviy, S., & Normansell, L. (1984). The psychobiology of play: theoretical and methodological perspectives. *Neuroscience & Biobehavioral Reviews, 8*, 465–492.

Pellegrini, A. D. (1984). The social cognitive ecology of preschool children. *International Journal of Behavioral Development, 7*, 321–332.

Pellegrini, A. D. (1987). Rough-and-tumble play: developmental and educational significance. *Educational Psychologist, 22*, 23–43.

Pellegrini, A. D. (1988a). Elementary-school children's rough-and-tumble play and social competence. *Developmental Psychology, 24*, 802–806.

Pellegrini, A. D. (1988b). What is a category? The case of rough-and-tumble play. *Ethology and Sociobiology, 10*, 331–341.

Pellegrini, A. D. (1989a). Elementary school children's rough-and-tumble play. *Early Childhood Research Quarterly, 4*, 245–260.

Pellegrini, A. D. (1989b). Categorizing children's rough-and-tumble play. *Play and Culture, 2*, 48–51.

Pellegrini, A. D. (1992). Rough-and-tumble play and social problem solving flexibility. *Creativity Research Journal, 5*, 13–26.

Pellegrini, A. D. (1993). Boys' rough-and-tumble play, social competence and group composition. *British Journal of Developmental Psychology, 11*, 237–248.

Pellegrini, A. D., & Smith, P. K. (1998). Physical activity play: the nature and function of a neglected aspect of play. *Child Development, 69*, 577–598.

Pellis, S., & Pellis, V. (2009). *The playful brain: venturing to the limits of neuroscience.* Oxford, UK: Oneworld.

Piaget, J. (1962). *Play, dreams and imitation in childhood.* New York: W.W. Norton.

Potegal, M., & Einon, D. (1989). Aggressive behaviors in adult rats deprived of playfighting experience as juveniles. *Developmental Psychobiology, 22*, 159–172.

Power, T. G. (2000). *Play and exploration in children and animals.* Mahwah, NJ: Lawrence Erlbaum Associates.

Scott, E. (2001). Toward a play program to benefit children's attention in the classroom. Unpublished Ph.D. Dissertation. Bowling Green State University, Bowling Green, OH.

Scott, E., & Panksepp, J. (2003). Rough-and-tumble play in human children. *Aggressive Behaviour, 29*, 539–551.

Siviy, S. M., & Panksepp, J. (2011). In search of the neurobiological substrates for social playfulness in mammalian brains. *Neuroscience and Biobehavioral Reviews, 35*, 1821–1830.

Smith, P., & Boulton, M. (1990). Rough-and-tumble play, aggression and dominance: perception and behavior in children's encounters. *Human Development, 33*, 271–282.

Smith, P. K., & Connolly, K. J. (1980). *The ecology of preschool behavior.* Cambridge, UK: Cambridge University Press.

Smith, P. K., & Hagan, T. (1980). Effects of deprivation on exercise play in nursery school children. *Animal Behavior, 28*, 922–928.

Smith, P. K., & Lewis, K. (1985). Rough-and-tumble play, fighting, and chasing in nursery school children. *Ethology and Sociobiology, 6*, 175–181.

Sumpner, C., & Blatchford, P. (1998). What do we know about breaktime? Results from a national survey of breaktime and lunchtime in primary and secondary schools. *British Educational Research Journal, 24*, 79–94.

Sutton-Smith, B., & Kelly-Byrne, D. (1984). The phenomenon of bipolarity in play theories. In B. Sutton-Smith & D. Kelly-Byrne (Eds.), *Child's play: developmental and applied* (pp. 29–47). New Jersey: Lawrence Erlbaum.

Talmadge, J., & Barkley, R. A. (1983). The interactions of hyperactive and normal boys and their fathers and mothers. *Journal of Abnormal Child Psychology, 11*, 565–580.

van den Berg, C. L., Hol, T., Van Ree, J. M., Spruijt, B. M., Everts, H., & Koolhaas, J. M. (1999). Play is indispensable for an adequate development of coping with social challenges in the rats. *Developmental Psychobiology, 34*, 129–138.

Vanderschuren, L. J. M. J. (2010). How the brain makes play fun. *American Journal of Play, 2*, 315–337.

Chapter 3
Physical Activity, Cognition, and School Performance: From Neurons to Neighborhoods

Darla M. Castelli and Charles H. Hillman

This generation of children is less physically active and fit than their predecessors. The prevalence of overweight and obesity rates in children have increased dramatically over the last two decades (Pate et al., 2006), with approximately 16 % of the US children identified as obese and 32 % identified as overweight. Media, video gaming, and the Internet are currently identified as inhibitors to regular engagement in physical activity among children. Habitual physical activity begins in the home environment prior to schooling, as one-third of 5-year-olds entering Kindergarten are identified as overweight or obese (Ogden, Carroll, & Flegal, 2008). Schools have been called to assume a leadership role in promoting behaviors that will prevent the development of overweight and obesity (Pate et al., 2006). Without intervention, there will be further decline of student health resulting from modern inactive lifestyles, as physical inactivity leads to the development of several chronic diseases in later life. As such, the short- and long-term effects of this modern sedentary lifestyle on physical and cognitive health are of immediate concern.

Recently, the focus on physical activity benefits to brain and cognition has shifted from the study of adult cognition to that of children. Accordingly, researchers and practitioners have become interested in whether physical activity may serve to improve not only physical health conditions, but also cognitive health and function. Several interesting lines of research have developed which are aimed at understanding

D.M. Castelli (✉)
Department of Kinesiology & Health Education Physical Education Teacher Education,
Anna Hiss Gym 103, A2000, The University of Texas at Austin, 1 University Station,
Mail code D3700, Austin, TX 78712, USA
e-mail: dcastelli@mail.utexas.edu

C.H. Hillman
Departments of Kinesiology & Community Health, Psychology, and Internal Medicine,
Beckman Institute for Advanced Science and Technology, Urbana, IL, USA

Division of Neuroscience, Division of Nutritional Sciences,
University of Illinois at Urbana-Champaign,
317 Louise Freer Hall, 906 South Goodwin Avenue, Urbana, IL 61801, USA

A.L. Meyer and T.P. Gullotta (eds.), *Physical Activity Across the Lifespan*,
Issues in Children's and Families' Lives 12, DOI 10.1007/978-1-4614-3606-5_3,
© Springer Science+Business Media New York 2012

basic and applied benefits of physical activity to cognitive and brain health. The aim of such research is to improve health, enhance cognition, and provide benefits to effective functioning across the lifespan. Since 1975 when a seminal study was conducted by Spriduso comparing the cognitive performance of exercising versus non-exercising adults, researchers have been attempting to quantify the mind–body relationship in a meaningful way. This chapter describes the body of work to date on physical activity and cognitive health in school age children.

Prior to the onset of the industrial revolution, people were required to be considerably more active than we are today. Our ancestors were predominantly hunter–gatherers (Eaton & Konner, 1985), who were required to expend energy for survival. However, contemporary humans do not have the same requirements, as recent technological advancements have obviated the need for many aspects of physical activity that were once necessities in our lives (see Vaynman & Gomez-Pinilla, 2006 for review). Further, through the consumption of high fat and processed foods, caloric intake has increased, translating to an epidemic of poor physical health.

Physical activity is any bodily movement that causes you to work harder than normal. Unlike the inherent physical demands of yesterday, today's definition of physical activity includes low impact activities such as standing and walking up stairs. Technological advances have manifested a reduction in energy expenditure and when coupled with increased caloric consumption, have increased the incidence of disease such as obesity and type 2 diabetes. Behavioral changes have led to decreased physical fitness. Initially, the definition of physical fitness focused primarily on athletic performance and how individual traits contributed toward the refinement of motor skill. Since that time, governmental agencies have equated physical fitness more closely with health-related components such as cardiorespiratory endurance, muscular endurance, strength, flexibility, and body composition. The modern definition of physical fitness is believed to more accurately reflect its importance, given the changes in our physical demands.

Recently, research has demonstrated that cognitive aspects of health may be at risk due to the evolution of human behavior. A recognized connection between mind and body may be traced at least as far back as ancient Greek civilization. A glance at our more recent past indicates that researchers have been aware that physical activity may influence cognitive function since at least the 1930s. For the next few decades, links between physical fitness and reaction time (i.e., the time from the beginning of a discrete stimulus to the initiation of the response to it) were described with mixed results (Beise & Peaseley, 1937; Burpee & Stroll, 1936; Lawther, 1951; Pierson & Montoye, 1958). It was not until the 1970s when Spirduso and her colleagues began the systematic investigation of the relationship between fitness and cognitive function, that the beneficial influences of aerobic exercise on simple (i.e., the mapping of a single stimulus to a single response) and choice (i.e., the mapping of multiple stimuli to multiple responses) were documented. Importantly, Spirduso's work demonstrated that aerobic fitness was beneficial to older adults' motor performance, while no such relationship was established in younger adults (Baylor & Spirduso, 1988; Spirduso, 1975, 1980; Spirduso & Clifford, 1978). Accordingly, Spirduso's findings gave rise to the notion that physical activity may ameliorate or protect against the maladaptive effects of cognitive aging.

Given these findings, researchers began to focus their attention on the relationship between physical activity and older adults' cognitive function. Several studies emerged in the 1980s. Among them, two influential projects impacted the field. The first was a randomized control intervention with older adults that gave rise to several publications demonstrating increases in aerobic fitness were beneficial to a number of cognitive and motor processes on the behavioral and neuroelectric levels (Dustman et al., 1984; 1990). These data were some of the first to manipulate change in aerobic fitness and demonstrate concomitant change in cognition selectively for aerobically trained older adults relative to non-exercising and strength-trained individuals. The second project to influence the field was a review of the extant literature by Tomporowski and Ellis (1986). This paper is credited with producing the first comprehensive review in which the authors' concluded that the 27 published studies presented insufficient information to posit the relationship between physical activity, fitness, and cognitive performance, thus shaping the focus of researchers in this field for the next 10–15 years.

During the late 1990s and into the new millennium, the investigation of physical activity on adult cognition continued. An influential meta-analysis examining over 107 published research papers (Etnier et al., 1997) supported the earlier empirical and descriptive findings that had been demonstrated a decade earlier and concluded that physical activity has a small, but positive impact on sensory, cognitive, and motor processes. A second published meta-analysis (Colcombe & Kramer, 2003), along with several empirical studies (e.g., Colcombe et al., 2004; Kramer et al., 1999), extended the earlier notion that physical activity benefited older adults' cognition, but indicated that the relationship was more complex. Specifically, convergent evidence by Kramer and his colleagues indicated that physical activity was generally beneficial to cognition, but that it had a selective and disproportionately large effect on an aspect of cognition known as executive control. Executive control refers to a subset of goal-directed cognitive processes involved in the selection, scheduling, and coordination of perception, memory, and action.

Concurrently, nonhuman animal research was evidencing beneficial effects of exercise on cellular and molecular alterations in brain. Greenough and his colleagues (Black, Isaacs, Anderson, Alcantara, & Greenough, 1990), observed differential effects of aerobic exercise and motor learning on the cerebellar cortex among trained and untrained rats. Since then, exercise effects on brain using nonhuman animal models have demonstrated benefits in neurogenesis (growth of new brain cells; van Praag, Kempermann, & Gage, 1999), including angiogenesis (growth of new blood vessels) and synaptogenesis (formation and enhancement of synapses; Isaacs, Anderson, Alcantara, Black, & Greenough, 1992); enhanced the production of neurochemicals such as brain-derived neurotrophin factor (Cotman & Berchtold, 2002; Neeper, Gomez-Pinilla, Choi, & Cottman, 1995; Vaynman & Gomez-Pinilla, 2006), insulin-like growth factor 1 (which plays an important role in brain development during childhood; Carro, Trejo, Busiguina, & Torres-Aleman, 2001), and monoamines (enhancement of brain function through an increased the presence of amino acids; Dishman et al., 1997); and regional changes in cerebral blood flow (Delp et al., 2001), to name a few.

Overview of Brain Development

To grasp the development of perception, cognition, and action, it is necessary to understand the development of underlying brain structure and function. The brain endures significant changes in both its structural architecture and functional organization across the human lifespan, but the most dramatic growth is evidenced in the first few years of life. During maturation, the brain exhibits substantial change, with its weight doubling during the first year of life resulting in a cortical surface area similar to the adult brain by the second year of life (Taylor, 2006). By 6 years of age, the developing brain is approximately 90 % the size of a fully mature adult brain (Casey, Galvan, & Hare, 2005), with dynamic changes continuing throughout the course of development until maturation is complete, and a functional peak achieved around the age of 21.

Accompanying such modifications in brain size are changes in metabolism. During the first year of life, the metabolic demands of the infant brain increase dramatically, with oxygen consumption being at least double to that of the adult brain (Morgan & Gibson, 1991). This increase in metabolism undoubtedly occurs in support of the alterations in gray and white matter volume. Maturation of the myelination process (i.e., white matter) has been routinely associated with brain development (Taylor, 2006) and is considered a rough index of regional brain development (Konner, 1991). Myelin, a dielectric fatty white sheath surrounding neuronal axons, allows for rapid and effective conduction of electrical signals through the nervous system. The myelination process, much like maturation in general, occurs throughout the course of development with myelination beginning prenatally in certain structures such as the spinal cord; while other structures such as the frontal lobes continue to demonstrate increased myelination into the fifth decade of life (Bartzokis et al., 2001) and beyond (Colcombe et al., 2006).

The development of gray matter volume also varies by brain region, with the majority demonstrating increases in volume through the preadolescent and adolescent years, after which point decreases due to loss or pruning of redundant connections are observed (Giedd et al., 1999). However, the decreases in gray matter are accompanied by increases in white matter, resulting in stability of brain volume (Taylor, 2006). Thus, both regressive (gray matter) and progressive (white matter) processes develop in concert to enhance neural efficiency underlying sensory, cognitive, and motor function (Casey et al., 2005a).

Accordingly, the efficiency of various cognitive functions is dependent upon the maturational timing of the underlying neural tissue and pathways mediating specific functions. For example, brain regions subserving primary sensory and motor functions are some of the earliest to mature (Casey, Tottenham, Liston, & Durston, 2005b), with the peak overproduction of synapses occurring during the first year of life in the visual cortex, and the pruning process complete during the next few years (Huttenlocher, 1979). By comparison, the prefrontal cortex (PFC), a region of the brain subserving more complex cognitions, exhibits peak overproduction about 1 year following birth, with the gradual retraction of synapses continuing into late adolescence (Shonkoff & Phillips, 2000). This latter region (i.e., PFC) is especially interesting because of its involvement with high-order cognitive functions such as executive control, which underlie scholastic performance (e.g., reading comprehension, mathematics, problem solving, etc.) and are some of the more protracted aspects of cognition to mature (Casey et al., 2005a; Casey, Giedd, & Thomas, 2000; Diamond, 2006). Some would suggest this is like the analogy *you cannot teach an old dog new tricks*; however, recent research on physical activity and cognition suggests otherwise.

Experience Shapes Neural Development

Certain aspects of brain development have been linked with experience, indicating an intricate interplay between genetic programming and external environmental influences. Gray matter, and the organization of synaptic connections in particular, appear to be dependent upon experience (Shonkoff & Phillips, 2000; Taylor, 2006), with the brain exhibiting a remarkable ability to reorganize itself in response to input from sensory systems, other cortical systems, or insult (Huttenlocher & Dabholkar, 1997). During normal development, following the excess growth of synaptic connections, experience shapes the pruning process, through the strengthening of neural networks that support relevant thoughts and actions and the elimination of unnecessary or redundant connections.

Greenough and his colleagues (Black & Greenough, 1986; Greenough & Black, 1992) distinguish between experience-expectant and experience-dependent influences upon brain development. Experience-expectant influences refer to situations or environments that are typical to a species, which are required for normal organization of the nervous system to occur. That is, normal development of the brain relies upon typical exposure to these aspects of the environment. For example, the genetic program for the visual cortex requires exposure to light and patterned visual information (Shonkoff & Phillips, 2000). When these aspects of the environment are not afforded, permanent deprivation of the visual cortex can occur, severely altering cognition and action. Experience-dependent influences refer to nontypical aspects (i.e., idiosyncratic experiences) of the environment that stimulate new brain growth and/or the sculpting of neural networks in support of these unique experiences. In this manner, experience-dependent processes shape the individual's adaptations to the environment on neural, and consequently behavioral, levels.

As such, the brain responds to experience in an adaptive or "plastic" manner, resulting in the efficient and effective adoption of thoughts, skills, and actions relevant to one's interactions within their surroundings. Examples of neural plasticity in response to unique environmental interaction have been demonstrated in human neuroimaging studies of music (Chan, Ho, & Cheung, 1998; Elbert, Pantev, Wienbruch, Rockstroh, & Taub, 1995; Münte, Kohlmetz, Nager, & Altenmüller, 2001) and sports participation (Aglioti, Cesari, Romani, & Urgesi, 2008; Hatfield & Hillman, 2001), thus supporting the educational practice of providing music education and opportunities for physical activity to children. More generally, the educational experience and quality of the education would be expected to influence neural growth and development in an experience-dependent manner, leading to idiosyncratic differences in development as a result of the particular educational environment.

Executive Control Function

As discussed earlier, the history of the field of physical activity and cognition was primarily focused on cognitive aging. Accordingly, several high profile review papers (e.g., Hillman, Erickson, & Kramer, 2008; Tomporowski & Ellis, 1986) and meta-analyses (Colcombe & Kramer, 2003; Etnier et al., 1997; Etnier, Nowell, Landers, & Sibley, 2006) described the beneficial relationship between physical activity and cognitive function in adult populations, along with a host of empirical studies using a variety of measures from behavioral assessments (Hillman et al., 2006; Kramer et al., 1999) to sophisticated neuroimaging techniques (Colcombe et al., 2004; Themanson, Hillman, & Curtin, 2006). Among these publications, a landmark study by Kramer et al. (1999) followed by a meta-analysis (Colcombe & Kramer, 2003) provided a new perspective, shaping the field of research on physical activity and cognitive functions. Specifically, Kramer and his colleagues observed that physical activity exhibited a generally beneficial relationship to multiple aspects of cognition that was selectively larger for tasks or task components requiring greater amounts of executive control. That is, their meta-analysis examined 18 randomized control trials in older adults, and found that the treatment group (i.e., those randomly assigned to exercise) demonstrated general improvements in cognition, which were observed across a variety of cognitive tasks (e.g., speeded response tasks, visuospatial, controlled processing). However, the findings also revealed that the largest improvement in cognition was observed when individuals were challenged with executive control tasks, indicating that in addition to the generalized benefit of physical activity on cognition, there was a disproportionately greater benefit for executive control (Colcombe & Kramer, 2003). Importantly, no such improvements in cognition were observed in the control groups, who did not receive physical activity interventions (Colcombe & Kramer, 2003). These findings, which have now been replicated across independent laboratories, have guided our thinking regarding the types of cognition that may be most improved in everyday life by physical activity participation.

Executive control describes a subset of goal-directed, self-regulatory cognitive operations involved in the selection, scheduling, and coordination of computational processes underlying perception, memory, and action. Core cognitive processes collectively termed "executive control" or "cognitive control" include; inhibition, working memory, and cognitive flexibility (Diamond, 2006). Inhibition (often termed "inhibitory control") refers to the ability to override a strong internal or external pull to appropriately act within environmental constraints (Davidson, Amso, Anderson,

& Diamond, 2006). Working memory refers to the ability to mentally represent information, manipulate stored information, and act upon it (Davidson et al., 2006). Cognitive flexibility refers to the ability to quickly and flexibly switch perspectives, focus attention, and adapt behavior for the purposes of goal directed action (Blair, Zelazo, & Greenberg, 2005; Davidson et al., 2006; Diamond, 2006).

Executive control exhibits protracted development relative to other cognitive processes (Casey et al., 2000b; Diamond, 2006) with efficient and effective allocation of executive function occurring during the latter stages of adolescence. The protracted development exhibited for executive control is tied to the protracted development of the neural tissue that mediate such functions, namely the frontal lobes (Bunge, Dudukovic, Thomason, Vaidya, & Gabrieli, 2002; Casey et al., 2000a, 2005b; Rueda et al., 2004; Segalowitz & Davies, 2004; van der Molen, 2000). Diamond's (1988, 1990, 2006) extensive observations of early executive control in young children has led to the understanding of the developmental processes of this area of cognition. She observed executive control function in 8–12-month-old children through the use of "detoured reaching," which requires retention of a goal, planning, and inhibition of a prepotent response. Interestingly, changes in the structure and function of the dorsolateral PFC between 7.5 and 12 months of age including increased dendritic growth of pyramidal neurons in layer III (Koenderink, Ulyings, & Mrzljiak, 1994), increased glucose metabolism (Chugani & Phelps, 1986), and increased dopamine levels (Brozoski, Brown, Rosvold, & Goldman, 1979), coincided with the early development of executive control on goal-directed reaching tasks, as well as the A-not-B task, requiring inhibitory control (Diamond, 2006). During the second year of life, improvements in the ability to make connections between physically linked items in the environment and the deduction of abstract rules has been linked to changes in the frontal cortex (i.e., inferior PFC; Diamond, 2006). Substantial improvements in executive control are observed between 3 and 7 years of age, especially related to inhibition and cognitive flexibility.

Late childhood and adolescence represent a time of development in the frontal lobes leading to greater functioning of the executive system (Travis, 1998). Younger children, whose frontal lobes are still immature, are more inclined to interference from irrelevant stimuli and have greater difficulty focusing attention on relevant stimuli (Ridderinkhof & van der Molen, 1995). With maturation comes the ability to control interference via increased efficiency of executive processes (Travis), and the ability to mentally hold two or more pieces of information while inhibiting a response tendency (Diamond & Taylor, 1996). The development of inhibitory processes is evidenced in children as young as age 4 (Dowsett & Livesey, 2000), although most improvement is seen by age 6 (Diamond & Taylor; Klenberg, Korkman, & Lahti-Nuuttila, 2001). However, such inhibitory processes continue to develop throughout childhood and adolescence, with children routinely demonstrating less ability to withhold inappropriate responses than adults (Bunge et al., 2002; Luciana & Nelson, 1998; Luna, Garver, Urban, Lazar, & Sweeney, 2004; Mezzacappa, 2004). The question remains how brief and continuous engagement in physical activity effects the refinement of executive control.

Physical Activity and Cognitive Development

Despite the interesting findings observed for physical activity benefits on adults' executive control functioning, and the knowledge that executive control processes exhibit protracted development, the initial study of physical activity in children and adolescents did not examine executive control aspects of cognition. As such, the study of physical activity and cognitive development is arguably in its very early stages, with the majority of published studies employing a correlational approach and thus offering only a description of the relationship between physical activity and cognition during development. More rigorous experimental designs, affording causal explanations have yet to emerge in the literature (see Hillman, Pontifex, Raine, Castelli, Hall, & Kramer, 2009b for an exception).

To characterize the early literature, Sibley and Etnier (2003) conducted a meta-analysis to better understand the relationship between physical activity and cognitive function in school-age children. They observed that physical activity participation was positively related to cognitive performance along eight measurement categories consisting of perceptual skills, intelligent quotient, achievement, verbal tests, mathematics tests, memory, developmental level/academic readiness, and a category that they termed as "other." Their findings suggested a beneficial relationship of physical activity on all categories, with the exception of memory (Sibley & Etnier 2003). Further, this effect was found for all age groups, but was stronger for children in the 4–7 and 11–13 year groupings, compared to the 8–10 and 14–18 year groupings. Although this meta-analysis offered a consolidation of the field at that time, the lack of experimental rigor and *a-theoretical* perspectives of the many studies included produced as many new questions as there were answers.

While basic science is the gold standard in determining merit of our scientific hypotheses, randomized controlled designs, and clinical trials are not always feasible or directly applicable to authentic contexts. Therefore, examination of physical activity and academic achievement is usually limited by the use of quasi-experimental and cross-sectional designs. In schools, cognitive function is most commonly measured by performance on standardized tests, as the results determine the effectiveness of the educational setting (i.e., a teacher's work with an individual learner; programmatic value; or as public record of the school's performance in delivering the curriculum).

Since 2003, several new lines of research have emerged that have employed greater experimental rigor, included sophisticated neuroimaging measures, and pursued theory-driven questions. Specifically, at the University of Illinois at Urbana-Champaign, work in the Neurocognitive Kinesiology Laboratory has produced several studies aimed at elucidating the physical activity-cognitive development area. An initial study examined 7–12-year-old children who completed a paper and pencil version of the Stroop Color-Word task, which requires executive control functioning among other cognitive processes, and the *Fitnessgram*; a field test of physical fitness (Buck, Hillman, & Castelli, 2008). Results indicated that better performance on each of the three Stroop conditions (i.e., color words presented in congruent color ink, e.g., "green" presented in green ink; arrays of symbols presented in various ink colors; color words presented in alternate color ink, e.g., "green" presented in the color red) was associated with better performance on the aerobic test (i.e., the number of laps run on the PACER test) of the *Fitnessgram*. That is, higher levels of aerobic fitness were associated with correctly naming more colors during each Stroop condition, independently of other factors such as age, gender, or intelligence. Although it is possible that the relationship between these variables can be explained by an environmental variable that predicts both cognitive function and physical activity (e.g., involved parenting) these initial findings suggest that increased levels of aerobic fitness may benefit cognitive processes underlying executive control function during preadolescent maturation.

Subsequent attempts in this laboratory have employed neuroelectric measurement to better understand some of the potential underlying mechanisms for the observed behavioral benefits observed in more physically active children. In particular, they have utilized event-related brain potentials (ERPs) to study aspects of the neuroelectric system that are thought to support task-relevant interactions. ERPs allow for the greater understanding of which cognitive processes occurring between stimulus engagement and response execution may be influenced by aerobic fitness. Embedded within stimulus-driven ERPs, the P3 component, an endogenously potential reflecting the allocation of attentional resource toward the stimulus environment, has demonstrated considerable utility in understanding fitness-related differences in cognition. Specifically, two cross-sectional studies aimed at fitness differences among groups of children (Hillman, Castelli, & Buck, 2005; Hillman, Buck, Themanson, Pontifex, & Castelli, 2009a) on the P3 potential have provided convergent evidence to suggest that higher amounts of aerobic fitness enhanced attentional processing of environmental information. In each of these studies, larger P3 amplitude was observed for more fit children relative to less fit children, respectively. Behavioral data from these studies corroborated the P3 findings with increased task performance (i.e., higher accuracy) in the higher fit group (Hillman et al., 2005; 2009a). Of interest, the tasks selected for these studies tap aspects of inhibition and working memory, which constitute core cognitive processes involved in executive control operations.

A second class of ERPs, which are linked to individuals' actions, have also demonstrated fitness-related benefits. Specifically, the error-related negativity (ERN) potential reflects the evaluation and monitoring of one's own actions. The ERN is modulated by response conflict that may be engendered by uncertainty in which response mapping is correct, being forced to override a habitual response in favor of a less established response, or more commonly through error production. That is, individuals are thought to monitor their actions within their environment (see Botvinick, Braver, Barch, Carter, & Cohen, 2001 for review), and the ERN is believed to represent the evaluation of conflict between stimulus-driven intended actions and actual behavioral responses (Gehring, Goss, Coles, Meyer, & Donchin, 1993; Falkenstein, Hohnsbein, Hoormann, & Blanke, 1991). Researchers have demonstrated through various neuroimaging techniques that the neural generator for ERN is at or very near the dorsal anterior cingulate cortex (Carter et al., 1998;

Miltner et al., 2003; van Veen & Carter, 2002), which has rich projections with the prefrontal and parietal cortices.

A study of the ERN potential in preadolescent children demonstrated that higher amounts of fitness were associated with smaller ERN amplitude following errors of commission on a speeded choice response task (Hillman et al., 2009a), corroborating several studies in young and older adults (Themanson & Hillman, 2006; Themanson, Hillman, & Curtin, 2006). These findings suggest that greater amounts of fitness are beneficial to the conflict monitoring system through a more efficient allocation of conflict monitoring processes or a reduced threshold with which to begin the cascade of processes underlying the upregulation of cognitive control following incorrect action. Support for the notion of a reduction in ERN amplitude underlying greater cognitive control stems from two other findings. First, behavioral data on the trial immediately following an error indicates greater accuracy in higher-fit individuals, suggesting that cognitive control processes aimed at correcting incorrect actions may be allocated more flexibly and effectively (Hillman et al., 2009a). Second, independent neuroimaging work in older adults has demonstrated reduced activation of the ACC in more fit individuals (Colcombe et al., 2004), supporting the reduced ERN potential observed in the higher-fit preadolescent children.

In summary, convergent ERP evidence has suggested that higher amounts of fitness may be related to better integrity of stimulus evaluation and response execution processes through more effective regulation of cognitive control. Although ERPs are not capable of definitively tying cognition to specific brain regions, their findings along with those from more sophisticated neural imaging measures, provide evidence to suggest that neural networks involving the frontal regions of the brain may benefit from increases in physical activity participation. Further, these interesting neurocognitive findings are supported by task performance differences demonstrating greater speed and accuracy of responding with greater amounts of physical activity. Accordingly, other research has focused on extrapolating the basic performance benefits observed in the laboratory to real-world cognitive challenges such scholastic performance and academic achievement.

Physical Activity and Academic Achievement

Seminal work examining physical activity and learning was conducted during the 1950s in Vanves, France where the daily academic schedule was reduced to allocate time for physical activities such as gymnastics and swimming. Findings suggested that elementary-aged children who participated in the physical activity opportunities had better academic performance than those who did not, despite the reduction in time spent in academic subjects such as mathematics and reading. Although these findings may be positive and lead us to believe that a relationship exists between academics and physical activity engagement, this study was never published in a peer-reviewed journal (Trudeau & Shephard, 2008).

It was not until the 1970s that an experimental design was used to examine the effects of increased physical activity time on academic performance. In Trois-Rivieres, Canada, the initial study was conducted over a 7-year period with 546 participants reporting mixed results, as those who were given more access to physical activity time had better test scores in mathematics, but not in English. Shephard and Trudeau (2005) performed a retrospective study of class cohorts from the Trois-Rivieres program, investigating the effects of daily, quality physical education on the cognitive development. Initially, the researchers demonstrated that the control group had better academic performance than the experimental group, but over time the experimental group performance was superior to that of the control group. As a follow-up to the original study, some 20 years after participation in the intervention, 32 males and 32 females were found to have better static balance than control group counterparts; however, there were no significant differences among the other physical and cognitive variables (Trudeau et al., 2000). As such, the physical activity intervention demonstrated immediate, but not lasting effects on physical fitness and cognitive performance, perhaps suggesting that the design of the intervention did not result in a permanent change in physical activity behavior. Unlike this study, modern interventions directly target the determinants of physical activity engagement and attempt to sustain the initial responses to training. The determinants of physical activity are those factors, when present, that have the greatest likelihood of resulting sustained engagement. In children, those who are most active usually spend time out-of-doors, exhibit self-efficacy toward physical activity, have access to facilities, and are enrolled in at least one formal physical activity program (Sallis, Prochaska, & Taylor, 2000).

The School Health, Academic Performance and Exercise (SHAPE) study examined the effects of a 14-week physical activity intervention on physical fitness and skinfold measures among South Australian youth (Dwyer, Coonan, Leitch, Hetzel, & Baghurst, 1983).

There was no difference in academic achievement (e.g., mathematics and reading standardized test scores) despite the intervention students spending 60 min of in-school time engaging in regular physical education. Although it is difficult for these findings to be directly compared to the Trois-Rivieres intervention, it can be concluded that the increased duration in physical education did not negatively influence academic achievement in either context.

Since the completion of these studies, the definition of academic achievement has been broadened to include not only performance on standardized tests, but also grades in school, attendance, behavioral office referrals, and attention. A large-scale study by the California Department of Education [CDE] examined the relationship between students' (fifth, seventh, and ninth graders in California) academic performance and their physical fitness by comparing the SAT scores and Fitnessgram test results (i.e., shuttle run for endurance, push-ups, sit-ups, and body composition). The findings identified that students with higher levels of fitness scored better on the SAT in mathematics and reading, and that the students who met minimum fitness levels in three or more of the six physical fitness areas measured by Fitnessgram also had the greatest academic gains (California Department of Education, 2001). Additionally, it was demonstrated that females exhibited higher academic achievement than males, especially at higher fitness levels (CDE, 2001). These findings have since been replicated in student populations from Illinois (Castelli, Hillman, Buck, & Erwin, 2007), Massachusetts (Chomitz et al., 2009), and Texas (The Cooper Institute, 2009). Although, these findings are positive and widespread, we cannot infer that improved physical fitness caused an improvement in academic achievement because of the constraints imposed by the quasi-experimental research design.

Participation in physical activity within the school day, such as that provided by physical education classes, has been associated with better academic performance (Coe, Pivarnik, Womack, Reeves, & Malina, 2006; Shephard, 1997) and increased on-task behaviors during academic instruction (Mahar et al., 2006). SPARK (Sports, Play, and Active Recreation for Kids curriculum) examined the relationship between physical activity, physical fitness, and the impact of health-related physical education on academic achievement (Sallis et al., 1999). Metropolitan Achievement Tests (MAT6 and MAT7) served as the measurement of academic achievement. Fourth and fifth graders were randomly assigned to one of two treatments or a control group. Similar to the Dwyer study in Australia, findings suggest that increased time for physical education does not have negative effects on academic achievement of elementary school students. More importantly, the results confirmed the value of having trained specialists (i.e., physical education teachers) to deliver programming aimed at increased physical activity engagement and improved health-related fitness knowledge. Further study of the physical education setting revealed that participation may be more cognitively advantageous for girls than boys, as females who were vigorously engaged did better in school (Carlson et al., 2008).

Single sessions of physical activity. According to the *Physical Activity Guidelines for Americans* (U.S. Department of Health and Human Services [USDHHS], 2008), children should engage in at least 60 min of physical activity each day, with schools providing quality physical education for at least 150 min and 225 min per week for elementary and secondary schools, respectively. The expectation is that during each physical education class at least 50 % of the time should be spent engaged in physical activity (National Association for Sport and Physical Education, 2009a, 2009b, 2009c), thus accounting for at least half of the recommended physical activity in a child's day. Yet, because of current economic and curricular constraints only 3.8 % of elementary schools, 7.9 % of middle schools, and 2.1 % of high schools provide daily physical education (U.S. Centers for Disease Control and Prevention, 2006). Across the country less than 10 % of the students, regardless of educational level are afforded an opportunity to enhance their skills, knowledge, abilities, and affect (i.e., self-efficacy toward specific physical activities) in health-related topics on a daily basis.

In a given school day, state and local policies as well as the formal class schedules dictate the amount, frequency, and duration of physical activity for each child. How these physical activity opportunities are provided has been creative and varied as some schools offer morning rituals in which all students simultaneously exercise for 10 min in their classroom via telecommunications or together in the gymnasium during an assembly. These sessions are typically a game of follow the leader attempting to elevate heart rate. Other schools have gone to the extreme by providing balance balls for seats and tread desks for use during seatwork. The aftereffects of such bouts of physical activity are still in question. For example, little is known about how literacy may improve, if reading lessons were conducted on a stationary bicycle placed in an elementary classroom. It is commonly acknowledged that if the intensity of exercise is too high, then it can be counter-productive to do academic work (see Pontifex & Hillman, 2007 for electrophysiological model); however, when the activity is low or moderate in nature and the child is allowed to recover (heart rate returns to near resting values) it may be impactful.

Using a within-subjects design, Hillman et al. (2009b) had 20 preadolescent children walk on a treadmill to record its potential effects on cognitive performance. The initial hour following a single bout of moderately intense walking resulted in enhanced allocation of attention, which improved response accuracy on a computer task and increased performance on academic testing, over baseline measures. These findings have ramifications for educators, as single, brief bouts of physical activity may improve attention and learning.

Further, as developed by the Activity Promotion Laboratory at East Carolina University, *Energizers* are short classroom-based physical activities that help get students healthy and active during academic instruction. Mahar et al. (2006) employed *Energizers* during academic instruction to evaluate the effects of the classroom-based physical activity program on children's on-task behavior. The findings demonstrated that a classroom-based physical activity program was effective in improving on-task behavior during academic instruction.

Coles and Tomporowski (2008) evaluated the effects of a brief bout of moderate aerobic exercise on executive function and short- and long-term memory of young adults. The study employed a set-switching test and a free-recall memory test, revealing that after exercise, participants recalled significantly more items during delayed free-recall tests than in the control groups, while individual bouts of aerobic exercise did not influence visual short-term memory of the experimental group. The study concluded that exercise-induced arousal may help to improve long-term memory and learning (Coles & Tomporowski, 2008). Further, physical activity may be a valuable means of enhancing specific aspects central to cognitive development. These effects in children also held true in young soccer players; however in this case, cognitive performance was measured as decision making during game play, which was enhanced after a period of intermittent training (i.e., exercise, rest, exercise, rest; McMorris & Graydon, 1997).

Despite these positive trends, some data continues to emerge suggesting that the short-term effects of physical activity may have negative consequence, as high intensity physical activity may have detrimental effects on performance (see Tomporowski, 2003 for review). Researchers have failed to identify a clear relation between highly intense, anaerobic exercise and information processing (see Tomporowski (2003) for review), as these types of exercise produce fatigue and initially, a reduction in cognitive performance. Intense exercise reduced concentration (McMorris & Keen, 1994) and inhibited the refinement of motor skills in learners (Dwyer, 1984). These mixed results are likely attributed to variations in exercise intensity and teacher implementation of curricula. Moreover, poorly selected outcome measures and variability of responses by children may be influential (Tomporowski, Davis, Miller, & Naglieri, 2008).

Additionally, brain-based learning or educational activities in which students use both sides of their brain during light physical activity, has become a popular trend among elementary classroom teachers. Unfortunately, despite its current popularity, it is likely that these brain-based activities have been developed from a liberal and perhaps inaccurate interpretation of the animal research (Goswami, 2006). As of the writing of this chapter, no single brain-based curricula or instruction has been empirically justified as a means of directly enhancing academic performance. Extrapolating justification for brain-based activities from the studies described here would be an embellishment of existing findings. In our translation of neurons to neighborhoods, we must judiciously scrutinize each application to the education setting.

Physical Activity Interventions

A study utilized a randomized controlled design, in which 94 sedentary children were assigned to no exercise, 20-, or 40-min of physical activity in an afterschool intervention. After 15 weeks, the active groups significantly outperformed the inactive group in fitness tests and the 40 min group had higher scores on the cognitive task than the inactive group (Davis et al., 2007), thus moving a step closer to the identification of a cause and effect relationship. Little is known about the impact of afterschool programming on physical activity and fitness, as a recent meta-analysis found that only eight studies have investigated its effects on the rate of physical activity engagement (Beets, Beighle, Erwin, & Huberty, 2009).

Additional work at the Neurocognitive Kinesiology Laboratory involves conducting a randomized control design entitled Fitness Improves Thinking (FIT Kids) afterschool program. Data collected during the program development suggested that both males and females can achieve the recommended daily step counts through afterschool programming. Additionally, third and fourth graders can be taught to accurately monitor their own step count rate as a means of meeting national physical activity guidelines as the minimal amount of activity needed for maintaining health (Hirsch, Hirsch, Castelli, Oh, & Goss, 2010). Further, boys completed more physical activity homework than did girls. Although it was believed that worksheets and homework generated from the afterschool program would likely increase physical activity over the weekend when the program was not in session, this study found no identifiable effect on engagement (Oh, Hirsch, Hirsch, Castelli, & Goss, 2010). Clearly, further research is warranted. The cognitive measures conducted in this study have yet to be analyzed at the time of publication.

Given that there is a casual relationship between physical activity and cognitive performance in adult humans and nonhuman animals, we intuitively believe that 1 day a similar effect will be confirmed in children. The ideal *dose* or amount and type of physical activity that is needed to elicit cognitive benefits among children have eluded researchers to now. This is particularly due to unrefined measures of cognition and the variability associated with growth and development. However, given our societal desire to augment student knowledge and prevent disease, it is currently the initiative of many researchers to more precisely define this relationship.

Best Practice Recommendations

From our understanding of the material discussed in this chapter and our own words in this area we believe: (a) trained specialists should provide children with opportunities to learn about and be active in physical activity; (b) formal and community interventions should be focused on the determinants associated with sustained physical activity and the national guidelines; (c) physical activity does not harm academic achievement and therefore has a place in the school curriculum; (d) age-related effects of physical activity on cognitive performance should be considered, and (e) everyone needs to help children increase their engagement in physical activity.

In 2007, the authors were invited to write an article for physical educators providing suggestions how their efforts could foster cognitive benefits (Castelli & Hillman, 2007) and they used the acronym, REACH to organize their recommendations for teachers (see Table 3.1). The underlying premises of REACH are five verbs (reach, enjoy, advocate, craft, and help) serving as action steps, specifically targeting best practice and maximizing the potential benefits for children. In this summary, the authors would like to broaden that proposal for public use.

Trained specialists. The best way to increase the probability of setting and *reaching* attainable goals related to understanding and performance of health-related fitness content, is through trained professionals. Research involving SPARK has clearly documented the value of certified physical education teachers and their role in achieving health-related fitness goals (Sallis et al., 1999), as children who worked with them outperformed those who worked with untrained or minimally trained (one-day workshop) individuals. Based upon these findings policy makers have begun to mandate that physical education and other in-school physical activity programs be delivered by certified individuals. The percentage of states that require newly hired staff who teach physical education at the elementary school level to

Table 3.1 Physical activity leaders can help children REACH their potential

REACH

- *Reach* attainable personal goals related to the understanding and performance of health-related fitness content.
- *Enjoy* human movement with your students.
- *Advocate* for physical activity breaks throughout the school day that connect with opportunities to active outside of school.
- *Craft* lessons that are largely active, promote success, and efficiently use learning time.
- *Help* children prepare for a lifetime of regular physical activity.

Source: Castelli and Hillman (2007)

have undergraduate and/or graduate training in physical education has increased from 51.1 % in 2000 to 64.7 % in 2006 (U.S. Centers for Disease Control and Prevention, 2006).

Reference to the National Association for Sport and Physical Education Appropriate Practices documents (2009a, 2009b, 2009c; see elementary, middle, and high school at www.naspeinfo.org) makes the rationale for this recommendation apparent. Certified physical education teachers spend at least 4 years preparing to enhance the knowledge, skills, abilities, and affect of children ages 5–18. The standards-based approach to teaching identifies grade level criteria for achievement specifically related to physical activity engagement and fitness. Physical education teachers are mandated by state level standards to track these variables across the school experience. Recently, there has been a call for the role of physical education teachers to move beyond the delivery of the single subject matter and embrace the responsibility of physical activity director (Castelli & Beighle, 2007; Beighle, Erwin, Castelli & Ernest, 2009). Utilizing a Coordinated School Health approach, a physical education teacher would help to organize all physical activity opportunities that take place before, during, or after school. For example, the physical education teacher may identify some parents to create a neighborhood walking school bus (children walk to school together each day), organize a recess runner's club, and offer intramurals afterschool, while teaching quality, formal physical education classes. Implementing this type of system increases the likelihood that each child will meet the daily recommendation of 60 min of moderate to vigorous physical activity each day, which based upon the evidence presented in this chapter would be contributory to enhanced learning.

Physical activity determinants. Interest and *enjoyment*, among other factors, are related to the regular engagement in physical activity. Rigid, adult-like activities, such as running on a treadmill at a steady pace are inappropriate for children. Instead, intermittent, play-oriented activities should be offered routinely and spontaneously. Since motor performance and perceptions of motor ability (Dwyer, 1984; Stodden, Langendorfer, & Robertson, 2009) as well as psychosocial characteristics such as self-efficacy are closely tied to physical activity engagement, these variables must be considered when designing physical activity interventions for children.

Interventions outside of the educational setting should build a support system within the family and community providing access to facilities and programs. Specifically, interventions of this type should involve current community organizations in the planning; enhance land use, welcome low-income and minority groups; and give parents a responsibility (role modeling, setting limits on screen time, developing household rules). Implementations of these types of family and community interventions have the potential to increase both physical activity engagement and fitness through augmented *enjoyment* and fun.

Physical activity and schools. Arguably, one of the most robust findings in this research is the idea that there are no known negative effects of reducing academic time during the school day to offer physical education or other physical activities. Yet, because of the frequency of standardized testing utilized as a mechanism to hold schools accountable for a high level of academic achievement, many schools have removed children from physical activity (i.e., recess, physical education class) for the purpose of remediation. These types of practices are contrary to the expansive literature outlined in this chapter and therefore this practice should be discouraged and discontinued. Instead, we should *advocate* for physical activity breaks during academic time such as the *Energizers* or *Take 10!* curriculum described earlier in this chapter. It is apparent that these "brain breaks" can actually improve student attention and readiness to learn.

The effects of physical activity and fitness are different by age. With birth, we begin to age, and at different time points across the lifespan it is more important and valuable than others to be engaged in physical activity for the purpose of improving mental and cognitive health; particularly during childhood and later life. We should *craft* age-appropriate activities for children and adults to regularly engage. These opportunities should be largely active, promote success, and efficiently use activity time; thus spending more than 50 % of the activity time in moderate to vigorous intensity. When the physical activity elicits fatigue among the children, then there should be time to dedicated for recovery, through an active cool-down, before sent into the academic setting.

All hands on deck! In order to reverse the effects of the obesity pandemic, it is going to require that everyone get involved in some way. No single entity can serve as the source for changing the behaviors of children that were developed in the home environment and continued into the educational setting. Child care providers, parents, teachers, psychologists, policy makers alike need to be active for their own health as well as to *help* children achieve physical and cognitive health. Ways in which individuals can help range from promoting the adoption of public policy enhancing infrastructure (i.e., sidewalks, safe routes to schools, bicycle lanes) to building self-efficacy in a single child by encouraging them to learn to ride a bicycle. The benefits of your help is varied and expansive, as children who are fit and physically active will be more successful in school. Providing testimony at one local school board or advocating for physical activity during a parent–teacher association meeting can aid in the creation of a single policy affecting hundreds of children in their prevention of disease by establishing healthy habits and improved performance in schools. In your neighborhood, you can facilitate advanced neurological function in both adults and children, simply by engaging in and encouraging others to join you in physical activity.

References

Aglioti, S. M., Cesari, P., Romani, M., & Urgesi, C. (2008). Action anticipation and motor resonance in elite basketball players. *Nature Neuroscience, 11,* 1109–1116.
Bartzokis, G., Beckson, M., Lu, P. H., Nuechterlein, K. H., Edwards, N., & Mintz, J. (2001). Age-related changes in frontal and temporal lobe volumes in men: a magnetic resonance imaging study. *Archives of General Psychiatry, 58,* 461–465.

Baylor, A. M., & Spirduso, W. W. (1988). Systematic aerobic exercise and components of reaction time in older women. *Journal of Gerontology, 43*, 121–126.

Beets, M. W., Beighle, A., Erwin, H. E., & Huberty, J. L. (2009). After-school program impact on physical activity and fitness. *American Journal of Preventive Medicine, 36*(6), 527–537.

Beighle, A., Erwin, H., Castelli, D., & Ernest, M. (2009). Preparing physical educators for the role of physical activity director. *Journal of Physical Education, Recreation, and Dance, 80*(4), 1–58.

Beise, D., & Peaseley, V. (1937). The relationship of reaction time, speed, and agility of big muscle groups and certain sport skills. *Research Quarterly, 8*, 133–142.

Black, J. E., & Greenough, W. T. (1986). Induction of pattern in neural structure by experience: implications for cognitive development. In M. E. Lamb, A. L. Brown, & B. Rogoff (Eds.), *Advances in developmental psychology* (Vol. 4, pp. 1–50). Hillsdale, NJ: Lawrence Erlbaum Associates.

Black, J. E., Isaacs, K. R., Anderson, B. J., Alcantara, A. A., & Greenough, W. T. (1990). Learning causes synaptogenesis, whereas motor activity causes angiogenesis, in cerebellar cortex of adult rats. *Proceedings of the National Academy of Science of the United States of America, 87*, 5568–5572.

Blair, C., Zelazo, P. D., & Greenberg, M. T. (2005). The measurement of executive function in early childhood. *Developmental Neuropsychology, 28*, 561–571.

Botvinick, M. M., Braver, T. S., Barch, D. M., Carter, C. S., & Cohen, J. D. (2001). Conflict monitoring and cognitive control. *Psychological Review, 108*, 624–652.

Brozoski, T. J., Brown, R. M., Rosvold, H. E., & Goldman, P. S. (1979). Cognitive deficit caused by regional depletion of dopamine in prefrontal cortex of rhesus monkey. *Science, 205*, 929–932.

Buck, S. M., Hillman, C. H., & Castelli, D. M. (2008). Aerobic fitness influences on Stroop task performance in preadolescent children. *Medicine & Science in Sports & Exercise, 40*, 166–172.

Bunge, S. A., Dudukovic, N. M., Thomason, M. E., Vaidya, C. J., & Gabrieli, J. D. E. (2002). Immature frontal lobe contributions to cognitive control in children: Evidence from fMRI. *Neuron, 33*, 301–311.

Burpee, R. H., & Stroll, W. (1936). Measuring reaction time of athletes. *Research Quarterly, 7*, 110–118.

California Department of Education. (2001). *California physical fitness test: report to the governor and legislature*. Sacramento, CA: California Department of Education Standards and Assessment Division.

Carlson, S. A., Fulton, J. E., Lee, S. M., Maynard, M., Brown, D. R., Kohl, H. W., et al. (2008). Physical education and academic achievement in elementary school: data from the early childhood longitudinal study. *American Journal of Public Health, 98*(4), 721–727.

Carro, E., Trejo, L. J., Busiguina, S., & Torres-Aleman, I. (2001). Circulating insulin-like growth factor 1 mediates the protective effects of physical exercise against brain insults of different etiology and anatomy. *Journal of Neuroscience, 21*, 5678–5684.

Carter, C. S., Braver, T. S., Barch, D. M., Botvinick, M. M., Noll, D., & Cohen, J. D. (1998). Anterior cingulated cortex, error detection, and the online monitoring of performance. *Science, 280*, 747–749.

Casey, B. J., Galvan, A., & Hare, T. A. (2005a). Changes in cerebral functional organization during cognitive development. *Current Opinion in Neurobiology, 15*, 239–244.

Casey, B. J., Giedd, J. N., & Thomas, K. M. (2000a). Structural and functional brain development and its relation to cognitive development. *Biological Psychology, 54*, 241–257.

Casey, B. J., Thomas, K. M., Welsh, T. F., Badgaiyan, R. D., Eccard, C. H., Jennings, J. R., et al. (2000b). Dissociation of response conflict, attentional selection, and expectancy with functional magnetic resonance imaging. *Proceedings of the National Academy of Sciences, 97*, 8728–8733.

Casey, B. J., Tottenham, N., Liston, C., & Durston, S. (2005b). Imaging the developing brain: what have we learned about cognitive development. *Trends in Cognitive Sciences, 9*, 104–110.

Castelli, D. M., & Beighle, A. (2007). The physical education teacher as school activity director. *Journal of Physical Education, Recreation, and Dance, 78*(5), 1–58.

Castelli, D. M., & Hillman, C. H. (2007). Physical education performance outcomes and cognitive function. *Strategies, 21*(1), 26–31.

Castelli, D. M., Hillman, C. H., Buck, S. M., & Erwin, H. E. (2007). Physical fitness and academic achievement in 3rd and 5th grade students. *Journal of Sport & Exercise Psychology, 29,* 239–252.

Chan, A. S., Ho, Y.-C., & Cheung, M.-C. (1998). Music training improves verbal memory. *Nature, 396,* 128.

Chomitz, V. R., Slinning, M. M., McGowan, R. J., Mitchell, S. E., Dawson, G. F., & Hacker, K. A. (2009). Is there a relationship between physical fitness and academic achievement? Positive results from public school children in the Northeastern United States. *Journal of School Health, 79*(1), 30–37.

Chugani, H. T., & Phelps, M. E. (1986). Maturational changes in cerebral function in infants determined by 18FDG positron emission tomography. *Science, 231*(4740), 840–843.

Coe, D. P., Pivarnik, J. M., Womack, C. J., Reeves, M. J., & Malina, R. M. (2006). Effect of physical education and activity levels on academic achievement in children. *Medicine & Science in Sports & Exercise, 38,* 1515–1519.

Colcombe, S. J., Erickson, K. I., Scalf, P. E., Kim, J. S., Prakash, R., McAuley, E., et al. (2006). Aerobic exercise training increases brain volume in aging humans. *Journal of Gerontology: Medical Sciences, 61,* 1166–1170.

Colcombe, S. J., & Kramer, A. F. (2003). Fitness effects on the cognitive function of older adults: a meta-analytic study. *Psychological Science, 14,* 125–130.

Colcombe, S. J., Kramer, A. F., Erickson, K. I., Scalf, P., McAuley, E., Cohen, N. J., et al. (2004). Cardiovascular fitness, cortical plasticity, and aging. *Proceedings of the National Academy of Sciences of the United States of America, 101,* 3316–3321.

Coles, K., & Tomporowski, P. D. (2008). Effects of acute exercise on executive processing, short-term and long-term memory. *Journal of Sport Sciences, 26*(3), 333–344.

Cotman, C. W., & Berchtold, N. C. (2002). Exercise: a behavioral intervention to enhance brain health and plasticity. *Trends in Neuroscience, 25,* 295–301.

Davidson, M. C., Amso, D., Anderson, L. C., & Diamond, A. (2006). Development of cognitive control and executive functions from 4 to 13 years: evidence from manipulations of memory, inhibition, and task switching. *Neuropsychologia, 44,* 2037–2078.

Davis, C. L., Tomporowski, P. D., Boyle, C. A., Waller, J. L., Miller, P. H., & Naglieri, J. A. (2007). Effects of aerobic exercise on overweight children's cognitive functioning: a randomized controlled trial. *Research Quarterly for Exercise and Sport, 78*(5), 510–519.

Delp, M., Armstrong, R., Godfrey, D., Laughlin, M., Ross, C., & Wilkerson, M. (2001). Exercise increases blood flow to locomotor, vestibular, cardiorespiratory, and visual regions of the brain in miniature swine. *The Journal of Physiology, 533,* 849–859.

Diamond, A. (1988). The abilities and neural mechanisms underlying A-not-B performance. *Child Development, 59,* 523–527.

Diamond, A. (1990). Developmental time course in human infants and infant monkeys, and the neural bases of inhibitory control in reaching. *Annals of the New York Academy of Sciences, 608,* 394–426.

Diamond, A. (2006). The early development of executive functions. In E. Bialystok & F. I. M. Craik (Eds.), *Lifespan cognition: mechanisms of change* (pp. 70–95). Oxford, UK: Oxford University Press.

Diamond, A., & Taylor, C. (1996). Development of an aspect of executive control: development of the abilities to remember what I said and to "Do as I say, not as I do". *Developmental Psychobiology, 29,* 315–334.

Dishman, R. K., Renner, K. J., Youngstedt, S. D., Reigle, T. G., Bunell, B. N., Burke, K. A., et al. (1997). Activity wheel running reduces escape latency and alters brain monoamine levels after footshock. *Brain Research Bulletin, 42,* 399–406.

Dowsett, S. M., & Livesey, D. J. (2000). The development of inhibitory control in preschool children: effects of "executive skills" training. *Developmental Psychobiology, 36*, 161–174.

Dustman, R. E., Emmerson, R. Y., Ruhling, R. O., Shearer, D. E., Steinhaus, L. A., Johnson, S. C., et al. (1990). Age and fitness effects on EEG, ERPs, visual sensitivity, and cognition. *Neurobiology of Aging, 11*, 193–200.

Dustman, R. E., Ruhling, R. O., Russell, E. M., Shearer, D. E., Bonekat, H. W., Shigeoka, J. W., et al. (1984). Aerobic exercise training and improved neuropsychological function of older individuals. *Neurobiology of Aging, 5*, 35–42.

Dwyer, T. (1984). Influence of physical fatigue on motor performance and learning. *The Physical Educator, 41*, 130–136.

Dwyer, T., Coonan, W. E., Leitch, D. R., Hetzel, B. S., & Baghurst, R. A. (1983). An investigation of the effects of daily physical activity on the health of primary school students in South Australia. *International Journal of Epidemiology, 12*(3), 308–313.

Eaton, S. B., & Konner, M. (1985). Paleolithic nutrition: a consideration of its nature and current implications. *The New England Journal of Medicine, 312*, 283–289.

Elbert, T., Pantev, C., Wienbruch, C., Rockstroh, B., & Taub, E. (1995). Increased cortical representation of the fingers of the left hand in string players. *Science, 270*, 305–307.

Etnier, J. L., Nowell, P. M., Landers, D. M., & Sibley, B. A. (2006). A meta-regression to examine the relationship between aerobic fitness and cognitive performance. *Brain Research Reviews, 52*, 119–130.

Etnier, J. L., Salazar, W., Landers, D. M., Petruzzello, S. J., Han, M., & Nowell, P. (1997). The influence of physical fitness and exercise upon cognitive functioning: a meta-analysis. *Journal of Sport & Exercise Psychology, 19*, 249–277.

Falkenstein, M., Hohnsbein, J., Hoormann, J., & Blanke, L. (1991). Effects of crossmodal divided attention on late ERP components: II. Error processing in choice reaction tasks. *Electroencephalography and Clinical Neurophysiology, 78*, 447–455.

Gehring, W. J., Goss, B., Coles, M. G. H., Meyer, D. E., & Donchin, E. (1993). A neural system for error detection and compensation. *Psychological Science, 4*, 385–390.

Giedd, J. N., Blumenthal, J., Jeffries, N. O., Castellanos, F. X., Liu, H., Zijdenbos, A., et al. (1999). Brain development during childhood and adolescence: a longitudinal MRI study. *Nature Neuroscience, 2*, 861–863.

Goswami, U. (2006). Neuroscience and education: from research to practice? *Nature Reviews. Neuroscience, 10*, 2–7.

Greenough, W. T., & Black, J. E. (1992). Induction of brain structure by experience: substrates for cognitive development. In M. R. Gunnar & C. A. Nelson (Eds.), *Developmental behavior neuroscience* (Vol. 24, pp. 155–200). Hillsdale, NJ: Lawrence Erlbaum Associates.

Hatfield, B. D., & Hillman, C. H. (2001). The psychophysiology of sport: a mechanistic understanding of the psychology of superior performance. In R. N. Singer, H. A. Hausenblaus, & C. M. Janelle (Eds.), *Handbook of sport psychology* (pp. 362–386). John Wiley: New York, NY.

Hillman, C. H., Buck, S. M., Themanson, J. T., Pontifex, M. B., & Castelli, D. M. (2009a). Aerobic fitness and cognitive development: Event-related brain potential and task performance indices of executive control in preadolescent children. *Developmental Psychology, 45*, 114–129.

Hillman, C. H., Castelli, D. M., & Buck, S. M. (2005). Aerobic fitness and neurocognitive function in healthy preadolescent children. *Medicine and Science in Sports and Exercise, 37*, 1967–1974.

Hillman, C. H., Erickson, K. I., & Kramer, A. F. (2008). Be smart, exercise your heart: exercise effects on brain and cognition. *Nature Reviews. Neuroscience, 9*, 58–65.

Hillman, C. H., Motl, R. W., Pontifex, M. B., Posthuma, D., Stubbe, J. H., Boomsma, D. I., et al. (2006). Physical activity and cognitive function in a cross-section of younger and older community-dwelling individuals. *Health Psychology, 25*, 678–687.

Hillman, C. H., Pontifex, M. B., Raine, L. B., Castelli, D. M., Hall, E. E., & Kramer, A. F. (2009b). The Effect of acute treadmill walking on cognitive control and academic achievement in preadolescent children. *Neuroscience, 159*, 1044–1054.

Hirsch, A., Hirsch, J., Castelli, D. M., Oh, J., & Goss, D. (2010). FIT Kids: a step in the right direction. *Research Quarterly for Exercise and Sport, 81*(1), A-53.

Huttenlocher, P. R. (1979). Synaptic density in human frontal cortex—developmental changes and effects of aging. *Brain Research, 163*, 195–205.

Huttenlocher, P. R., & Dabholkar, A. S. (1997). Regional differences in synaptogenesis in human cerebral cortex. *The Journal of Comparative Neurology, 387*, 167–178.

Isaacs, K. R., Anderson, B. J., Alcantara, A. A., Black, J. E., & Greenough, W. T. (1992). Exercise and the brain: Angiogenesis in the adult rat cerebellum after vigorous physical activity and motor skill learning. *Journal of Cerebral Blood Flow and Metabolism, 12*, 110–119.

Klenberg, L., Korkman, M., & Lahti-Nuuttila, P. (2001). Differential development of attention and executive functions in 3-12 year old Finnish children. *Developmental Neuropsychology, 20*, 407–428.

Koenderink, M. J. T., Ulyings, H. B. M., & Mrzljiak, L. (1994). Postnatal maturation of the layer III pyramidal neurons in the human prefrontal cortex: a quantitative Golgi analysis. *Brain Research, 653*, 173–182.

Konner, M. (1991). Universals of behavioral development in relation to brain myelination. In K. R. Gibson & A. C. Petersen (Eds.), *Brain maturation and cognitive development* (pp. 181–223). New York: Aldine deGruyter.

Kramer, A. F., Hahn, S., Cohen, N. J., Banich, M. T., McAuley, E., Harrison, C. R., et al. (1999). Aging, fitness and neurocognitive function. *Nature, 400*, 418–419.

Lawther, J. D. (1951). *Psychology of coaching*. Englewood Cliffs, NJ: Prentice-Hall.

Luciana, M., & Nelson, C. A. (1998). The functional emergence of prefrontally-guided working memory systems in four- to eight-year-old children. *Neuropsychologia, 36*, 273–293.

Luna, B., Garver, K. E., Urban, T. A., Lazar, N. A., & Sweeney, J. A. (2004). Maturation of cognitive processes from late childhood to adulthood. *Child Development, 75*, 1357–1372.

Mahar, M. T., Murphy, S. K., Rowe, D. A., Golden, J., Shields, A. T., & Raedeke, T. D. (2006). Effects of a classroom-based program on physical activity and on-task behavior. *Medicine & Science in Sports & Exercise, 38*, 2086–2094.

McMorris, T., & Graydon, J. (1997). The effect of exercise on cognitive performance in soccer-specific tests. *Journal of Sports Sciences, 15*, 459–468.

McMorris, T., & Keen, P. (1994). Effect of exercise on simple reaction time of recreational athletes. *Perceptual and Motor Skills, 78*, 123–130.

Mezzacappa, E. (2004). Alerting, orienting, and executive attention: developmental properties and sociodemographic correlates in an epidemiological sample of young, urban children. *Child Development, 75*, 1373–1386.

Miltner, W. H. R., Lemke, U., Weiss, T., Holroyd, C., Scheffers, M. K., & Coles, M. G. H. (2003). Implementation of error-processing in the human anterior cingulated cortex: a source analysis of the magnetic equivalent of the error-related negativity. *Biological Psychology, 64*, 157–166.

Morgan, B. G., & Gibson, K. R. (1991). Nutritional and environmental interactions in brain development. In K. R. Gibson & A. C. Petersen (Eds.), *Brain maturation and cognitive development* (pp. 91–106). New York: Aldine deGruyter.

Münte, T. F., Kohlmetz, C., Nager, W., & Altenmüller, E. (2001). Superior auditory spatial tuning in conductors. *Nature, 409*, 580.

National Association for Sport and Physical Education [NASPE]. (2009a). *Appropriate instructional practice guidelines for elementary school physical education* (3rd ed.). Reston, VA: Author.

National Association for Sport and Physical Education [NASPE]. (2009b). *Appropriate instructional practice guidelines for middle school physical education* (3rd ed.). Reston, VA: Author.

National Association for Sport and Physical Education [NASPE]. (2009c). *Appropriate instructional practice guidelines for high school physical education* (3rd ed.). Reston, VA: Author.

Neeper, S., Gomez-Pinilla, F., Choi, J., & Cottman, C. (1995). Exercise and brain neurotrophins. *Nature, 373*, 109.

Ogden, C. L., Carroll, M. D., & Flegal, K. M. (2008). High body mass index for age among US children and adolescents, 2003–2006. *Journal of the American Medical Association, 299*(20), 2401–2405.

Oh, J., Hirsch, J., Hirsch, A., Castelli, D., & Goss, D. (2010). FIT Kids: using homework and worksheets to increase physical activity. *Research Quarterly for Exercise and Sport, 81*(1), A64.

Pate, R. R., Davis, M. G., Robinson, T. N., Stone, E. J., McKenzie, T. L., & Young, J. C. (2006). Promoting physical activity in children and youth. *Circulation, 114*, 1214–1224.

Pierson, W. R., & Montoye, H. J. (1958). Movement time, reaction time, and age. *Journal of Gerontology, 13*, 418–421.

Pontifex, M. B., & Hillman, C. H. (2007). Neuroelectric and behavioral indices of interference control during acute cycling. *Clinical Neurophysiology, 118*, 570–580.

Ridderinkhof, K. R., & van der Molen, M. W. (1995). A psychophysiological analysis of developmental differences in the ability to resist interference. *Child Development, 66*, 1040–1056.

Rueda, M. R., Fan, J., McCandliss, B. D., Halparin, J. D., Gruber, D. B., Lercari, L. P., & Posner, M. I. (2004). Development of attentional networks in childhood. *Neuropsychologia, 42*, 1029–1040.

Sallis, J. F., McKenzie, T. L., Kolody, B., Lewis, M., Marshall, S., & Rosengard, P. (1999). Effects of health-related physical education on academic achievement: Project SPARK. *Research Quarterly for Exercise and Sport, 70*(2), 127–134.

Sallis, J. F., Prochaska, J. J., & Taylor, W. C. (2000). A review of correlates of physical activity in children and adolescents. *Medicine and Science in Sport and Exercise, 32*(5), 963–975.

Segalowitz, S. J., & Davies, P. L. (2004). Charting the maturation of the frontal lobe: an electrophysiological strategy. *Brain and Cognition, 55*, 116–133.

Shephard, R. J. (1997). Curricular physical activity and academic performance. *Pediatric Exercise Science, 9*, 113–126.

Shephard, R. J., & Trudeau, F. (2005). Contribution of school programmes to physical activity levels and attitudes in children and adults. *Sports Medicine, 35*(2), 89–105.

Shonkoff, J. P., & Phillips, D. A. (2000). *From neurons to neighborhoods: the science of early childhood development* (pp. 182–217). Washington, DC: National Academies Press.

Sibley, B. A., & Etnier, J. L. (2003). The relationship between physical activity and cognition in children: a meta-analysis. *Pediatric Exercise Science, 15*, 243–256.

Spirduso, W. W. (1975). Reaction and movement time as a function of age and physical activity level. *Journal of Gerontology, 30*, 435–440.

Spirduso, W. W. (1980). Physical fitness, aging, and psychomotor speed: a review. *Journal of Gerontology, 6*, 850–865.

Spirduso, W. W., & Clifford, P. (1978). Replication of age and physical activity effects on reaction and movement times. *Journal of Gerontology, 33*, 26–30.

Stodden, D., Langendorfer, S., & Robertson, M. A. (2009). The association between motor skill competence and physical fitness in young adults. *Research Quarterly for Exercise and Sport, 80*(2), 223–229.

Taylor, M. J. (2006). Neural bases of cognitive development. In E. Bialystok & F. I. M. Craik (Eds.), *Lifespan cognition: mechanisms of change* (pp. 15–26). Oxford, UK: Oxford University Press.

The Cooper Institute (March, 2009). *Texas education agency newsletter*. Retrieved from The Cooper Institute web site: http://www.cooperinstitute.org/news/eventDetail.cfm?news_id=47. Accessed 17 Aug 2009.

Themanson, J. R., & Hillman, C. H. (2006). Cardiorespiratory fitness and acute aerobic exercise effects on neuroelectric and behavioral measures of action monitoring. *Neuroscience, 141*, 757–767.

Themanson, J. R., Hillman, C. H., & Curtin, J. J. (2006). Age and physical activity influences on action monitoring during task switching. *Neurobiology of Aging, 27*, 1335–1345.

Tomporowski, P. D. (2003). Effects of acute bouts of exercise on cognition. *Acta Psychologica, 112*, 297–324.

Tomporowski, P. D., Davis, C. L., Miller, P. H., & Naglieri, J. A. (2008). Exercise and children's intelligence, cognition, and academic achievement. *Educational Psychology Review, 20*(2), 111–131.

Tomporowski, P. D., & Ellis, N. R. (1986). Effects of exercise on cognitive processes: a review. *Psychological Bulletin, 99*, 338–346.

Travis, F. (1998). Cortical and cognitive development in 4th, 8th, and 12th grade students: the contribution of speed of processing and executive functioning to cognitive development. *Biological Psychology, 48*, 37–56.

Trudeau, F., Espindola, R., Laurencelle, L., Dulac, F., Rajic, M., & Shephard, R. J. (2000). Follow-up of participants in the Trois-Rivieres growth and development study: examining their health-related fitness and risk factors as adults. *American Journal of Human Biology, 12*, 207–213.

Trudeau, F., & Shephard, R. J. (2008). Physical education, school physical activity, school sports and academic performance. *International Journal of Behavioural Nutrition and Physical Activity, 5*(10), 1–12.

U.S. Centers for Disease Control and Prevention (2006). *School health policies and programs study 2006: overview.* http://www.cdc.gov/healthyyouth/shpps/2006/factsheets/pdf/FS_Overview_SHPPS2006. Accessed 4 Jan 2009.

U.S. Department of Health and Human Services (2008). *Physical activity guidelines for Americans.* http://www.health.gov/Paguidelines/pdf/paguide.pdf. Accessed 4 Jan 2010.

van der Molen, M. W. (2000). Developmental changes in inhibitory processing: evidence from psychophysiological measures. *Biological Psychology, 54*, 207–239.

van Praag, H., Kempermann, G., & Gage, F. H. (1999). Running increases cell proliferation and neurogenesis in the adult mouse dentate gyrus. *Nature Neuroscience, 2*, 266–270.

van Veen, V., & Carter, C. S. (2002). The timing of action-monitoring processes in the anterior cingulated cortex. *Journal of Cognitive Neuroscience, 14*, 593–602.

Vaynman, S., & Gomez-Pinilla, F. (2006). Revenge of the "sit": how lifestyle impacts neuronal and cognitive health though molecular systems that interface energy metabolism with neuronal plasticity. *Journal of Neuroscience Research, 84*, 699–715.

Chapter 4
Influences of Social and Built Environments on Physical Activity in Middle-Aged and Older Adults

Fuzhong Li

Introduction

With advancing age come physiological changes that result in loss of muscle mass, which leads to progressive weakening in strength, endurance, and balance, as well as cardiopulmonary and cognitive function (Spirduso, Francis, & MacRae, 2005). Declines in body systems attributable to aging, accompanied by unhealthy lifestyles (physical inactivity, poor diet, substance use) ultimately become risk factors for developing various chronic health conditions such as heart disease, cancer, stroke, diabetes, high blood pressure, and mental distress (National Center for Health Statistics [NCHS], 2007). Currently, chronic diseases are the leading causes of death for US adults aged 65 or older (Centers for Disease Control and The Merck Company Foundation, 2007). Approximately 80 % of older Americans are living with at least one chronic condition, and 50 % have at least two (Centers for Disease Control and Prevention [CDC], 2003). Chronic diseases in older adults can lead to disability and limitations in daily activities (NCHS, 2007), thus reducing health-related quality of life and independence (CDC and Merck, 2007). At the social level, this increases the burden on the nation's health care system, with a projected average increase of 7 % each year from 2010 to 2018 in Medicare spending (Thorpe, Ogden, & Galactionnova, 2010) and an increase of 25 % in health care spending by 2030 (Agency for Healthcare Research and Quality [AHRQ] & CDC, 2002).

However, many health-related issues, such as chronic and degenerative illnesses, poor mental health, and substance abuse, in older adults can be prevented or improved through physical activity. Participation in regular physical activity has been shown to elicit a number of favorable responses that contribute to improved physical and mental health, quality of life, and independence in this population (Chodzko-Zajko et al., 2009;

F. Li(✉)
Oregon Research Institute, 1715 Franklin Blvd., Eugene, OR 97403, USA
e-mail: fuzhongl@ori.org

A.L. Meyer and T.P. Gullotta (eds.), *Physical Activity Across the Lifespan*,
Issues in Children's and Families' Lives 12, DOI 10.1007/978-1-4614-3606-5_4,
© Springer Science+Business Media New York 2012

Haskell et al., 2007; Mazzeo et al., 1998; U.S. Department of Health and Human Services, 1996; 2008). Thus, physical activity should be considered essential for healthy aging and one of the most important lifestyle components for preventing age-related decline in overall physical capability and well-being (Bouchard, Blair, & Haskell, 2007). However, national data indicate that a sedentary lifestyle remains common among older adults (AHRQ, 2002), and data from the 2007 Behavioral Risk Factor Surveillance System indicate that, among all age groups, people aged 65+ have the highest prevalence of physical inactivity ("inactive" = 23.7 %; "no leisure-time physical activity" = 32.7 %, respectively) (CDC, 2009a). Overall, physical activity is one behavioral health indicator for persons aged 65 and older that has not met the target set by *Healthy People 2010* (CDC & Merck, 2007). Contributing factors to physical inactivity are multifactorial and include personal, social, and environmental influences.

This chapter focuses on social and built environment factors associated with physical activity, an important behavioral lifestyle outcome. These issues are relevant to people of all ages (Sallis & Kerr, 2006), ranging from school children and adolescents (American Academy of Pediatrics [AAP], 2009) to adults (Brownson, Hoehner, Day, Forsyth, & Sallis, 2009; Humpel, Owen, & Leslie, 2002) and older adults (Li, Fisher, Bauman et al., 2005a; Yen, Michael, & Perdue, 2009). This chapter is specifically concerned with adults age 50+ because they are the most physically inactive, are at higher risk for health problems, and are the primary population targeted for physical activity promotion (Robert Wood Johnson Foundation [RWJ], 2001).

Place and Health: Why Is the Neighborhood Environment Relevant?

The increasing trend in urbanization and the anticipated growth in the prevalence of baby-boomers and aging populations for the coming decades have made place-and-health a relevant public health topic and an area of scientific inquiry. With ever-increasing land development and unmanaged growth leading to urban sprawl, there is increasing concern over the impact of the built environment on public health and quality of life for people in their communities.

Some recent evidence points directly to the influence of neighborhood social and built environment characteristics on various aspects of older adults' health. For example, older adults living in a poor neighborhood environment have been shown to have greater risk of functional loss over time (Balfour & Kaplan, 2002); similarly, residents of socioeconomically disadvantaged or psychosocially hazardous neighborhoods are associated with a higher likelihood of being obese (Glass, Rasmussen, & Schwartz, 2006; Grafova, Freedman, Kumar, & Rogowski, 2008). As far as the built environment is concerned, living in neighborhoods with low walkability has been found to be associated with depression (Berke, Gottlieb, Vernez Moudon, & Larson, 2007) and hypertension (Li, Harmer, Cardinal, & Vongjaturapat, 2009c) in older adults. Clearly, the kind of neighborhood environment in which older adults live has direct relevance to their health, making it important to understand the neighborhood effects on all aspects of health and health-related behaviors.

Relevance of Environmental Settings to Physical Activity

Physical activity often takes place in a person's community or neighborhood (Li, Fisher, Bauman et al., 2005a). For example, older adults frequently participate in physical activity programs offered through local community organizations (e.g., parks and recreation agencies, senior service providers, health departments, or private foundations) (Hooker, 2002; Orsega-Smith, Payne, & Godbey, 2003; Stewart et al., 1997). The most prevalent forms of physical activity in middle-aged and older adults, walking and jogging (Crespo, Keteyian, Heath, & Sempos, 1996; Eyler, Brownson, Black, & Housemann, 2003), typically occur in the immediate vicinity of the individual's residence (Fisher & Li, 2004; Li, Fisher, Bauman et al., 2005a). Thus, these outdoor behavioral phenomena have made the neighborhood context relevant for research into understanding physical activity behavior in older adults.

Physical activity is, however, a complex behavior that may be influenced by multiple factors within environmental, social/cultural, and psychological/cognitive domains. The two most salient and researched dimensions are social and built environments because they present opportunities for, and barriers to, participation in physical activity, thereby influencing older adults' decisions of whether or not to exercise. Within the context of this chapter, we define the social environment in terms of social capital/social cohesion, social support, and socioeconomic position (status) that affect physical activity (Li, Fisher, Bauman et al., 2005a; McNeill, Kreuter, & Subramanian, 2006). The built environment refers to man-made features, including buildings, land-use patterns, streets, and transportation (Ewing, 2004; Handy, Boarnet, Ewing, & Killingsworth, 2002) that have been linked to levels of, and opportunities for, physical activity.

Conceptual Frameworks and Empirical Studies of Social and Built Environment Influences on Physical Activity

Conceptual Frameworks

Research on the influences of social and built environments on physical activity has predominantly been driven by social–cognitive (Bandura, 2001) and/or social ecological models (King, Stokols, Talen, & Brassington, 2002; Sallis & Owen, 2002). The social–cognitive model emphasizes the importance of social and environmental factors providing feedback about behaviors, opportunities, and consequences. From this perspective, physical activity behaviors are likely to be shaped by the social influences to which older adults are exposed and the environmental settings in which they find themselves. Social ecological models take into account multiple levels of influences involving individual, social, physical environment, and policy factors. Recent studies of social and neighborhood environments involve sociologically based concepts of social cohesion and social capital (Kawachi & Berkman, 2000,

2003). The differing models have provided the means to study social and built environments and physical activity in various domains (e.g., leisure, social, transportation, household). In light of the multiple behaviors and levels of influence, many scholars have called for integration of theories and concepts across disciplines, including public health, behavioral sciences, urban planning, transportation, leisure studies, and landscape architecture (King et al., 2002; Lee & Vernez Moudon, 2004; Sallis, Frank, Saelens, & Kraft, 2004), and a multilevel analysis approach that allows researchers to disentangle the different (level-specific) sources of variations in levels of physical activity (Li, Fisher, Bauman et al., 2005a).

Social Environment

Because physical activity by older adults occurs in community settings (i.e., their neighborhoods), it provides great potential for social networking and personal and social interactions with others (Li, Fisher, Bauman et al., 2005a). Therefore, the degree to which older adults engage in physical activity may help build social ties, thereby reducing social isolation and increasing social cohesion and social capital in their neighborhood communities. Social cohesion, which generates social capital, has been defined as the "extent of connectedness and solidarity among groups in society" (Kawachi & Berkman, 2000). Social capital, in turn, refers to levels of interpersonal trust between citizens, connectedness, reciprocity, and social bonding, which facilitate cooperation for mutual benefit (Kawachi & Berkman, 2000).

In general, research has indicated that walkable, mixed-used neighborhoods encourage enhanced levels of social and community engagement (i.e., social capital) and that those living in walkable neighborhoods are more likely to know their neighbors, participate politically, trust others, and be socially engaged (Leyden, 2003). This important neighborhood social dimension has also been linked to levels of physical activity. For example, older adults who perceived their neighborhoods as having high social cohesion report high levels of physical activity or walking (Fisher, Li, Michael, & Cleveland, 2004; King, 2008). King further indicates that social cohesion may mediate the relationship between certain neighborhood factors (e.g., yard maintenance, litter) and physical activity. Similarly, social participation (a dimension of social capital) is related to leisure time physical activity in neighborhoods (Lindström, Moghaddassi, & Merlo, 2003), and perceptions of social protective factors such as social networks, participation, social cohesion, informal social control, sense of community, reciprocity, trust, and safety are associated with an increased likelihood of meeting general recommendations for physical activity in adults (Brennan, Baker, Haire-Joshu, & Brownson, 2003).

Social support, which may include sources of support from family members and friends, is also an important correlate of physical activity and walking (Eyler et al., 1999, 2003). In two studies that involve older adults, those who perceived high support from friends and family were associated with being more physically active compared to those perceiving low social support (Booth et al., 2000), and the support mechanism was shown to be important for engaging in frequent physical activity in later life (Kaplan, Newsom, McFarland, & Lu, 2001). To date, social support is often constructed at the individual level (i.e., perceived support from immediate family members or friends), and there have been no studies that have examined whether perceptions of community support (e.g., perceived support from local neighborhood associations, community coalitions or organizations, etc.) would facilitate participation in physical activity by older adults.

Neighborhood Socioeconomic Status

As with other built environmental factors, neighborhood socioeconomic status is a significant contributor to physical activity, although the direction of the relationship to physical activity varies across studies. For example, a regional study in Pittsburgh, Pennsylvania, involving postmenopausal women living in a neighborhood classified as low socioeconomic status reported high levels of physical activity (King et al., 2005), possibly because in these neighborhoods there is limited access to transportation, resulting in walking as a necessity. On the other hand, Tucker-Seeley, Subramanian, Li, and Sorensen (2009) surveyed a national representative sample of US adults aged ≥50 and found that older adults living in high socioeconomic neighborhoods reported a higher level of leisure-time physical activity.

Built Environment

Research has shown that multifaceted, built environment factors are associated with levels of physical activity in middle-aged and older adult populations. Both qualitative and quantitative analyses reveal important descriptive features of neighborhood environments, including the presence or absence of sidewalks, street lights, enjoyable scenery, heavy traffic, access and proximity to local facilities, and levels of crime or fear about safety, that can either support or act as a barrier to physical activity (Centers for Disease Control and Prevention, 1999; Berke, Koepsell, Vernez Moudon, Hoskins, & Larson, 2007; Booth et al., 2000; King, 2008; Strath, Isaacs, & Greenwald, 2007; Tucker-Seeley et al., 2009). These reoccurring factors show that the immediate environment (i.e., neighborhood) matters when people make decisions about being physically active.

In multilevel studies where the influence of neighborhood-level factors above and beyond those of individual-level factors is examined, evidence suggests that a host of built environment factors are related to physical activity. For example, older adult residents of neighborhoods with a high density of places of employment and households, greater numbers of street intersections, and green and open spaces for recreation, are more likely to engage in walking activity (Li, Fisher, Brownson, & Bosworth, 2005c). Similarly, certain street characteristics, such as path continuity and the presence of curb cuts and crosswalks, are associated with frequency of walking for errands (King, 2008). In predicting change in walking activity, Li, Fisher, and Brownson (2005b) show that, although levels of walking were reduced over a 1-year study period, neighborhoods with greater access to physical activity facilities were associated with a lower decline in walking over time.

Land use patterns or urban form are likewise associated with levels of physical activity. In a study (Li et al., 2008) involving a population inclusive of the immediate pre-Baby Boom/early-Baby Boom generations (adults aged 50–75 years), high mixed-use land and street connectivity were found to be associated with greater levels of various types walking activities (neighborhood walking, walking for transportation, walking for errands) and meeting physical activity recommendations. Density of public transit stations has also been associated with high levels of walking for transportation (Li et al., 2008). Other research has indicated that a greater density of neighborhood destinations, proximity to businesses and facilities, and residential density were related to more walking among middle-aged or older adults (Gauvin et al., 2008; Nagel, Carlson, Bosworth, & Michael, 2008; King et al., 2005; Rodríguez, Evenson, Diez Roux, & Brines, 2009; Satariano et al., 2010). King et al., (2005) further observed that living in a neighborhood with homes built between 1950 and 1960 (representing an urban form that is more pedestrian-friendly) was associated with more walking.

Impact of the Environment on Public Health

Collective findings from current research have ramifications for public health. First, in the coming decades, there will be a significant increase in the aging population, with nearly one in five Americans expected to be 65 years or older (88.5 million) by 2030, more than double the 2008 distribution (38.7 million) (U.S. Census Bureau, 2009). This increase, coupled with the high proportion of chronic diseases and sedentary lifestyles in the population, makes understanding the social and built environment one of the most urgent issues in urban and suburban health.

Increases in urban and suburban sprawl, which pull people and resources away from the center of cities or towns, will affect the way people act and interact. Communities that are stressful, unsafe, and poorly designed with low walkability are likely to limit physical activity and foster sedentary lifestyles. Sedentary living habits contribute to poor health outcomes because they are a significant factor in the incidence of overweight and obesity. Among adults, obesity prevalence doubled from 1980 to 2004, and recent data indicate that an estimated 33 % of US adults are overweight and 34 % are obese, with nearly 6 % extremely obese (defined as BMI ≥ 40.0) (CDC, 2008). Obesity is a known major risk factor for cardiovascular disease, certain cancers, and Type 2 diabetes. The literature clearly indicates that the built environment contributes to overweight and obesity (Ewing, Schmid, Killingsworth, Zlot, & Raudenbush, 2003; Feng, Glass, Curriero, Stewart, & Schwartz, 2010; Hill, Wyatt, Reed, & Peters, 2003; Li et al., 2008; Li, Harmer, Cardinal, Bosworth, & Johnson-Shelton, 2009a; Li et al., 2009b; Papas et al., 2007).

The expected increase in the population age 65 and older will present great challenges in designing contemporary urban centers and suburban subdivisions optimally configured for the growing older population. The dominant trend of suburban sprawl and deurbanization, as opposed to the traditional urban form (represented by more pedestrian-friendly neighborhoods), will create more environmental barriers for older adults. This is especially true for those in vulnerable subgroups (e.g., people with disabilities, frail elderly) who are often ignored in public policy and land development practices (Glass & Balfour, 2003), thus impeding their potential to remain productive and socially engaged through activities of daily living, such as getting from place to place or accessing basic facilities where health care and social services are provided.

Future Research

From both a scientific and public health perspective, a better understanding of social and built environment influences on physical activity is critical. Although there have been significant advances in the use of Geographic Information System-based measures to capture attributes of the built environment, not much has been done to assess social aspects of neighborhood environments related to physical activity. Given the lack of gold-standard measures in this area, multiple sources of multilevel data (i.e., self-report, census, public data, GIS-based measures) are needed. A recent methodological review by Brownson et al. (2009) clearly indicated that further work is needed to develop valid and psychometrically sound measures that allow better assessment of both social and built environments.

The majority of research examining environment and physical activity relationships is cross-sectional in design, making it difficult to draw causal inference. To assign causality, longitudinal studies are needed to explicitly examine changes in physical activity in relation to either static or dynamic measures of social and built environment characteristics. Quasi-experiment research is also needed to examine change as a result of policy initiatives in natural community settings. Community-based intervention studies are rare (Sallis & Kerr, 2006), and more of them are needed (e.g., Fisher & Li, 2004) to examine various types of community land-use features in relation to physical activity.

To better understand how neighborhood context affects physical activity in the older adult population, there is a need to consider mechanisms and pathways through which neighborhood characteristics affect physical activity (King et al., 2002; Li, Fisher, Bauman et al., 2005a). This may involve mediation and moderation analyses among independent (exposure) variables of interest. There have been a handful of studies that reflect these efforts. For example, Li et al. (2005c) examined the interaction between the number of street intersections and older adults' perceptions of safety from traffic on neighborhood walking, and Tucker-Seeley et al. (2009) examined socioeconomic status as a moderator of the relationship between older adults' perceptions of neighborhood safety and leisure-time physical activity.

Research to date has predominately focused on urban or suburban areas. However, it is quite conceivable that social and built environments differ significantly between urban and rural settings, resulting in different facilitators and barriers for physical activity. In an early study comparing rural and urban older women, Wilcox, Castro, King, Housemann, and Brownson (2000) found that caregiving duties was the main barrier to leisure-time physical activity for rural women, whereas urban women reported lack of time as the barrier. When asked about environmental barriers to physical activity, rural women experienced more barriers, such as the absence of sidewalks and streetlights, high crime, and lack of access to recreational facilities. There is a paucity of research from which to draw inferences about these different environments. Similarly, research that focuses on the relationship between the built environment and health behaviors among socially disadvantaged subgroups (Casagrande, Whitt-Glover, Lanscaster, Odoms-Young, & Gary, 2009), such as low-income, African Americans, or Latinos, is needed.

Given that the mission of public health is to promote population health, environmental and policy research is required to develop effective policies and practices to increase physical activity (Dannenberg et al., 2003; Heath, Brownson, Kruger, & Services Task Force on Community Preventive Services, 2006; Schmid, Pratt, & Witmer, 2006). In this regard, the Centers for Disease Control and Prevention has provided such strategies (CDC, 2009b), including the Active Community Environments Initiative, which encourages environmental and policy interventions to increase physical activity and improve public health by promoting walking, bicycling, and the development of accessible recreation facilities.

As mentioned previously, it is critical to realize that social and built environment influences on activity are not restricted to middle-aged and older adults. For example, the previously discussed features of social and built environments are also relevant for children and adolescents in regard to their ability to walk to and from school and opportunities for play and active lifestyles (AAP, 2009). What is lacking in the literature are studies on the extent to which social and built environments may affect the amount of time that parent–child or grandparent–child groupings spend in engaging in physical activity. Environment-specific features that may operate differentially to affect levels of physical activity among youth and adults are also unclear. To understand how built environment features, such as walkability and neighborhood safety, may have differential associations by age groups, we need a developmental or lifespan approach that links early emergence in physical activity or health behaviors to adulthood.

Practical Implications

There are a number of practical implications that can be derived from the existing literature that may be especially relevant for city planners; public health administrators; researchers in the areas of epidemiology, behavioral/leisure sciences, and sociology; transportation professionals; community leaders; and other health advocates and public health decision makers whose goals are centered on understanding and promoting public health and developing highly livable communities.

Neighborhood Social Support and Social Capital

Providing social support and fostering social cohesion within a community can promote physical activity among older adults. One approach for developing social cohesion and neighborhood social capital is to increase civil engagement or participation in social activity and cooperation among neighborhood residents, including local political action groups or neighborhood associations. Doing so may ultimately lead to increased activity levels in older adults (Fisher et al., 2004). To strengthen this approach, policy-based interventions should emphasize community or social support to help older adults in the community develop healthier behaviors (Heath et al., 2006).

It has also been shown that positive features of urban design can enhance social capital (Leyden, 2003). Neighborhoods that are well mixed (in terms of land use) and walkable are more conducive to enhanced levels of social cohesion and social capital among residents, thereby encouraging physical activity. From urban design and zoning policies perspectives, discouraging urban sprawl and embracing traditional neighborhood designs (e.g., mixed land-use, good public transportation systems, pedestrian-oriented streets) can foster social engagement and civil activities (e.g., participating in church activities, walk-a-thons, community events) and, ultimately, promote neighborhood walking and other forms of physical activity.

Perceptions of the Neighborhood Environment

Promoting neighborhood physical activity may need to take into account individuals' perceptions about their social and built environment. For example, studies show that street connectivity facilitates walking but only when older adults perceive traffic conditions near their residences as safe (Li et al., 2005c). Higher levels of perceived neighborhood safety in this regard are associated with high levels of physical activity (CDC, 1999). This also suggests that neighborhood communities should be designed around the needs of people where they live rather than meeting the needs of automobiles. Similarly, the association between built environmental factors and physical activity may be mediated through older adults' perceptions of their neighborhood social cohesion and safety from crime (King, 2008). Such findings would seem to argue for using designs associated with traditional neighborhoods, which are connected by networks of intersecting streets and well-maintained sidewalks that are easy to get to and safe to walk. Results from various studies point to the importance of older adults' perceptions of the quality of their neighborhood when promoting physical activity in this population. The same is for the design and use of retirement communities.

Neighborhood Designs and Walkability

City planners, transportation developers, and architects should integrate issues of public health into their urban planning and development and consider changing existing zoning or building codes to encourage multiuse land-development patterns. Changes should facilitate opportunities and remove environmental barriers so that older adults can be more active in their communities. Evidence to date suggests that neighborhoods containing high land-use mix, better street connectivity, walkable distances to facilities, and greater amounts of green and open spaces for recreation are associated with increased likelihood of urban mobility, including walking among residents.

Planning for retirement communities should encourage physical activity by emphasizing walkability and accessibility to facilities that are used daily. Common environmental enabling factors likely to promote physical activity and facilitate neighborhood walking for various purposes (e.g., utilitarian, leisure, social) include grocery stores and senior services within walking distance of older adults' homes, the presence of sidewalks, well-lit streets, easy access to parks, enjoyable scenery, and low neighborhood levels of crime. Given that many older adults face physical impairments or functional decline due to aging, emphasis should be placed on encouraging building and site design that is accessible for those with mobility impairments. This can be accomplished by eliminating uneven sidewalks and high curbs and increasing street lighting and signaled crosswalks, thus reducing safety concerns about traffic and crime.

Improvements in neighborhood walkability may help increase levels of physical activity and consequently reduce health risk factors for older adults. A longitudinal study in Oregon, for example, found that older adults who lived in walkable neighborhoods and engaged in high levels of physical activity were likely to maintain a healthy weight over time (Li et al., 2009b), while those who were not meeting physical activity guidelines, combined with frequent visits to local fast-food restaurants and low efficacy of eating fruits and vegetables, had an increased risk of being obese. Similarly, when compared to those living in low-walkable neighborhoods, older adults living in high-walkable neighborhoods were associated with reduced levels of systolic and diastolic blood pressure over time (Li et al., 2009c).

Policy Considerations

The impact of social and built environments on health and health behaviors is apparent, and the challenges facing those with the responsibility for ensuring the health and quality of life of older Americans are clear. The challenges are greater in suburban or rural settings because they entail more environmental barriers to mobility and accessibility.

The need for enlightened environmental policies and interventions is evident in the literature (AAP, 2009; CDC, 2009c; Heath et al., 2006; Orleans, Kraft, Marx, &

McGinnis, 2003; Sallis & Kerr, 2006; Task Force on Community Preventive Services, 2002) and the recognition of the value of this approach is reflected in movements and initiatives, at the national and regional level, that advocate mixed land use and pedestrian-friendly neighborhood designs. For example, the Smart Growth movement supports limiting urban sprawl and promoting better design, planning, and development of land to make cities and towns across America "more livable" (Smart Growth America, 2010). Similarly, Active Living by Design (http://www.activelivingbydesign.org/), supported by Robert Wood Johnson Foundation (2001), promotes better communities through "community-led change by working with local and national partners to build a culture of active living and healthy eating." At the regional level, a similar concept has been adopted in Portland, Oregon, with the 2040 Growth Concept plan from the Metro Regional Government (MRG, 2010). This plan aims to promote regional development that focuses on mixed land-use, accessibility to facilities, and a walkable neighborhood environment with a well-supported public transit system.

Most of the social and built environment variables influencing physical activity can be modified through interventions or public policy changes at the national, regional, and local level, thus improving neighborhood walkability, increasing physical activity, and subsequently improving health in the population. Changes in community social and built environments, however, need to be made through the joint effort of individuals from multidisciplinary fields, including public health, urban planning, transportation planning, landscape architecture, epidemiology/sociology, and behavioral/leisure/nutrition sciences (Lee & Vernez Moudon, 2004; Sallis et al., 2004; Schmid et al., 2006). A good example of this type of collaboration is the previously mentioned Active Living by Design, an initiative in which professionals work together collaboratively and effectively to influence public health and environmental policies.

There is a growing consensus that existing evidence-based findings are sufficient to justify environment and policy changes (Heath et al., 2006; Sallis & Kerr, 2006; Transportation Research Board and Institute of Medicine, 2005). However, many of the social and built environment factors identified here may vary in importance across settings; therefore, appropriate community-specific tailoring or adjustments will be needed (Brownson, Baker, Housemann, Brennan, & Bacak, 2001).

Conclusions

While it is premature to draw definite conclusions regarding a causal relationship from the current research findings, the accumulating evidence demonstrates considerable consistency of an observable association between social and built environment characteristics and levels of physical activity in middle-aged and older adult populations. That is, the amount of physical activity is facilitated or impeded by a host of social and built environment characteristics. By extension, these characteristics should play an important role in guiding environmental and policy approaches to promoting healthy aging by increasing levels of physical activity. Fortunately, most of the environmental variables are modifiable through changes in urban planning and zoning policies to promote physical activity.

Because physical activity is a significant determinant of health and quality of life for older adults, it is of great urgency that we acknowledge its public health significance and consider various evidence-based environmental issues in policymaking. We must adopt and implement multilevel policies that influence the social and built environment, which will in turn improve health, increase physical activity, and prevent obesity. The overarching goal of these policies should be to design and develop sustainable communities that are convenient, safe, and attractive, where middle-aged and older adults can be physically active, live well, and maintain life independence.

Acknowledgment The work presented in this paper is supported by a research grant from the National Institute of Environmental Health Sciences, National Institutes of Health (Grant #1R01ES014252).

References

Agency for Healthcare Research and Quality and the Centers for Disease Control and Prevention (2002). *Activity and older Americans: benefits and strategies.* Retrieved May 11, 2010 from http://www.ahrq.gov/ppip/activity.htm.

American Academy of Pediatrics. (2009). The built environment: designing communities to promote physical activity children. *Pediatrics, 123*, 1591–1598.

Balfour, J. L., & Kaplan, G. A. (2002). Neighborhood environment and loss of physical function in older adults: evidence from the Alameda County Study. *American Journal of Epidemiology, 155*, 507–515.

Bandura, A. (2001). Social cognitive theory: an agentic perspective. *Annual Review of Psychology, 52*, 1–26.

Berke, M. E., Gottlieb, L. M., Vernez Moudon, A., & Larson, E. B. (2007). Protective association between neighborhood walkability and depression in older men. *Journal of American Geriatrics Society, 55*, 526–533.

Berke, E. M., Koepsell, T. D., Vernez Moudon, A., Hoskins, R. E., & Larson, E. B. (2007). Association of the built environment with physical activity and obesity in older persons. *American Journal of Public Health, 97*, 486–492.

Booth, M. L., Owen, N., Bauman, A., Clavisi, O., & Leslie, E. (2000). Social-cognitive and perceived environment influences associated with physical activity in older Australians. *Preventive Medicine, 31*, 15–22.

Bouchard, C., Blair, S. N., & Haskell, W. L. (2007). *Physical activity and health.* Champaign, IL: Human Kinetics.

Brennan, L. K., Baker, E. A., Haire-Joshu, D., & Brownson, R. C. (2003). Linking perceptions of the community to behavior: are protective social factors associated with physical activity? *Health Education and Behavior, 30*, 740–755.

Brownson, R. C., Baker, E. A., Housemann, R. A., Brennan, L. K., & Bacak, S. J. (2001). Environmental and policy determinants of physical activity in the United States. *American Journal of Public Health, 91*, 1995–2003.

Brownson, R. C., Hoehner, C. M., Day, K., Forsyth, A., & Sallis, J. F. (2009). Measuring the built environment for physical activity: state of the science. *American Journal of Preventive Medicine, 36*(4S), S99–S123.

Casagrande, S. S., Whitt-Glover, M. C., Lanscaster, K. J., Odoms-Young, A. M., & Gary, T. L. (2009). Built environment and health behaviors among African Americans: a systematic review. *American Journal of Preventive Medicine, 36*, 174–181.

U.S. Census Bureau (2009). *An older and more diverse nation by midcentury.* Retrieved September 3, 2009 from http://www.census.gov/Press-Release/www/releases/archives/population/012496. html.

Centers for Disease Control and Prevention. (1999). Neighborhood safety and the prevalence of physical inactivity—selected States, 1996. *Morbidity and Mortality Weekly Report, 48*(07), 143–146.

Centers for Disease Control and Prevention. (2003). Public health and aging: trends in aging— United States and worldwide. *Morbidity and Mortality Weekly Report, 52*(06), 101–106.

Centers for Disease Control and Prevention. (2008). *Prevalence of overweight, obesity, and extreme obesity among adults: United States, Trends 1976–80 through 2005–2006.* Hyattsville, MD: US Department of Health and Human Services, National Center for Health Statistics, CDC.

Centers for Disease Control and Prevention (2009a). *U.S. physical activity statistics.* Retrieved August 2009 from http://apps.nccd.cdc.gov/PASurveillance/DemoCompareResultV.asp?State =0&Cat=1&Year=2007&Go=GO.

Centers for Disease Control and Prevention (2009b). *Active environments.* Retrieved May 11, 2010 from http://www.cdc.gov/nccdphp/dnpa/physical/health_professionals/active_environments/ index.htm.

Centers for Disease Control and Prevention (2009c). *About healthy places.* Retrieved May 11, 2010 from http://www.cdc.gov/HEALTHYPLACES/about.htm.

Centers for Disease Control and Prevention and The Merck Company Foundation. (2007). *The state of aging and health in America 2007.* Whitehouse Station, NJ: The Merck Company Foundation.

Chodzko-Zajko, W. J., Proctor, D. N., Fiatarone Singh, M. A., Minson, C. T., Nigg, C. R., Salem, G. J., et al. (2009). Exercise and physical activity for older adults. *Medicine and Science in Sports and Exercise, 41*, 1510–1530.

Crespo, C. J., Keteyian, S. T., Heath, G. W., & Sempos, C. T. (1996). Leisure-time physical activity among US adults. *Archives of Internal Medicine, 156*, 93–98.

Dannenberg, A. L., Jackson, R. J., Frumkin, H., Schieber, R. A., Pratt, M., Kochtizky, C., et al. (2003). The impact of community design and land-use choices on public health: a scientific research agenda. *American Journal of Public Health, 93*, 1500–1508.

Ewing, R. (2004). Can the physical environment determine physical activity levels? *Exercise Sport Science Review, 33*, 69–75.

Ewing, R., Schmid, T., Killingsworth, R. E., Zlot, A., & Raudenbush, S. (2003). Relationship between urban sprawl and physical activity, obesity, and morbidity. *American Journal of Health Promotion, 18*, 47–57.

Eyler, A. A., Brownson, R. C., Black, S. J., & Housemann, R. A. (2003). The epidemiology of walking for physical activity in the United States. *Medicine and Science in Sports and Exercise, 35*, 1529–1536.

Eyler, A. A., Brownson, R. C., Donatelle, R. J., King, A. C., Brown, D. R., & Sallis, J. F. (1999). Physical activity social support and middle- and older-aged minority women: results from a US survey. *Social Science and Medicine, 49*, 781–789.

Feng, J., Glass, T. A., Curriero, F. C., Stewart, W. F., & Schwartz, B. S. (2010). The built environment and obesity: a systematic review of the epidemiologic evidence. *Health and Place, 16*, 175–190.

Fisher, K. J., & Li, F. (2004). A community-based walking trial to improve neighborhood quality of life in the elderly: a multilevel analysis. *Annals of Behavioral Medicine, 28*, 186–194.

Fisher, K. J., Li, F., Michael, Y., & Cleveland, M. (2004). Neighborhood level influences on physical activity among older adults: a multilevel analysis. *Journal of Aging and Physical Activity, 11*, 49–67.

Gauvin, L., Viva, M., Barnett, T., Richard, L., Lynn Craig, C., Spivock, M., et al. (2008). Association between neighborhood active living potential and walking. *American Journal of Epidemiology, 167*, 944–953.

Glass, T. A., & Balfour, J. L. (2003). Neighborhoods, aging, and functional imitations. In I. Kawachi & L. Berkman (Eds.), *Neighborhoods and health* (pp. 303–334). New York: Oxford University Press.

Glass, T. A., Rasmussen, M. D., & Schwartz, B. S. (2006). Neighborhoods and obesity in older adults: the Baltimore Memory Study. *American Journal of Preventive Medicine, 31*, 455–463.

Grafova, I. B., Freedman, V. A., Kumar, R., & Rogowski, J. (2008). Neighborhoods and obesity in later life. *American Journal of Public Health, 98*, 2065–2071.

Handy, S., Boarnet, M., Ewing, R., & Killingsworth, R. (2002). How the built environment affects physical activity: views from urban planning. *American Journal of Preventive Medicine, 23*, 64–73.

Haskell, W. L., Lee, I.-M., Pate, R. R., Powell, K. E., Blair, S. N., Franklin, B. A., et al. (2007). Physical activity and public health: updated recommendation for adults from American College of Sports Medicine and the American Heart Association. *Medicine and Science in Sports and Exercise, 39*(8), 1423–1434.

Heath, G., Brownson, R., Kruger, J., & Services Task Force on Community Preventive Services. (2006). The effectiveness of urban design and land use and transport policies and practices to increase physical activity: a systematic review. *Journal of Physical Activity and Health, 3*(suppl. 1), S55–S76.

Hill, J. O., Wyatt, H. R., Reed, G. W., & Peters, J. C. (2003). Obesity and the environment: where do we go from here? *Science, 299*, 1371–1374.

Hooker, S. P. (2002). California active aging project. *Journal of Aging and Physical Activity, 10*, 354–359.

Humpel, N., Owen, N., & Leslie, E. (2002). Environmental factors associated with adults' participation in physical activity: a review. *American Journal of Preventive Medicine, 22*, 188–199.

Kaplan, M. S., Newsom, J. T., McFarland, B. H., & Lu, L. (2001). Demographic and psychosocial correlates of physical activity in late life. *American Journal of Preventive Medicine, 21*(4), 306–312.

Kawachi, I., & Berkman, L. F. (2000). Social cohesion, social capital, and health. In L. Berkman & I. Kawachi (Eds.), *Social epidemiology* (pp. 174–190). New York: Oxford University Press.

Kawachi, I., & Berkman, L. F. (2003). *Neighborhood and health*. New York, NY: Oxford University Press.

King, D. (2008). Neighborhood and individual factors in activity in older adults: results from the neighborhood and senior health study. *Journal of Aging and Physical Activity, 16*, 144–170.

King, W. C., Belle, S. H., Brach, J. S., Simkin-Silverman, L. R., Soske, T., & Kriska, A. M. (2005). Objective measures of neighborhood environment and physical activity in older women. *American Journal of Preventive Medicine, 28*, 461–469.

King, A. C., Stokols, D., Talen, E., & Brassington, G. S. (2002). Theoretic approaches to the promotion of physical activity. *American Journal of Preventive Medicine, 23*, 15–25.

Lee, C., & Vernez Moudon, A. (2004). Physical activity and environment research in the health field: implications for urban and transportation planning practice and research. *Journal of Planning Literature, 19*, 147–181.

Leyden, K. M. (2003). Social capital and the built environment: the importance of walkable neighborhoods. *American Journal of Public Health, 93*, 1546–1551.

Li, F., Fisher, K. J., Bauman, A., Ory, M. G., Chodzko-Zajdo, W., Harmer, P., et al. (2005a). Neighborhood influences on physical activity in older adults: a multilevel perspective. *Journal of Aging and Physical Activity, 13*, 32–58.

Li, F., Fisher, K. J., & Brownson, R. C. (2005b). A multilevel analysis of change in neighborhood walking activity in older adults. *Journal of Aging and Physical Activity, 13*, 145–159.

Li, F., Fisher, K. J., Brownson, B. C., & Bosworth, M. (2005c). Multilevel modeling of built environmental characteristics in relation to neighborhood walking activity in older adults. *Journal of Epidemiology and Community Health, 59*, 558–564.

Li, F., Harmer, P., Cardinal, B. J., Bosworth, M., Acock, A., Johnson-Shelton, D., et al. (2008). Built environment, adiposity and physical activity in adults aged 50-75. *American Journal of Preventive Medicine, 35*, 38–46.

Li, F., Harmer, P., Cardinal, B. J., Bosworth, M., & Johnson-Shelton, D. (2009a). Obesity and the built environment: does the density of neighborhood fast-food outlets matter? *American Journal of Health Promotion, 23*(3), 203–209.

Li, F., Harmer, P., Cardinal, B. J., Bosworth, M., Johnson-Shelton, D., Moore, J. M., et al. (2009b). Built environment and 1-year change in weight and waist circumference in middle-aged and older adults: Portland Neighborhood Environment and Health Study. *American Journal of Epidemiology, 169*, 401–408.

Li, F., Harmer, P., Cardinal, B. J., & Vongjaturapat, N. (2009c). Built environment and changes in blood pressure in middle aged and older adults. *Preventive Medicine, 48*, 237–241.

Lindström, M., Moghaddassi, M., & Merlo, J. (2003). Social capital and leisure time physical activity: a population based multilevel analysis in Malmö, Sweden. *Journal of Epidemiology and Community Health, 57*, 23–28.

Mazzeo, R. S., Cavanagh, P., Evans, W. J., Fiatarone, M., Hagberg, J., McAuley, M., et al. (1998). Exercise and physical activity for older adults. *Medicine and Science in Sports and Exercise, 30*, 992–1008.

McNeill, L. H., Kreuter, M. W., & Subramanian, S. V. (2006). Social environment and physical activity: a review of concepts and evidence. *Social Science and Medicine, 63*, 1011–1022.

Metro Regional Government (2010). *Metro*. Retrieved May 20, 2010 from http://www.oregon-metro.gov/index.cfm/go/.

Nagel, C. L., Carlson, N. E., Bosworth, M., & Michael, E. L. (2008). The relation between neighborhood built environment and walking activity among older adults. *American Journal of Epidemiology, 168*, 461–468.

National Center for Health Statistics (2007). *Health, United States, 2007, with chartbook on trends in the health of Americans*. Retrieved May 11, 2010 from www.cdc.gov/nchs/data/hus/hus07.pdf.

Orleans, C. T., Kraft, M. K., Marx, J. F., & McGinnis, J. M. (2003). Why are some neighborhoods active and others not? Charting a new course for research on the policy and environmental determinants of physical activity. *Annals of Behavioral Medicine, 25*, 77–79.

Orsega-Smith, E., Payne, L. L., & Godbey, G. (2003). Physical and psychosocial characteristics of older adults who participate in a community-based exercise program. *Journal of Aging and Physical Activity, 11*, 516–531.

Papas, M. A., Alberg, A. J., Ewing, R., Helzlsouer, K. J., Gary, T. L., & Klassen, A. C. (2007). The built environment and obesity. *Epidemiologic Reviews, 29*, 129–143.

Robert Wood Johnson Foundation. (2001). National blueprint for increasing physical activity among adults age 50 and older: creating a strategic framework and enhancing organization capacity for change. *Journal of Aging and Physical Activity, 9*, S5–S12.

Rodríguez, D. A., Evenson, K. R., Diez Roux, A. V., & Brines, S. J. (2009). Land use, residential density, and walking: the multi-ethnic study of atherosclerosis. *American Journal of Preventive Medicine, 37*, 397–404.

Sallis, J. F., Frank, L. D., Saelens, B. E., & Kraft, M. K. (2004). Active transportation and physical activity: opportunities for collaboration on transportation and public health research. *Transportation Research Part A: Policy and Practice, 38*, 249–268.

Sallis, J.F., & Kerr, J. (2006). *Physical activity and the built environment*. President's Council on Physical Fitness and Sports, Washington, DC. Retrieved 1 August 2009 from http://www.fitness.gov/digests/December2006Digest.pdf.

Sallis, J. F., & Owen, N. (2002). Ecological models of healthy behavior. In K. Glanz, F. M. Lewis, & B. K. Rimer (Eds.), *Health behavior and health education: theory, research and practice* (3dth ed., pp. 462–484). San Francisco, CA: Jossey-Bass.

Satariano, W. A., Ivey, S. L., Kurtovich, E., Kealey, M., Hubbard, A. E., Bayles, C. M., et al. (2010). Lower-body function, neighborhoods, and walking in an older population. *American Journal of Preventive Medicine, 38*, 419–428.

Schmid, T. L., Pratt, M., & Witmer, L. (2006). A framework for physical activity policy research. *Journal of Physical Activity and Health, 3*, S20–S29.

Smart Growth America. (2010) *Who we are*. Retrieved March 28, 2009 from http://smart-growthamerica.org/whoweare.html.

Spirduso, W. W., Francis, K. L., & MacRae, P. G. (2005). *Physical dimensions of aging*. Champaign, IL: Human Kinetics.

Stewart, A. L., Mills, K. M., Sepsis, P. G., King, A. C., McLellan, B. Y., Roitz, K., et al. (1997). Evaluation of CHAMPS, a physical activity promotion program m for older adults. *Annals of Behavioral Medicine, 19*, 353–361.

Strath, S., Isaacs, R., & Greenwald, M. J. (2007). Operationalizing environmental indictors for physical activity in older adults. *Journal of Aging and Physical activity, 15*, 412–424.

Task Force on Community Preventive Services. (2002). Recommendations to increase physical activity in communities. *American Journal of Preventive Medicine, 22*(4), 67–72.

Thorpe, K. E., Ogden, L. L., & Galactionnova, K. (2010). Chronic conditions account for rise in Medicare spending from 1987 to 2006. *Health Affairs, 29*, 718–724.

Transportation Research Board and Institute of Medicine (2005). *Does the built environment influence physical activity? Examining the evidence*. Retrieved August 2009 from http://online-pubs.trb.org/onlinepubs/sr/sr282.pdf.

Tucker-Seeley, R. D., Subramanian, S. V., Li, Y., & Sorensen, G. (2009). Neighborhood safety, socioeconomic status, and physical activity in older adults. *American Journal of Preventive Medicine, 37*, 207–213.

U.S. Department of Health and Human Services. (1996). *Physical activity and health: a report of the surgeon general*. Atlanta, GA: U.S. Department of Health and Human Services, Centers for Disease Control and Prevention.

U.S. Department of Health and Human Services (2008). *2008 physical activity guidelines for Americans*. Retrieved January 10, 2009 from http://www.health.gov/paguidelines/guidelines/default.aspx.

Wilcox, S., Castro, C., King, A. C., Housemann, R., & Brownson, R. C. (2000). Determinants of leisure time physical activity in rural compared with urban older and ethnically diverse women in the United States. *Journal of Epidemiology and Community Health, 54*, 667–672.

Yen, I. H., Michael, Y. L., & Perdue, L. (2009). Neighborhood environment in studies of health of older adults: a systematic review. *American Journal of Preventive Medicine, 37*, 455–463.

Chapter 5
Physical Activity as Depression Treatment

Lynette L. Craft

The Importance of Treating Depression in Youth and Adolescents

Clinical depression affects millions of young people each year. During youth and adolescence, depression is associated with a variety of psychological and social difficulties. For example, youth and adolescents with depression often experience low self-esteem and confidence, impaired social and interpersonal skills, poor school performance and achievement, social withdrawal, and difficult family and peer relationships (Bylund & Reed, 2007; Mehler-Wex & Kolch, 2008). Treatment for this disorder is vital because experiencing an episode of major depressive disorder (MDD) during adolescence greatly increases the likelihood that the child will develop another depressive episode (5 year recurrence rates are in excess of 70 %) or will develop substance abuse during young adulthood (Lewinsohn & Clarke, 1999; Mehler-Wex & Kolch, 2008). Finally, untreated depression is associated with suicidal ideation and suicide is the third leading cause of death among adolescents in the United States (Klomek & Stanley, 2007).

Individuals with depression commonly engage in unhealthy lifestyle behaviors such as poor quality diet, smoking, and being physically inactive (Chuang, Mansell, & Patten, 2008). In adults, depression is now recognized as a risk factor for several chronic diseases that generally start in young adulthood, such as cardiovascular disease, diabetes, and obesity (Arroyo et al., 2004; Carnethon, Kinder, Fair, Stafford, & Fortmann, 2003; Chapman, Perry, & Strine, 2005; Ferketich & Frid, 2001). Consequently, the physical health complications associated with depression further contribute to the overall health impact of this disorder, with even subclinical depressive symptoms negatively affecting physical health and associated with morbidity

L.L. Craft(✉)
Department of Preventive Medicine, Feinberg School of Medicine, Northwestern University,
680 N. Lake Shore Drive, Suite 1400, Chicago, IL, USA
e-mail: lynette-craft@northwestern.edu

A.L. Meyer and T.P. Gullotta (eds.), *Physical Activity Across the Lifespan*,
Issues in Children's and Families' Lives 12, DOI 10.1007/978-1-4614-3606-5_5,
© Springer Science+Business Media New York 2012

(Wells et al., 1989). As a result, depression signifies a threat to the psychological, physical, and social well-being of millions of young people. Thus, efficacious treatments for this disorder are needed so that psychological and physical health are not negatively affected during youth and adolescence, and to lessen the potential for poor health outcomes in adulthood.

Traditional Treatments and Their Limitations

Great strides have been made in the treatment of adult depression, but research on the treatment of depression in youth and adolescence lags behind. Recently, however, this has become a very active area of research with new information emerging about appropriate treatment options for young people with depression. Treatment for depression in youth and adolescence generally include various forms of psychotherapy and pharmacological therapies. Specifically, research has shown that cognitive behavioral therapy (CBT) and some of the newer antidepressant medications may be beneficial in treating childhood and adolescent depression (Lewinsohn & Clarke, 1999; Milin, Walker, & Chow, 2003; Reinecke, Ryan, & DuBois, 1998; Waslick, Schoenholz, & Pizarro, 2003) and that, for some, the combination of the two is the best approach (Vitiello, 2009). However, these therapies are not without criticism. For some, they are ineffective or are associated with unpleasant side effects such as nausea, loss of appetite, headaches, sleep disturbances, and sexual dysfunction (Mehler-Wex & Kolch, 2008). There also remains concern about the potential for an increased risk of suicidal ideation in young people taking some types of antidepressant medications (Hammad, Laughren, & Racoosin, 2006; Mehler-Wex & Kolch, 2008). As a result, researchers and clinicians continue to investigate alternative, efficacious treatment strategies that can be used alone or in combination with traditional therapies to treat depression.

Exercise represents one such alternative strategy, and while most of the research examining the use of exercise to alleviate symptoms of clinical depression has been conducted with adult samples, there remains reason to be optimistic about its potential use in the treatment of youth and adolescent depression. This chapter discusses physical activity as a depression intervention component, potential mechanisms underlying the exercise and depression relationship, and reviews evidence-based interventions incorporating exercise into the treatment of clinical depression. Most of this work has been done with adults, our discussion focuses on findings in adult samples and how they may generalize to younger individuals.

Physical Activity as a Significant Intervention Component

The relationship between exercise and depression has been studied for well over 100 years. Although methodological concerns (e.g., small samples, lack of random assignment, lack of control groups) initially dampened enthusiasm for this body of research, contemporary researchers have addressed these design issues, and presently there are multiple studies utilizing experimental designs or randomized clinical trial approaches that demonstrate the antidepressant effects of exercise (e.g., Blumenthal et al., 2007, 1999; Dimeo, Bauer, Varahran, Proest, & Halter, 2001; Dunn, Trivedi, Kampert, Clark, & Chambliss, 2005; McNeil, LeBlanc, & Joyner, 1991; Singh et al., 2005). As a result, clinicians and researchers are now interested in incorporating exercise into the treatment of depression and understanding the ways in which it effectively alleviates depressive symptoms.

In many ways, exercise accomplishes several of the therapeutic goals of hallmark treatments like psychotherapy and pharmacological interventions. There are several psychological, sociological, and neurochemical changes that occur with exercise that might play an important role. As mentioned previously, specific types of psychotherapy, such as CBT, are thought to work through treatment elements that promote active problem solving, monitoring thoughts, feelings, and behaviors, and using behavioral techniques and cognitive strategies to address clinical problems (Lewinsohn & Clarke, 1999; Waslick et al., 2003). Exercise may mirror many of these treatment components. For example, monitoring exercise behavior and setting and achieving exercise goals both enhances self-regulatory skills and improves self-efficacy. Exercise can be used as a mood regulator and thus contributes to one's confidence to manage one's symptoms of depression. If the depressed person is exercising under the guidance of an exercise professional, many aspects of the therapist–client relationship are utilized (empathy, support, both structured and unstructured interaction) and the activity offers an opportunity to receive positive feedback, boosting confidence, and to practice and improve social interaction and support skills. Even therapy components such as cognitive restructuring and communication skills can be taught and practiced within the context of exercise.

Pharmacological treatments for depression impart changes in brain neurochemistry to alter depressive symptoms. Many of the newer selective serotonin reuptake inhibitors (SSRIs) effectively work by altering the availability of important brain chemicals, such as serotonin, norepinephrine, and dopamine that are associated with depression. There is some evidence, particularly in studies of animals, that exercise alters these brain chemicals as well (Dishman, 1997a; 1997b; Jacobs, 1994; Meeusen, Piacentini, & DeMeirleir, 2001; Ransford, 1982). In addition, these drugs work to effectively aid the generation of new neurons in the brain, improving the transmission of brain messages and the use of brain chemicals (Elder, DeGasperi, & Gama Sosa, 2006). In studies of animals, exercise promotes the precursors of this neurogenesis (Carro, Nunez, Busiguina, & Torres-Aleman, 2000; Duman, Schlesinger, Russell, & Dunam, 2008).

Potential Mechanisms Underlying the Exercise and Depression Relationship

Gaining a better understanding of the ways in which exercise reduces symptoms of clinical depression is an important step in deciding whether exercise should be incorporated as an intervention in the treatment of depression. There have been many theories proposed about how exercise works to alleviate depressive symptoms including neurobiological, psychological, and social–cognitive approaches.

Physiological Mechanisms

The monoamine hypothesis appears to be one of the most promising of the proposed neurobiological mechanisms. This hypothesis proposes that exercise leads to an increase in the availability of brain neurotransmitters (e.g., serotonin, norepinephrine, and dopamine) that are diminished with depression. These neurotransmitters increase in plasma and urine following exercise, but whether exercise leads to an increase in neurotransmitters in the brain remains unknown (Ebert, Poste, & Goodwin, 1972; Tang, Stancer, Takahashi, Shephard, & Warsh, 1981). Animal studies suggest that exercise increases serotonin, dopamine, and norepinephrine in various brain regions such as parietal lobe, striatum, spinal cord, and frontal cortex but, to date, this relationship has not been studied in humans (Dishman, 1997b; Dunn, Reigle, Youngstedt, Armstrong, & Dishman, 1996; Meeusen et al., 2001). Mechanistically, this is consistent with the way in which antidepressant medications work to lessen depressive symptoms, but methodological difficulties have prevented this line of research from advancing. Invasive procedures are required to assess these brain chemicals and test this hypothesis and samples obtained from blood or other bodily fluids may not directly reflect the activity of these compounds in the brain (Dishman, 1997a; 1997b; Martinsen, 1987). Hopefully, newer neuroimaging techniques will aid researchers in examining whether exercise leads to the neurochemical changes in the brain predicted by this hypothesis.

The hippocampal neurogenesis hypothesis is a newer neurobiological theory proposed to explain how exercise alleviates depression. It is known that individuals with chronic, recurrent depression have significant atrophy of the hippocampal region of the brain (Russo-Neustadt, Ha, Ramirez, & Kesslak, 2001; Sheline et al., 1996). And traditional treatments for depression (both pharmacological and non-pharmacological) enhance hippocampal neurogensis. The time it takes for the promotion of neurogenesis by pharmacological interventions (e.g., SSRIs) mirrors the delay in clinical efficacy of antidepressant medications (Elder et al., 2006; Malberg, 2004) Thus, it is believed that one way in which traditional treatments work to reduce depression is by promoting neuron growth in the hippocampus, an area that is damaged by the chronic effects of depression. Researchers now believe that exercise also has this effect in the brain. Exercise is thought to increase neurogenesis through an increase in B-endorphins and growth factors such as brain derived neurotrophic factor (BDNF), vascular endothelial growth factor, and intracellular growth factor-1 that promote neurogenesis (Elder et al., 2006; Duman et al., 2008; Meeusen, et al., 2001). A study by Russo-Neustadt and colleagues compared the effects of exercise, antidepressant medication, and the combination on BDNF expression in an animal model. They found that both exercise and medication led to an increase in BDNF and that the combination of exercise and medication led to greater increases than either treatment alone (Russo-Neustadt et al., 2001).

Thus, while these results are promising, debate remains as to whether the observed increase in growth factors and neurogenesis associated with exercise actually results in functioning neurons. As this work continues, we again look to the newer, less invasive, imaging techniques to shed light on the utility of this hypothesis.

Psychological Mechanisms

The enhancement of self-efficacy through exercise involvement may be one psychological mechanism by which exercise exerts its antidepressant effects. Self-efficacy refers to the belief that one possesses the necessary skills to complete a task as well as the confidence that the task can actually be completed with the desired outcome obtained. Depressed individuals often feel inefficacious to bring out positive desired outcomes in their lives and have low efficacy to cope with the symptoms of their depression (Bandura, 1997). This can lead to negative self-evaluation, negative ruminations, and faulty styles of thinking. It has been suggested that exercise may enhance self-efficacy based on its ability to provide the individual with a meaningful mastery experience. Research examining the association between physical activity and self-efficacy in the general population has focused predominantly on the enhancement of physical self-efficacy and efficacy to regulate exercise behaviors. The relationship between exercise and self-efficacy in the clinically depressed has received far less attention. The findings of the few studies that have examined this relationship have been equivocal as to whether exercise leads to an enhancement of generalized feelings of efficacy (Brown, Welsh, Labbe, Vitulli, & Kulkarni, 1992; Martinsen, Hoffart, & Solberg, 1989). We have examined the relationship between involvement in an exercise program and enhanced feelings of coping self-efficacy (i.e., confidence to copy with one's symptoms of depression, rather than general feelings of efficacy) in depressed women. We found that exercise was associated with enhanced feelings of coping self-efficacy, which, in turn, were inversely related to and the best predictor of symptoms of depression (Craft, 2005).

The use of exercise to regulate affect may play a key role in how exercise alleviates depressive symptoms. As described in the upcoming chapter on depression prevention, acute or individual bouts of exercise can improve negative mood and may act to provide temporary symptom relief. Bartholomew, Morrison and Ciccolo (2005) found that a single bout of moderate-intensity exercise significantly improved negative aspects of mood and elevated feelings of general well-being and vigor in adults diagnosed with MDD. Mood was assessed for 60 min following the exercise bout and the mood benefits endured for the entire 60 min period. Thus, exercise may lessen depressive symptoms by allowing patients a means to more immediately regulate their mood and to experience brief periods of relief from their depression. This may be particularly important as those with depression often choose less healthy mood management strategies such alcohol, tobacco, and drugs (Bartholomew et al., 2005).

Behavioral activation may also explain the antidepressant effects of exercise. Depressed individuals often engage in maladaptive coping strategies such as inactivity and withdrawal. Behavioral activation is a therapy component in which individuals are asked to begin replacing their inactive and passive activities with more active, enjoyable, and pleasurable activities (Hopki, Lejuez, Ruggiero, & Eifert, 2003). This theory suggests that exercise is an action that is inconsistent with the natural tendencies associated with depression and thus, it is thought that exercise represents an activity that has the potential to be rewarding and enjoyable, providing a sense of accomplishment. Consequently, depressive symptoms may be alleviated as the individual begins to replace passive activities with exercise and other more enjoyable activities. There is no research to date that has explicitly tested this hypothesis, but it is consistent with what is known about the benefits of including behavioral activation in the treatment of depression.

More research is needed to determine which, if any, of the mechanisms described in this chapter underlie the exercise effect. It is highly likely that a combination of biological, psychological, and sociological factors influence the relationship between exercise and depression. This is consistent with current treatments for depression in which the effects of pharmacotherapy and psychotherapy on depression are often additive and address biological, psychological, and sociological aspects of the patient. However, until we gain a better understanding of how exercise alleviates the symptoms of depression, we will likely continue to encounter difficulty in achieving a permanent place for exercise in mainstream depression treatment.

Review of Evidence Based Interventions Incorporating Physical Activity

Our best understanding of the use of exercise to alleviate depressive symptoms comes from randomized clinical trials (RCT). While it is not possible to exhaustively review the RCT literature within the context of this chapter, several studies are highlighted to offer the reader a basic understanding of the types of experiments supporting evidence-based interventions. As mentioned previously, nearly all of this work has been conducted in adults with depression. One published RCT was located that examined the effect of an exercise program on depressive symptoms among adolescents with a clinical diagnosis and is discussed first. Additional examples of experimental studies (in adults) examining the efficacy of exercise to alleviate the symptoms of clinical depression follow.

Exercise as Treatment for Adolescent Depression

In the early 1990s, Brown and colleagues examined the effect of a 9-week aerobic exercise program as an adjunct to standard treatment in a sample of institutionalized adolescents (Brown et al., 1992). Participants in that study were volunteers who were residing at a private psychiatric facility and were diagnosed with dysthymia and conduct disorder. Twenty-seven adolescents started the study, but only 11 participants completed the entire 9-week program. In addition to their usual care, participants were randomly assigned to either a 3×/week running/aerobic exercise program or control condition. At study entry, 4½ weeks, and completion of the 9-week program, the participants completed a self-report of depressive symptoms and self-efficacy. Results indicated that depression was reduced after 4½ weeks, with the effect strongest among girls. However, by 9 weeks, all participants in the exercise program had decreased depression, and the difference was not significantly different between boys and girls. Similarly, those in the exercise program reported increases in feelings of self-efficacy across the 9-week program, while those in the control condition reported decreases in self-efficacy. While this study is limited by a very small sample size, participants with mixed diagnoses, and a large number of dropouts (due to discharge from the facility), it offers initial support for the use of exercise in an adolescent population.

Exercise Compared to Medication

In adults, our strongest support for the use of exercise to treat depression comes from studies that have compared exercise to antidepressant medication. One example of a seminal RCT comparing exercise to medication was conducted by Blumenthal et al. (1999). That study compared the efficacy of supervised aerobic exercise, medication (Zoloft), and the combination of exercise and medication in a sample of 156 moderately depressed older men and women. Results indicated that while medication worked more quickly to reduce symptoms of depression, by the end of the 16 week intervention, all groups had experienced significant reductions in depression and that remission rates in the groups did not differ significantly.

A follow-up to that study found that 10 months after study completion, those in the exercise group were significantly less likely to have experienced a depression relapse than those in the medication group (Babyak et al., 2000). A second RCT by that group compared supervised aerobic exercise, home-based aerobic exercise, medication (Zoloft), and a placebo pill in the treatment of 202 depressed middle-aged older adults (Blumenthal et al., 2007). Results replicated and extended previous findings in that those in both exercise and medication groups achieved significantly higher rates of remission than those in the control group, results for the exercise group were comparable to and not significantly different from medication, and supervised and home-based exercise were similarly effective in reducing depression.

Exercise as an Adjunct to Medication

Exercise appears to benefit older adults who are already taking antidepressant medications but remain depressed. Mather et al. (2002) randomized 86 men and women, aged 53 years and older, to either a 10-week exercise intervention or health education control group. Those in the exercise intervention attended a 45-min exercise class that consisted of aerobic endurance, muscular strength and stretching activities. Exercise participants attended the class 2×/week. All participants continued to take their antidepressant medication throughout the trial. Depression was assessed at study entry, 10 weeks, and 34 weeks. At 10 weeks, a significantly larger percentage (55 %) of those in the exercise group than those in the health education group (33 %) had achieved a treatment response (defined as ≥30 % reduction in their depression score from baseline). By 34 weeks, both groups reported reductions in depression score. The findings of this study suggest that, in adults, exercise might provide some additional antidepressant benefit for individuals who have had an incomplete response to antidepressant medication.

Exercise and a Dose–Response Relationship

Researchers have been curious as to whether a dose–response relationship exists between exercise and depression. That is, do the antidepressant benefits increase with increasing levels or intensity of physical activity? Dunn et al. (2005) randomly assigned 80 adults, aged 20–45 years, with mild-to-moderate depression to one of five conditions: a group that did a low dose of exercise 3 days/week, a group that did the public health recommended dose of exercise 3 days/week, a group that did a low dose of exercise 5 days/week, a group that did the public health recommended dose 5 days/week, or an exercise placebo control group (3 days/week of flexibility training). Those in exercise groups completed aerobic exercise on a treadmill or stationary bicycle in a supervised laboratory for 12 weeks. Depression was assessed weekly across the study and the primary outcome of interest was change in depression score from baseline to 12 weeks. Results indicated that the public health dose was significantly more effective in reducing depression than either the low dose or the control condition. On average, the depression scores of those in the public health dosage groups were reduced by approximately 47 %, as compared to only 30 % reduction in the low dose group, and 29 % reduction in the control group. Further, 42 % of those in the public health dose groups experienced a 50 % or greater reduction in their symptoms. Results did not differ by number of exercise bouts per week (3 vs. 5), indicating that the largest antidepressant effects were seen with the public health dose, regardless of whether the exercise was completed on 3 or 5 days/week.

Previous research has demonstrated similar antidepressant effects for nonaerobic types of activities. Singh et al. (2005) attempted to determine if a dose–response relationship exists between resistance training and alleviation of depressive symptoms. That study compared high-intensity weight training, low-intensity weight training, and general practitioner care in 60 community dwelling older adults meeting criteria for clinical depression. Results of the 8-week study indicate that high-intensity resistance training is superior to low-intensity resistance training and general practitioner care in alleviating depressive symptoms, supporting the possibility of a dose–response relationship.

Supervised Exercise as Compared to Home-Based Exercise

Researchers have investigated whether exercise needs to be done while supervised, in a lab or hospital based setting, in order to be effective. Blumenthal et al. (2007) compared lab-based to home-based activity in older adults with depression. The results of that study demonstrated that home-based and lab-based activity were equally effective in alleviating symptoms of depression. A study by Craft, Freund, Culpepper and Perna (2007) compared home-based to lab-based exercise in a predominantly minority sample of adult women with depression. Thirty-two women, with moderate symptoms of depression, were randomly assigned to either a lab- or home-based exercise intervention with assessments at baseline and 3-months. In both intervention groups, participants completed three, moderate-intensity exercise sessions/week, approximately 30–45 min per session. For the first month of the study, those assigned to the lab-based intervention completed two supervised aerobic exercise sessions each week at the lab and were asked to complete one additional exercise session/week at home. The women were then transitioned to home-based activity and asked to continue their exercise program at home for the remaining 8 weeks of the study. Those assigned to the home-based intervention completed their exercise sessions at home for the entire 12-weeks of the study. Results indicated that both exercise programs were associated with significant reductions in depressive symptoms and increased physical activity participation, suggesting that even a home-based program can benefit women with depressive symptoms. Findings such as these are important as long-term adherence to an exercise program (and, in this case, depression treatment) is likely to be enhanced among individuals who are able to exercise at home or in their communities, as opposed to completing exercise at a hospital or research facility.

Aerobic Compared to Nonaerobic Exercise

Few studies have directly compared aerobic forms of exercise (e.g., jogging, biking, walking) to nonaerobic forms of exercise (e.g., strength training). And while the majority of studies have utilized aerobic forms of activity, studies that have examined the antidepressant effects of exercise following nonaerobic exercise programs also demonstrate antidepressant effects. For example, one trial randomized a group of community dwelling older adults with clinical depression to either a resistance training program or a health education control group (Singh, Clements, & Singh, 2001). The progressive resistance training program was 20 weeks in length. Those in the resistance training group experienced significantly larger reductions in depression than those in the control group and, at follow-up (26 months later), the antidepressant effect remained for those in the resistance training group and approximately 30 % were still maintaining a regular program of resistance training. Likewise, as described previously, the dose–response study examining the effects of two different strength training programs (compared to a standard care control) found support for the antidepressant effects of nonaerobic activity (Singh et al., 2005). Therefore, each of these studies provides support for the use of nonaerobic forms of exercise to alleviate depressive symptoms. This may be particularly important as some individuals will find strength training programs more enjoyable and easier to initiate and maintain than aerobic exercise programs.

Meta-Analytic Studies

Meta-analysis provides a statistical method for quantifying the results of many individual studies. One advantage to this method of summarizing studies is that it allows the researcher to statistically compare subgroups or conditions across studies. For example, a researcher could examine the effects of an exercise program on depressive symptoms for men as compared to women, even if all of the individual studies did not make this direct comparison. This technique is often used to statistically summarize the findings from areas of research where many studies have been done. Within the exercise and depression literature, several meta-analyses have been conducted. The findings from five frequently cited meta-analyses are discussed below (Craft & Landers, 1998; Lawlor & Hopker, 2001; North, McCullagh, & Tran, 1990; Rethorst, Wipfli, & Landers, 2009; Strathopoulou et al., 2006). As each of these meta-analyses utilized slightly different criteria for including primary research articles, varying numbers of effect sizes were calculated which resulted in different overall effect size estimates. Further, only the Craft and Landers (1998) and Rethorst et al. (2009) meta-analyses examined variables that potentially moderate the effect of exercise on depression.

Overall results from these five meta-analyses indicate that exercise interventions have a large impact on depression, with between groups effect sizes (ES), ranging from −0.72 to −1.4. That is, those in exercise groups were approximate 3/4 to 1½ of a standard deviation less depressed following an exercise intervention as compared to control groups who did not exercise. Converting these ES values to a clinical indicator of treatment success, one finds that exercise results in an approximately 67–79 % reduction in depressive symptoms (Rosenthal, 1984). Clinically significant reductions in depression are generally defined as a 50 % or greater decline in symptoms. Therefore, even according to a more clinically relevant and stringent definition of treatment success, exercise is an effective antidepressant.

Further, when examining the types of person and exercise characteristics that moderate the effect of exercise on depression, results are again favorable among a variety of patient subgroups and exercise program types (Craft & Landers, 1998; Rethorst et al., 2009). That is, patients with both moderate and more severe depression appear to benefit similarly and, among adults, exercise is equally effective for men and women across a wide range of ages. When comparing exercise to more traditional treatments, we find that exercise effects are comparable to and not significantly different from psychotherapy and pharmacological treatment (Craft & Landers, 1998; Rethorst et al., 2009).

Exercise program characteristics have also been examined and it appears that factors such as exercise duration, intensity, frequency, and mode (i.e., aerobic or nonaerobic) do not moderate the effects of exercise on depression. Similarly, it is not necessary for the individual to improve his/her cardiovascular fitness in order to achieve reductions in depression. However, the length of the exercise program is a significant moderator, with programs 9–10 weeks or longer associated with larger reductions in depression (Craft & Landers, 1998; Rethorst et al., 2009). Conversely, emerging experimental research demonstrates that a dose–response relationship may exist with more exercise associated with larger reductions in depression (Dunn et al., 2005; Singh et al., 2005). However, few studies to date have directly examined this and more research is needed. The meta-analysis conducted by Rethorst examined dose–response as a potential moderator of the exercise effect and failed to find support for a dose–response relationship (Rethorst et al., 2009). Thus, while it is clear that an exercise bout need not be lengthy or intense to promote positive changes in depressive symptoms, it may be the case that individuals who can exercise at public health recommended doses will experience even larger benefits.

It is important to note that dropout from exercise trials is roughly 14–19 %. This is similar to dropout from pharmacological trials (Rethorst et al., 2009; Strathopoulou et al., 2006), suggesting that exercise may be a viable treatment adjunct for many patients.

Finally, a meta-analysis has recently been conducted to examine the effect of exercise in the prevention and treatment of anxiety and depression among children and young people (Larun et al., 2006). The majority of the studies included in that meta-analysis were prevention studies and the treatment studies that were included were predominantly conducted among children and adolescents in the general population, rather than those actually having a diagnosis of depression. The authors conclude that there is some evidence to support a small effect of exercise on anxiety and depression in the general population of youth but that there is insufficient research in clinical populations to ascertain whether exercise has a favorable effect.

Summary of Research Findings

Research conducted among adult samples provides strong support for the antidepressant effects of exercise. Exercise appears to be effective across a variety of patient subgroups, is as effective as medication and psychotherapy for some, and basic exercise program characteristics such as the type of activity, the intensity of the program, and the duration of the exercise bout do not seem to be important in promoting the effect. Our understanding of how exercise works to lesson depressive symptoms is lacking, yet proposed mechanisms are theoretically consistent with the ways in which medication and psychotherapy work to alleviate symptoms. While these findings are hopeful for adults, there is a paucity of research utilizing youth or adolescent samples. Intuitively, one could speculate that exercise promotes similar psycho-social and neurobiological changes in young persons. However, youth and adolescence are times of considerable physical and psychosocial growth. As such, it is not clear if exercise is associated with the same type or magnitude of antidepressant effect that is seen in adults. Consequently, empirical investigation is warranted.

Best Practice

When contemplating the best exercise prescription to combat depressive symptoms, clinicians and researchers are challenged by a lack of studies directly comparing different types of exercise programs. Consequently, our recommendations come from the meta-analytic data and those exercise characteristics that produced the largest effect sizes. In general, 30 min of moderate-intensity activity, 3–5×/week should be an adequate exercise dose. The type of activity is unimportant, so we recommend picking an activity that is perceived as enjoyable. It is important to keep in mind that antidepressant benefits are garnered even if the exercise is brief, of light-intensity, and a few times per week. As a result, for those initiating an exercise program, we recommend starting slowly. While the research remains equivocal, there is some support for a dose–response relationship. Therefore, for those who can progress to the public health recommended dose of physical activity (30 min, moderate-intensity, 5–7×/week) even larger benefits may be obtained.

It is likely that the symptoms of depression may impart additional challenges to beginning an exercise program. That is, a lack of motivation, feelings of lethargy, inability to find pleasure in activities, and psychomotor retardation may all make the initiation of an exercise program more challenging for depressed individuals. Research examining barriers to and correlates of physical activity in adult women with self-reported depressive symptoms (Craft, Perna, Freund, & Culpepper, 2008) found that the most frequently reported barriers to exercise were feeling too tired, a lack of time, feeling self-conscious about one's looks when exercising, and not having an exercise partner. Seventy percent of the women indicated that they had three or more barriers that "sometimes," "often," or "very often" interfered with their attempts to exercise. After controlling for factors known to be associated with both depression and leisure-time activity (age, severity of depressive symptoms, and family income), the number of barriers to exercise ($\beta=-0.31$, $p=0.05$), education level ($\beta=0.43$, $p=0.01$), and length of current depressive episode ($\beta=-0.32$, $p=0.07$) were the best determinants of time spent in exercise, accounting for 28.5 % of the variance. The women in that study also reported low levels of self-efficacy for exercise and low friend and family social support for exercise. Thus, it may be particularly important to help individuals with depression recognize and address perceived barriers to exercise, as well as to identify appropriate social support for their exercise attempts.

Several practical approaches may facilitate the adoption of exercise programs in depressed youth and adolescents. Specifically, this may include exercising with the young person or making exercise a family activity. Planning family activities around exercise sessions or incorporating physical activities into the family's daily routine can also encourage exercise initiation. Keeping an exercise log, setting achievable goals, and self-monitoring progress may help to enhance feelings of self-efficacy. It may also be important to provide positive feedback when exercise has been completed. Keeping track of mood both before and after an exercise bout can provide additional reinforcement that exercise is "working."

It is important to start an exercise program slowly, with an activity that is perceived as enjoyable. It is generally recommended that the young person first work on the frequency of the activity, making exercise (even short, light bouts) a habit. Once exercise is occurring on a regular basis, next focus on gradually increasing the duration of each exercise bout (still not being too concerned about intensity). Exercise intensity should be the final exercise variable that is adjusted, with individuals working toward moderate intensity. It is important to keep in mind that antidepressant benefits can be derived from short bouts of light-to-moderate intensity. Thus, doing something on most days is far better than abandoning an exercise bout because one does not feel like working out "long" or "hard."

Future Directions

While there is overwhelming support for the use of exercise in the treatment of clinical depression in adults, much remains unknown about its utility among young people. Almost no RCT research exists examining the effects of exercise on clinical depression in children and adolescents. As researchers and clinicians continue to try and determine best treatment approaches for depression in the young, exercise needs to be investigated as a possible treatment component. Depression may differ across the lifespan or among individuals from differing racial/ethnic backgrounds. Consequently, research is needed to determine if exercise programs are effective in alleviating symptoms of depression in various age and racial/ethnic groups, the types of programs that are most effective, and the types of exercise programs that lead to long-term adherence.

Identifying and understanding the mechanisms underlying the exercise–depression relationship remains another principal challenge for researchers in this field. Until we better understand how exercise works, and the mechanisms by which it might augment existing therapies, it will be difficult to gain acceptance of exercise into mainstream treatments for depression. More work is also needed to examine a potential dose–response relationship. Research suggests that even minimal amounts of exercise have antidepressant effects, yet it is imperative that we understand what dose of exercise leads to optimal depression treatment. It also remains unclear how long-lasting the effects of exercise are on depressive symptoms, and research in this area is also warranted. Finally, it is now recognized that depression has many serious physical health consequences. Regular exercise is well known to invoke many positive physical health benefits and reduce the risk of developing many chronic diseases. More research is needed to determine whether treating depression with exercise can also concurrently impart positive physical health benefits and reduce chronic disease risk in individuals with depression.

References

Arroyo, C., Hu, F. B., Ryan, L. M., Kawachi, I., Colditz, G. A., Speizer, F. E., et al. (2004). Depressive symptoms and risk of type 2 diabetes in women. *Diabetes Care, 27,* 129–133.

Babyak, M., Blumenthal, J. A., Herman, S., Khatri, P., Doraiswamy, M., Moore, K., et al. (2000). Exercise treatment for major depression: maintenance of therapeutic benefit at 10 months. *Psychosomatic Medicine, 62,* 633–638.

Bandura, A. (1997). *Self-efficacy: the exercise of control.* New York, NY: WH Freeman.

Bartholomew, J. B., Morrison, D., & Ciccolo, J. T. (2005). Effects of acute exercise on mood and well-being in patients with major depressive disorder. *Medicine and Science in Sports and Exercise, 37,* 2032–2037.

Blumenthal, J. A., Babyak, M. A., Doraiswamy, P. M., Watkins, L., Hoffman, B. M., Barbour, K. A., et al. (2007). Exercise and pharmacotherapy in the treatment of major depressive disorder. *Psychosomatic Medicine, 69,* 587–596.

Blumenthal, J. A., Babyak, M. A., Moore, K. A., Craighead, W. E., Herman, S., Khatri, P., et al. (1999). Effects of exercise training on older patients with major depression. *Archives of Internal Medicine, 159,* 2349–2356.

Brown, S. W., Welsh, M. C., Labbe, E. E., Vitulli, W. F., & Kulkarni, P. (1992). Aerobic exercise in the treatment of adolescents. *Perceptual and Motor Skills, 74,* 555–560.

Bylund, D. B., & Reed, A. L. (2007). Childhood and adolescent depression: why do children and adults respond differently to antidepressant drugs? *Neurochemistry International, 51,* 246–253.

Carnethon, M. R., Kinder, L. S., Fair, J. M., Stafford, R. S., & Fortmann, S. P. (2003). Symptoms of depression as a risk factor for incident diabetes: findings from the National Health and Nutrition Examination Epidemiologic Follow-up Study, 1971–1992. *American Journal of Epidemiology, 158,* 416–423.

Carro, E., Nunez, A., Busiguina, S., & Torres-Aleman, I. (2000). Circulating insulin-like growth factor I mediates effects of exercise on the brain. *Journal of Neuroscience, 20,* 2926–2933.

Chapman, D.P., Perry, G.S., & Strine, T.W. (2005). The vital link between chronic disease and depressive disorders. *Preventing Chronic Disease* [serial online] 2005 January, volume 2. Retrieved September 15, 2009 from http://www.cdc.gov/pcd/issues/2005/jan04_0066.html.

Chuang, H. T., Mansell, C., & Patten, S. B. (2008). Lifestyle characteristics of psychiatric outpatients. *Canadian Journal of Psychiatry, 53,* 260–266.

Craft, L. L. (2005). Exercise and clinical depression: examining two psychological mechanisms. *Psychology of Sport and Exercise, 6,* 151–171.

Craft, L. L., Freund, K. M., Culpepper, L., & Perna, F. M. (2007). Intervention study of exercise for depressive symptoms in women. *Journal of Women's Health, 16,* 1499–1509.

Craft, L. L., & Landers, D. M. (1998). The effect of exercise on clinical depression and depression resulting from mental illness: a meta-analysis. *Journal of Sport and Exercise Psychology, 20,* 339–357.

Craft, L. L., Perna, F. M., Freund, K. M., & Culpepper, L. (2008). Psychosocial correlates of physical activity in women with self-reported depressive symptoms. *Journal of Physical Activity and Health, 5,* 469–480.

Dimeo, F., Bauer, M., Varahran, I., Proest, G., & Halter, U. (2001). Benefits from aerobic exercise in patients with major depression: a pilot study. *British Journal of Sports Medicine, 35,* 114–117.

Dishman, R. K. (1997a). The norepinephrine hypothesis. In W. P. Morgan (Ed.), *Physical activity and mental health* (pp. 199–212). Washington, DC: Taylor & Francis.

Dishman, R. K. (1997b). Brain monoamines, exercise, and behavioral stress: animal models. *Medicine and Science in Sports and Exercise, 29,* 63–74.

Duman, D. H., Schlesinger, L., Russell, D. S., & Dunam, R. S. (2008). Voluntary exercise produces antidepressant and anxiolytic behavioral effects in mice. *Brain Research, 1199,* 148–158.

Dunn, A. L., Reigle, T. G., Youngstedt, S. D., Armstrong, R. B., & Dishman, R. K. (1996). Brain norepinephrine and metabolites after treadmill training and whell running in rats. *Medicine and Science in Sports and Exercise, 28,* 204–209.

Dunn, A. L., Trivedi, M. H., Kampert, J. B., Clark, C. G., & Chambliss, H. O. (2005). Exercise treatment for depression: efficacy and dose response. *American Journal of Preventive Medicine, 28,* 1–8.

Ebert, M. H., Poste, R. M., & Goodwin, F. K. (1972). Effect of physical activity on urinary MHPG excretion in depressed patients. *Lancet, 2,* 766.

Elder, G. A., DeGasperi, R., & Gama Sosa, M. A. (2006). Research update: neurogenesis in adult brain and neuropsychiatric disorders. *Mount Sinai Journal of Medicine, 7,* 931–940.

Ferketich, A. K., & Frid, D. J. (2001). Depression and coronary heart disease: a review of the literature. *Clinical Geriatrics, 9,* 1–8.

Hammad, T. A., Laughren, T., & Racoosin, J. (2006). Suicidality in pediatric patients treated with antidepressant drugs. *Archives of General Psychiatry, 63,* 332–339.

Hopki, D. R., Lejuez, C. W., Ruggiero, K. J., & Eifert, G. H. (2003). Contemporary behavioral activation treatments for depression: procedures, principles, and progress. *Clinical Psychology Review, 23,* 699–717.

Jacobs, B. L. (1994). Serotonin, motor activity and depression-related disorders. *American Scientist, 82,* 456–463.

Klomek, A. B., & Stanley, B. (2007). Psychosocial treatment of depression and suicidality in adolescents. *CNS Spectrum, 12,* 135–144.

Larun, L., Nordheim, L. V., Ekeland, E., Hagen, K. B., & Heian, F. (2006). Exercise in prevention and treatment of anxiety and depression among children and young people. *Cochrane Database Systematic Reviews, 3,* CD004691, 1–52. Retrieved September 8, 2009 from http://mrw.interscience.wiley.com/cochrane/clsysrev/articles/CD004691/pdf_fs.html.

Lawlor, D. A., & Hopker, S. W. (2001). The effectiveness of exercise as an intervention in the management of depression: systematic review and meta-regression of randomized controlled trials. *British Medical Journal, 322,* 763–767.

Lewinsohn, P. M., & Clarke, G. N. (1999). Psychosocial treatments for adolescent depression. *Clinical Psychology Review, 19,* 329–342.

Malberg, J. E. (2004). Implications of adult hippocampal neurogenesis in antidepressant action. *Journal of Psychiatry and Neuroscience, 29,* 196–205.

Martinsen, E. W. (1987). The role of aerobic exercise in the treatment of depression. *Stress Medicine, 3,* 93–100.

Martinsen, E. W., Hoffart, A., & Solberg, O. (1989). Comparing aerobic and nonaerobic forms of exercise in the treatment of clinical depression: a randomized trial. *Comprehensive Psychiatry, 30,* 324–331.

Mather, A. S., Rodriguez, C., Guthrie, M. F., McHarg, A. M., Reid, I. C., & McMurdo, M. E. T. (2002). Effects of exercise on depressive symptoms in older adults with poorly responsive depressive disorder: randomized controlled trial. *British Journal of Psychiatry, 180,* 411–415.

McNeil, J. K., LeBlanc, E. M., & Joyner, M. (1991). The effect of exercise on depressive symptoms in the moderately depressed elderly. *Psychology of Aging, 6,* 487–488.

Meeusen, R., Piacentini, M. F., & DeMeirleir, K. (2001). Brain microdialysis in exercise research. *Sports Medicine, 31,* 965–983.

Mehler-Wex, C., & Kolch, M. (2008). Depression in children and adolescents. *Deutsches Aerzteblatt International, 105*, 149–155.

Milin, R., Walker, S., & Chow, J. (2003). Major depressive disorder in adolescence: a brief review of the recent treatment literature. *Canadian Journal of Psychiatry, 48*, 600–606.

North, T. C., McCullagh, P., & Tran, Z. V. (1990). Effects of exercise on depression. *Exercise and Sport Science Reviews, 18*, 379–415.

Ransford, C. P. (1982). A role for amines in the antidepressant effect of exercise: a review. *Medicine and Science in Sports and Exercise, 14*, 1–10.

Reinecke, M. A., Ryan, N. E., & DuBois, D. L. (1998). Cognitive-behavioral therapy of depression and depressive symptoms during adolescence: a review and meta-analysis. *Journal of the American Academy of Child and Adolescent Psychiatry, 37*, 26–34.

Rethorst, C. D., Wipfli, B. M., & Landers, D. M. (2009). The antidepressive effects of exercise: a meta-analysis of randomized trials. *Sports Medicine, 39*, 491–511.

Rosenthal, R. (1984). The evaluation of meta-analytic procedures and meta-analytic results, In: R. Rosenthal (Ed.) *Meta-analytic procedures for social research* (p. 132). Newbury Park, CA: Sage.

Russo-Neustadt, A., Ha, T., Ramirez, R., & Kesslak, J. P. (2001). Physical activity-antidepressant treatment combination: impact on brain-derived neurotrophic factor and behavior in an animal model. *Behavioural Brain Research, 120*, 87–95.

Sheline, Y. I., Wang, P. W., Gado, M. H., Csernannsky, J. G., & Vannier, M. W. (1996). Hippocampal atrophy in recurrent major depression. *Proceedings of the National Academy of Science of the Unites States of America, 93*, 3908–3913.

Singh, N. A., Clements, K. M., & Singh, M. A. F. (2001). The efficacy of exercise as a long-term antidepressant in elderly subjects: a randomized controlled trial. *Journal of Gerontology, 56A*, M497–504.

Singh, N. A., Stavrinos, T. M., Scarbek, Y., Galambos, G., Liber, C., & Fiatarone Singh, M. A. (2005). A randomized controlled trial of high versus low intensity weight training versus general practitioner care for clinical depression in older adults. *Journal of Gerontology, 6*, 768–776.

Strathopoulou, G., Powers, M. B., Berry, A. C., Smits, A. J., & Otto, M. W. (2006). Exercise interventions for mental health: a quantitative and qualitative review. *Clinical Psychology Science and Practice, 13*, 179–193.

Tang, S. W., Stancer, H. C., Takahashi, S., Shephard, R. J., & Warsh, J. J. (1981). Controlled exercise elevates plasma but not urinary MHPG and VMA. *Psychiatry Research, 4*, 13–20.

Vitiello, B. (2009). Combined cognitive-behavioural therapy and pharmacotherapy for adolescent depression: does it improve outcomes compared with monotherapy? *CNS Drugs, 23*, 271–280.

Waslick, B., Schoenholz, D., & Pizarro, R. (2003). Diagnosis and treatment of chronic depression in children and adolescents. *Journal of Psychiatric Practice, 9*, 354–366.

Wells, K. B., Stewart, A., Hays, R. D., Burnam, M. A., Rogers, W., Daniels, M., et al. (1989). The functioning and well-being of depressed patients. Results from the medical outcomes study. *Journal of the American Medical Association, 262*, 914–919.

Chapter 6
Physical Activity for the Prevention of Depression

Bethany M. Kwan, Kyle J. Davis, and Andrea L. Dunn

Mental, emotional, and behavior disorders, including depression, often begin in childhood and are the result of multiple etiologies (National Research Council and Institute of Medicine, 2009). Depression affects millions of people worldwide, and the identification and delivery of effective treatments is an ongoing challenge. An estimated 1 % of adults, or as many as 1.8 million new cases, develop major depressive disorder in the USA every year (Murphy et al., 2002). The lifetime prevalence of major depression is 16.2 %, with rates of treatment around 35.4 % during the onset of the disorder and, on average, a nearly 4 year delay for seeking treatment. It is estimated that less than one in four receive successful treatment, meaning remission of symptoms. Among adolescents, the lifetime prevalence of depressive illness is about 12 %, and less than half of teens with depression receive treatment (Office of Applied Studies, 2005). Given the total global impact of both major depression and subthreshold symptoms of depression, a substantial but largely unquantified problem, and the perpetual difficulties with and considerable costs of achieving full remission, an investment of resources into prevention efforts is warranted (National Research Council and Institute of Medicine, 2009).

Data suggest there is a 2–4 year window between the onset of the first symptom of depression and diagnosed illness during which prevention programs might be targeted (National Research Council and Institute of Medicine, 2009). Depression

B.M. Kwan (✉)
Colorado Health Outcomes Program,
13199 E. Montview Blvd, Mail Stop F443,
Aurora, CO 80045, USA
e-mail: bethany.kwan@ucdenver.edu

K.J. Davis
Department of Psychology, University of Colorado, 345 UCB,
Boulder, CO 80309, USA

A.L. Dunn
Klein Buendel, Inc., 1667 Cole Boulevard, Suite 225, Golden, CO 80401, USA

A.L. Meyer and T.P. Gullotta (eds.), *Physical Activity Across the Lifespan*,
Issues in Children's and Families' Lives 12, DOI 10.1007/978-1-4614-3606-5_6,
© Springer Science+Business Media New York 2012

is most likely to develop around vulnerable periods in life, such as adolescence, peripartum, and old age (American Psychiatric Association, 1994), and when stressful life events occur, such as major illness, divorce, loss of a loved one, or job loss (National Research Council and Institute of Medicine, 2009). The average age of onset of a first depressive episode is 14, with the first symptoms appearing several years earlier around the age of 11 (National Research Council and Institute of Medicine, 2009). There are a number of possible reasons for the emergence of depression around this time, such as changes in hormones and hormone receptors and changes in brain structure and function that affect socioemotional responding, motivation, and reward systems (Paus, Keshavan, & Giedd, 2008). Prevention of the first episode of depression can have lifelong implications, particularly when adequate treatment for an incident case would not subsequently be available (Akerblad, Bengtsson, von Knorring, & Ekselius, 2006; Kennard, Emslie, Mayes, & Hughes, 2006). Thus, depression prevention efforts would perhaps be best targeted at adolescents and young people (those between the ages of 10 and 24), to help foster healthy habits and skills to combat depression that can be carried into adulthood. As discussed in this chapter, promising evidence exists to support physical activity (including leisure-time, occupational and transportation physical activity, as well as more structured aerobic exercise and resistance training) as an effective method of prevention for depression throughout the lifespan.

It is possible that physical activity could play a role in the prevention of depression through the use of each of the study typologies recommended by the Institute of Medicine; these include universal, selective and preventive interventions (National Research Council and Institute of Medicine, 2009). These typologies clearly differentiate treatment from prevention, such that the goal of prevention is to reduce the development of diagnosed depression disorders and subthreshold symptoms. The major defining difference between prevention and treatment is the population included in the study. For instance, universal preventive interventions are aimed at the general public and not at those diagnosed with a depressive disorder. Physical activity interventions targeted to the general public may provide skills to better cope with stress and other psychological or biological risks associated with depression. Selective preventive interventions are aimed at individuals whose risk of developing depression is higher than the general public, e.g., children of divorce or children whose parents might suffer from depression. In this case, physical activity interventions might be included as part of a curriculum that teaches age-appropriate resilience skills. Finally, indicated preventive interventions are aimed at individuals who are at high risk for developing depressive disorders such as those who might have subclinical symptoms of depression but who do not meet the criteria for a major depressive episode.

In this chapter, we present the extant evidence (cross-sectional, prospective, and experimental) regarding the relationship between physical activity and incidence of depression, and discuss a number of hypothesized (although generally untested) mechanisms by which the relationship between exercise and depression might exist. We focus on the period of childhood and adolescence, due to the emergence of depression, developmental processes that may be particularly amenable to physical activity intervention, and the establishment of what could be lifelong physical activity habits during this time.

Standard Depression Prevention Interventions and Their Limitations

The prevention of depression is not a new goal. A meta-analysis of programs targeting children, adolescents, adults and older people found that depression prevention programs in general (e.g., using behavioral therapy) can reduce depressive symptoms by 11 % (Jane-Llopis, Hosman, Jenkins, & Anderson, 2003). This effect size did not appear to vary between age groups. Predictors of efficacy in these programs included quality of the research design, length of the program and duration of sessions, the number of components in the intervention (e.g., competence techniques), and whether or not the program was delivered by a healthcare professional rather than lay personnel. Another meta-analysis of 19 interventions for the prevention of depression was more recently conducted (Cuijpers, van Straten, Smit, Mihalopoulos, & Beekman, 2008). Age groups included in this analysis were both adolescents and adults, and a number of studies involved peripartum women. These interventions typically involved cognitive behavioral therapy or interpersonal therapy, and on average they reduced the incidence of depression by 22 %. There were indications from this analysis that universal efforts (incidence rate ratio (IRR) not significantly different from 1.0) were less effective than selective (IRR=0.72) and indicated (IRR=0.76) approaches.

Several depression prevention efforts have been undertaken with children and adolescent populations. For example, 718 children in the sixth through eighth grades from three middle schools were randomly assigned to the Penn Resiliency Program (PRP), which focused on teaching cognitive-behavioral and social problem-solving skills, the suspected active components (Gillham et al., 2007). This was compared to a control condition similar to the active intervention that was matched for adult attention, social support, peer contact and discussing depression, but did not include the suspected active components, and a no-contact control. In two of the schools, the PRP significantly reduced depressive symptoms at a 3-year follow-up relative to the control groups, while there were no effects on depression prevention in the third school. A school-based depression prevention program for New Zealand adolescents showed that a CBT-based placebo-controlled trial had small but significant and persistent effects on depression symptoms (Merry, McDowell, Wild, Bir, & Cunliffe, 2004). A recent Cochrane review of psychological and educational interventions for the prevention of depression in children and adolescents revealed mixed findings, with psychological interventions, especially those using targeted rather than universal efforts, generally leading to improved symptom reduction (Merry, McDowell, Hetrick, Bir, & Muller, 2004). The effects were inconsistent across genders and tended not to have long-term effects.

Rationale for Consideration of Physical Activity as an Approach for Depression Prevention

It therefore appears to be possible, using standard psychotherapeutic techniques, to prevent the onset of depression. There are a broad range of possible ways in which physical activity could prevent both the onset of depression and symptoms of depression, given its relevance to a number of physiological and neurobiological processes (e.g., endorphins and neurogenesis), social processes (e.g., group involvement and social support), physical processes (e.g., physical appearance and weight control), and psychological processes (e.g., emotion regulation and self-efficacy) that are associated with the development of depression. Physical activity or exercise may improve symptoms associated with depression disorders such as disordered sleep, fatigue, irritability, or feelings of sadness or worthlessness, thus preventing the onset of the full-blown disorder. Given the stigma, cost and time-commitment associated with therapy, and the broader range of positive effects of regular physical activity, interventions for depression prevention that focus on increasing physical activity may be more desirable than other types of therapy, should it prove to be effective.

Empirical Support for Physical Activity as a Method to Prevent Depression

Various methodological approaches have been used to test the hypothesis that physical activity is an effective method for reducing depressive symptoms or improving mood. The earliest, and still most common, are cross-sectional epidemiology studies, followed by prospective epidemiology studies. These studies typically entail asking participants to complete a survey in which they report their current, past and/or habitual level of physical activity and their current level of depressive symptoms or some other measure of mood. Quite often the measurement of physical activity and mood is vague, and may include only a single item. Better studies have used more well-validated scales or objective measures of physical activity (e.g., the Centers for Epidemiological Studies Depression scale and accelerometers). Analyses then typically involve calculation of correlation coefficients, comparison of mean values of depression scores across different levels of physical activity (many measures of PA are ordinal or even nominal in nature) using standard ANOVA procedures, or the use of logistic regression and calculation of odds ratios or Chi-squares to predict the odds of reaching a given threshold in depression scores (e.g., $CESD \geq 16$) at different levels of PA. Rarely is an actual clinical diagnostic assessment performed to determine the prevalence of depression in the sample. When such a relationship is found, the conclusion has been that physical activity aids in the prevention of depression.

The limitations of cross-sectional approaches are well-known, ranging from recall bias due to self-reports to the standard inability to determine the direction of the effect. While it is tempting to assume inactivity precedes (and in fact causes) the development of depressive symptoms and the onset of clinical depression, it is possible that it is just the opposite. Symptoms of depression, such as lack of energy and psychomotor retardation, can be manifested in decreased PA. There might also be a third variable confounding the relationship, such as age, disability or genetic factors. Even prospective or longitudinal designs, while an improvement on the cross-sectional design, are not immune to such alternative explanations. The assessment of PA at baseline and the subsequent assessment of depression at some later follow-up (even when substantially delayed) allows us to establish temporal precedence—a necessary but not sufficient criterion for causal inference. Given these caveats, a brief examination of cross-sectional and prospective studies is consistent in providing promising evidence that exercise could prevent the onset of symptoms and new cases of full-blown depression.

Correlational Evidence Regarding Physical Activity and Depression Symptoms

Correlational evidence has fairly convincingly established that there is an inverse relationship between physical activity and symptoms of depression, such that those who tend to report being more physically active also tend to report fewer and/or less severe symptoms of depression (Goodwin, 2003; Paffenbarger, Lee, & Leung, 1994; Teychenne, Ball, & Salmon, 2008b). Large epidemiological studies from the USA (Goodwin, 2003; Paffenbarger et al., 1994), Australia (Brown, Ford, Burton, Marshall, & Dobson, 2005), and other countries (Abu-Omar, 2004) have shown this effect, although it is often small and inconsistent across measurement of depression and physical activity, populations, and domains of physical activity. A review of eight cross-sectional studies from around the world that all had depression (or, at least, emotional distress) as a measured outcome revealed a significant relationship between regular physical activity and prevalence of depressive symptoms (Strohle, 2009), including one study reporting significant dose–response effects.

Several recent studies corroborate these past findings. Using recent population-based data from the 2006 US Behavioral Risk Factor Surveillance Survey (BRFSS), Strine et al. (2008) showed that physical inactivity was associated with incremental risk for depression, such that current physical inactivity (i.e., no participation in physical activities or exercise other than their regular job) was associated with higher odds of more severe current depression, in both men and women. In a large national sample of college students, increased physical activity (including strength training) was again associated with odds of self-reported depression (Adams, Moore, & Dye, 2007). In a sample of adults age 26–36, physical activity was assessed using both pedometers and the International Physical Activity Questionnaire

(IPAQ), and prevalence of depression in the past 12 months was assessed by diagnostic interview (CIDI) (McKercher et al., 2009). Pedometer data showed that women achieving at least 7500 steps per day had about 50 % lower prevalence of depression than women who were sedentary, a significant effect. Men achieving at least 12,500 steps per day also had a 50 % lower prevalence of depression than men who were sedentary, but this effect was not significant. Total physical activity, as assessed by the IPAQ, was not predictive of depression. However, greater leisure-time PA was associated with lower prevalence of depression while greater work PA was associated with higher prevalence of depression in women. These effects were not found in men, or for active commuting or yard/household PA. In a study of women age 18–65 in Australia, both moderate leisure-time PA and vigorous leisure-time PA was associated with decreased odds of depression symptoms, with a stronger effect for vigorous activity (Teychenne, Ball, & Salmon, 2008a). There were no such associations for work, domestic or transport PA.

Substantial cross-sectional evidence regarding the correlation between PA and depression in children and adolescents has been gathered in the last 10–15 years, with mixed findings. A study of 933 children age 8–12 found that parent and teacher ratings of whether or not a child was active or inactive was correlated with whether or not the child was experiencing symptoms of depression (Tomson, Pangrazi, Friedman, & Hutchison, 2003). Field, Diego and Sanders (2001) found that exercise explained 5 % of the variance in CESD scores when controlling for other factors such as affection from parents, and Norris, Carroll and Cochrane (1992) found a correlation of −0.18 between exercise and depression scores in adolescents. A large study ($N=11,828$) of US college students who were on average 21 years old revealed increased odds of depressive symptoms in students not meeting recommendations for vigorous PA (Harbour, Behrens, Kim, & Kitchens, 2008). The relative risk of depressive symptomatology was increased for boys, but not girls, rated as inactive by their parents, while the relative risk was increased for girls, but not boys, rated as inactive by their teachers.

A survey of 891 adolescents in Sri Lanka showed no association between physical activity level and CESD scores (Perera, Torabi, Jayawardana, & Pallethanna, 2006), and another study showed no correlation between participation in moderate-to-vigorous PA (assessed using physical activity diaries and calculations of METs) and depressive symptoms for girls or boys, although a significant relationship was detected for parental reports of sports participation and depressive symptoms for boys (Desha, Ziviani, Nicholson, Martin, & Darnell, 2007). A large Canadian study of 2,104 adolescents showed that PA in the previous week was weakly correlated ($r=-0.12$, $p<0.05$) with depression and anxiety scores, although the effect disappeared when controlling for age, gender, and SES (Allison et al., 2005). An American study of 4,734 adolescents revealed a significant negative correlation between hours of moderate-to-vigorous PA (measured with the Leisure Time Exercise Questionnaire) and depression symptoms for boys, but not girls (Fulkerson, Sherwood, Perry, Neumark-Sztainer, & Story, 2004).

Higher quality studies have used more rigorous methods of measuring PA and depression outcomes. For instance, Parfitt and Eston (2005) measured depression using the Childhood Depression Inventory and then collected pedometer data for 7 days with a sample 70 children (9–11 years old) from North Wales. The children were grouped into physical activity groups according to average steps per day according to the pedometer. They observed a strong, negative correlation between step count group and depression scores ($r=-0.60$), an effect that was similar for both boys and girls. Haarasilta et al. (2004) found that the odds of MDE (established by diagnostic interview) were significantly increased for young adults age 20–24 who never exercised relative to those who exercised daily. They saw no such effect in a sample of adolescents (ages 15–19). Most recently, Johnson et al. (2008) showed that there was no effect of PA (measured using accelerometers and 3-day physical activity recalls) on CESD scores or odds of reaching a diagnostically meaningful cutoff of 24 for a sample of sixth grade girls. There were small effects of sedentary behavior on depression outcomes, but this could be a type I error due to a large sample size.

Prospective Evidence Regarding the Relationship Between Physical Activity and Prevention of Depression

Prospective/longitudinal designs provide better evidence that PA can help prevent the onset of depression (Camacho, Roberts, Lazarus, Kaplan, & Cohen, 1991; Farmer et al., 1988; Mobily, Rubenstein, Lemke, Ohara, & Wallace, 1996; Paffenbarger et al., 1994; Strohle et al., 2007). These designs can help determine the direction of the effect, although causal inferences can still not be conclusively made. For example, Sagatun, Sogaard, Bjertness, Selmer and Heyerdahl (2007) detected small longitudinal effects of PA at age 15–16 on depression symptoms at age 18–19, effects that remained significant when adjusting for covariates, but only for boys. In an 8-year follow-up study of Finnish adults over the age of 65, Lampinen, Heikkinen and Ruoppila (2000) showed that maintaining or increasing exercise intensity predicted the likelihood of depression symptoms over time. Also in older adults, PA in 1994 predicted incidence of depression in 1999, even when controlling for a variety of covariates and eliminating those with a physical disability (Strawbridge, Deleger, Roberts, & Kaplan, 2002). A large study of a Dutch working population found that strenuous leisure time PA was associated with reduced odds of depression 3 years later, but only for workers that had sedentary jobs (Bernaards et al., 2006). Among a sample of women aged 45–50, levels of PA at baseline predicted odds of depressive symptoms (using the CESD-10 and the mental health subscale of the SF-36) at a 5-year follow-up (Brown et al., 2005). Furthermore, among those who reported low levels of PA at baseline, those who remained low at follow-up had increased odds of depression than those who increased their PA, effects that remained when adjusting for covariates. In a study of 35,224 African American women, less average vigorous PA (hours/week) in 1995 and 1997 was associated with increased odds of meaningful depression scores (CESD$\geq$16) in 1999 (Wise, Adams-Campbell, Palmer, & Rosenberg, 2006), whereas walking was associated with depression in obese women only, excluding participants who were depressed at baseline.

A prospective study of exercise behavior and depression symptoms during and after pregnancy revealed significant relationships in both early and later pregnancy, although effects were weaker for women who were more active pre-pregnancy (Downs, DiNallo, & Kirner, 2008).

Conversely, Sanchez-Villegas et al. (2008) found no associations between leisure-time PA (in MET h wk^{-1}) and incidence of depression (using diagnostic interview), or between sedentary lifestyles and incidence of depression in a large Spanish adult population. A 2-year prospective study of adolescents in the UK showed no association between activity levels (based on self-reports of exercising more or less than twice a week for an hour) and risk of depressive symptoms (Clark et al., 2007). A longitudinal study of primarily white male former medical students also showed no effects of PA on later odds of depression (Cooper-Patrick, Ford, Mead, Chang, & Klag, 1997). In a long-term study of depressed patients, baseline PA was associated with baseline depression, but not with changes in depression over time (at 1, 4, and 10 year follow-ups) (Harris, Cronkite, & Moos, 2006). There was, however, an apparent interaction between baseline PA and medical conditions and between baseline PA and negative life events on later depressive symptoms. Baseline PA lessened the effect of medical conditions and negative life events on future depression.

One benefit of a design with repeated measures is the diversity of statistical approaches that can be used to examine the relationship between PA and depression. For instance, using a latent-growth modeling (LGM) approach allows for the testing of relationships between baseline values of two variables, baseline values in one variable and changes over time in another variable, and changes over time between two variables. Motl, Birnbaum, Kubik, and Dishman (2004) used LGM to show a significant relationship between baseline levels of PA and depression symptoms, and between changes in PA and changes in depression symptoms over the course of 2 years in a sample of seventh and eighth graders. The effect was small, however. Birkeland, Torsheim, and Wold (2009) also used a LGM approach to test the relationship between yearly assessments of leisure-time PA and depression over the course of 10 years in adolescents from age 13 to 23. They also found weak correlations between changes in PA and changes in depression. They concluded that there was no evidence of either causal pathway—either that PA prevents future depression or that depression serves as a barrier to future exercise, as they found no association between baseline PA and changes in depression or between baseline depression and changes in PA.

Conclusions Based on Correlational and Prospective/Longitudinal Evidence

While the cross-sectional and prospective/longitudinal evidence appears favorable regarding a relationship between increased physical activity and decreased depression, there are studies that find no effect. We are not aware of any studies that show that PA is harmful and leads to worse depression outcomes. Based on this evidence, we currently lack the ability to make clear conclusions regarding types of PA that may be effective (e.g., leisure time vs. household or occupational activity), the dose of PA needed to prevent depression, and other mediators and moderators of this effect. Importantly, we are unable to make causal inferences. As noted previously, it may be that the relationship between PA and incidence of depression is in fact incidental to a third variable that makes an individual prone to both inactivity and depression. For example, De Moor et al. (2008) conducted a large twin study to rule out genetic factors. While they found correlations between voluntary leisure-time PA and symptoms of depression within a given twin, once the co-twin was added to the model to control for genetic factors, the correlation became nonsignificant. These findings add uncertainty to the potential causal effects of voluntary exercise on depression. Randomized intervention trials would help to clarify this relation.

Interventions to Prevent Depression through Physical Activity

A recent Cochrane review focused on the effectiveness of PA in the prevention and treatment of depression and anxiety in children and young people (Larun, Nordheim, Ekeland, Hagen, & Heian, 2006). With respect to the prevention of depression, they reviewed evidence using samples from the general (i.e., nonclinical) population of children. The studies reviewed were exclusively conducted in the 1980s and 1990s. In five studies comparing exercise to no intervention, there was a statistically significant effect on depression outcomes in favor of the intervention. In two studies comparing exercise to low intensity exercise or relaxation, there was no significant difference between groups in depression outcomes. Similarly, in two studies comparing exercise to a psychosocial intervention, no group differences were observed. The studies reviewed were considered to be of low methodological quality, and the evidence for PA for the prevention of depression in children was considered weak. A recent paper by Dunn and Weintraub (2008) discussed how this evidence might be improved. They specifically recommended that future studies specifically target prevention, and use the IOM framework that includes universal, selective, and indicated populations.

In one of several studies conducted in older populations, Motl et al. (2005) compared depressive symptoms in a walking group to a resistance/toning comparison group in a sample of 174 sedentary adults, age 60–75 years, with medical clearance for exercise. Depression symptoms decreased following a 6-month intervention, and these effects persisted for 5 years. However, there were no differences between the walking group and the resistance/toning group, which precludes causal inferences. It may be that a resistance/toning group was not a sufficient control group, as this still constitutes physical activity and beneficial effects of strength training on depressive symptoms in older adults have been demonstrated elsewhere (e.g., Sims, Hill, Davidson, Gunn, & Huang, 2006; Singh, Clements, & Fiatarone, 1997). A large Finnish RCT ($N=632$) of adults age 75–81 revealed no main effect of a PA counseling intervention on CESD scores, although there was an interaction with baseline CESD scores (Pakkala et al., 2008). The intervention did decrease CESD scores, but only for those with minor depression symptoms at baseline. A review of exercise interventions in nonclinical older populations found mixed results, with effects often only significant among men and for those with higher levels of baseline depression (Sjosten & Kivela, 2006).

An older review of exercise interventions in nonclinically depressed populations reported mixed findings; for example, there were beneficial effects of exercise leading to improved depression symptoms for moderate (but not high) intensity exercise (Paluska & Schwenk, 2000). They concluded that PA as a preventive factor for depression was not as certain as PA as treatment for depression, and that, at the time, no experimental data had shown that PA can prevent the onset of depression. It continues to be a limitation that PA intervention studies do not use clinical diagnosis of new cases of depression as a primary or even secondary outcome. While a reduction in symptoms of depression is likely to have a significant public health impact, without establishing a conclusive link between PA and clinically diagnosed incidence of MDD/MDE the preventive capability of PA will be called into question.

Exercise Interventions in Those Specifically at Risk for Depression

Targeted interventions to prevent depression in populations suspected to be at risk for depression are also valuable. Patients undergoing treatment for cancer, patients recovering from stroke, and patients with hypertension are all at increased risk for depression. Culos-Reed, Carlson, Daroux, and Hately-Aldous (2006) conducted a small pilot study ($N = 38$) testing the effects of a yoga intervention on psychological outcomes in breast cancer survivors. There was a marginal effect of the intervention on improvements in depression (a change in the POMS depression score from 4.70 to 2.22), an effect not seen in the control group (change from 5.44 to 5.50). Burnham and Wilcox (2002) also conducted a small ($N = 18$) trial examining the effects of a 10-week supervised aerobic exercise program on psychological outcomes in cancer survivors. They found a nonsignificant decrease in depression score in the exercise group, and a nonsignificant increase in depression score in the control group. Similarly, Payne, Held, Thorpe, and Shaw (2008), studying 20 women with breast cancer, found no significant group differences in changes in CESD scores between an exercise intervention group and a control group, although trends suggested a favorable effect for the exercise group and no change for the control group. Participants in these studies were generally not clinically depressed at baseline. These studies are clearly limited by their small sample sizes, but the results suggest a trend in favor of exercise. A review of exercise interventions (mostly RCTs) during cancer treatment concluded that there were typically positive effects of the intervention on mental health outcomes, including depression (Courneya, 2001).

Exercise interventions have been conducted with patients in other clinical settings. In a sample of 100 patients recovering from stroke, a 3-month exercise intervention led to significantly lower depression scores on the Geriatric Depression Scale and lower rates of significant depressive symptoms compared to a usual care group (Lai et al., 2006). The effects were stronger for those with greater depressive symptoms at baseline. In a subset of nondepressed patients undergoing cardiac rehabilitation (education and exercise) following major coronary events ($N=269$), there were no changes in depression over the course of treatment, although there was no control group for comparison (Milani, Lavie, & Cassidy, 1996). However, they did find a significant decrease in depression for those who were already depressed at baseline ($N=69$). Similarly, an exercise intervention for patients with hypertension ($N=133$) lead to decreased depressive symptoms for those with higher levels of depressive symptoms at baseline, as compared to a wait-list control (Smith et al., 2007), an effect comparable to a weight loss condition. This effect was further moderated by changes in aerobic fitness (VO_2peak). In a sample of 60 adults with HIV, a 12-week aerobic exercise intervention lead to significant decreases in depressive symptoms according to the CESD and the POMS, and a marginal decrease according to the BDI, as compared to a wait-list control group (Neidig, Smith, & Brashers, 2003). About a third of this sample was considered depressed at baseline; however, the authors did not examine the effect of baseline depression on these findings.

Women who are pregnant or have recently given birth are at risk for prenatal and postpartum depression. While not specifically addressing prevention efforts, two reviews of exercise and depression in perinatal populations have been conducted. A review of five studies testing the effects of exercise on postpartum depression was inconclusive, although generally favorable (Daley, Jolly, & MacArthur, 2009). A review of six studies on PA and depression symptoms during pregnancy found that most studies show the typical inverse relationship between PA and depression symptoms (Poudevigne & O'Connor, 2006).

Conclusions Based on Experimental Evidence

Since 1994, evidence for preventing depression in pregnant women and adolescents has been demonstrated using cognitive behavioral interventions, but prevention studies using physical activity are somewhat rare and need to undergo efficacy and effectiveness trials (Merry et al., 2004). Remaining questions from this evidence base include the determination of the dose–response relationship and appropriate domains and types of exercise that might have protective effects for depression. A review of both observational and experimental studies of the relationship between PA and risk of depression in adults considered both dose and setting issues (Teychenne et al., 2008b). As much of the work in this area has found, the findings were mixed. The authors found no effects of duration of PA on depression outcomes. While some studies showed that vigorous PA was better than moderate intensity, others showed no differences for moderate vs. vigorous intensity. Two studies (both observational) suggested that only leisure-time PA, and not other domains such as household or occupational PA, was associated with improved depression outcomes. Similarly, another review of observational and experimental studies found no dose–response effects in young women (Azar, Ball, Salmon, & Cleland, 2008).

Given what appears to be a small effect size, unclear dose–response effects, and the need for large, heterogeneous samples, the purported global protective effect of PA for depression may be difficult to demonstrate conclusively. It remains to be seen whether or not a finite exercise intervention can prevent depression over the long term, as exercise may need to be maintained—which can be difficult to achieve for just 6 months, let alone 10–20 years—in order to observe significant effects. Exercise maintenance has been shown to be a factor in the prevention of symptoms of depression (Dunn, Cheng, Sinclair, Trivedi, & Kampert, 2003). At this point in the evidence base, our efforts may be most productively focused on the examination of mediators and moderators (other than gender and baseline depression since these are well known) of the PA-depression relationship. In terms of moderators, this might mean an examination of the population of interest (e.g., age, and particularly stage of development, at-risk populations, genetic predispositions), the types, domains and dose of PA, or social context in which physical activity is performed. As Kraemer and colleagues have described, the purpose is to determine the best treatment and its effects for specific groups of individuals (what treatment for whom) (Kraemer, Stice, Kazdin, Offord, & Kupfer, 2001; Kraemer, Wilson, Fairburn, & Agras, 2002; King, Ahn, Atienza, & Kraemer, 2008). It also means testing possible mediating pathways, which does not necessarily require a direct effect of PA on depression outcomes. The remainder of this chapter discusses what the mechanisms of change might be.

Potential Mechanisms for Physical Activity and Depression Prevention

The influence of physical activity in the prevention of depression likely draws from an array of physiological, neurobiological, social–cognitive, and physical effects of exercise. These potential mechanisms likely play similar roles in both prevention and treatment of depression; however, some may play a stronger role in prevention than in treatment. For instance, physical activity may be a resilience strategy that influences responsiveness to stress or, perhaps, causes neurobiological changes that affect the expression of genes associated with the tendency to develop symptoms of depression. In many cases, these proposed mechanisms are directly relevant to developmental processes occurring in adolescence and young adulthood (e.g., the formation of self-schemas and identities that are consistent with being a physically active person), and as such are associated with the establishment of lifelong exercise habits with the potential for enduring promotion of mental health.

The many potential effects of exercise might subsequently have any number of possible influences on the many causes and vulnerabilities associated with the incidence of depression. In fact, this multiple-mechanism/multiple-etiology explanation may be one reason for the inconsistent findings regarding the protective effect of physical activity on depression. It may not always be the case that the factors leading to depression in a given population (e.g., stressful life events) are necessarily ameliorated by the effects of physical activity in that population in that setting (e.g., physical activity leads to weight loss but not increased social support). Because of the wide range of proposed mechanisms, only a brief review of the hypothesized antidepressant mediators of physical activity is provided.

Physiological and Neurobiological Effects of Exercise

The potential physiological and neurobiological antidepressant mediators of physical activity may prevent the development of depression by maintaining a proper balance of neurotransmitters necessary for euthymic mood. The proposed physiological and neurobiological mediators of exercise are numerous and readers may wish to refer to papers that include general reviews of potential mediators (Daley, 2002). Similarly, interested readers may also refer to Ernst, Olson, Pinel, Lam, and Christie (2006), van Praag (2008), Dishman et al. (2006), and Dishman and O'Connor (2009) for reviews of potential neurobiological mediators. Proposed neurobiological theories of how physical activity influences mood include the following: the atrial natriuretic peptide (ANP) hypothesis (Strohle, Feller, Strasburger, Heinz, & Dimeo, 2006), the transient hypofrontality hypothesis (Dietrich, 2006), the endocannabinoid hypothesis (Dietrich & McDaniel, 2004), the endorphin hypothesis (Steinberg & Sykes, 1985), the neurogenesis hypothesis, and physical activity's role in regulating the stress response (Hill & Gorzalka, 2005). The ANP hypothesis proposes that ANP, produced in response to physical activity, has an anxiolytic effect that may reduce depression (Strohle et al., 2006). The transient hypofrontality hypothesis suggests that physical activity requires extensive neural activation in brain regions associated with physical movement, resulting in a transient decrease of neural activity in brain structures not related to physical activity (Dietrich, 2006). Specifically, decreased activation in areas such as the Ventral Medial Prefrontal Cortex, which has been associated with depression (Mayberg, 1997), may result in improved mood. The endocannabinoid hypothesis states that the pleasurable psychological state obtained after exercise can be attributed to increased serum concentrations of endogenous endocannabinoids and may result in increased affect (Dietrich & McDaniel, 2004) as well as an improved regulation of the stress response (Hill & Gorzalka, 2005). The endorphin hypothesis, or the often described "runner's high," proposes that the euphoric effects of physical activity are a result of endogenous opioids released in the brain (Steinberg & Sykes, 1985). Boecker et al. (2008) present some evidence for this hypothesis by demonstrating increased opiodergic activity in frontolimbic brain structures in response to sustained physical activity using positron emission topography (PET) scanning. This increased activation was correlated with feelings of euphoria (Boecker et al. 2008) and may help regulate mood. However, this study was done in trained runners who had reported feeling euphoric after running. As a recent review by Dishman and O'Connor (2009) points out, there is ambiguity in what is meant by the term "runners high" and many people never experience this feeling as a result of exercise. Endorphins may play a role in improved mood, but clearly more research is needed in this area.

Physical activity may also increase production of Brain Derived Neurotrophic Factor (BDNF), the nonacronymic neuropeptide VGF, Vascular Endothelial Growth Factor (VEGF), β-endorphins, and serotonin (5-HT), which have all been linked with decreased rates of depression (Ernst et al., 2006). While these relationships are poorly understood, we do know all of the factors listed above are associated with increased rates of neurogenesis, or the proliferation of neurons in the brain (see Ernst et al. for a review of BDNF, VEGF, β-endorphins, and 5-HT, and Thakker-Varia and Alder (2009) for a discussion of VGF). Physical activity may also have an antidepressant effect in aiding regulation of the Hypothalamic Pituitary Axis stress response (Droste et al., 2003; Wittert, Livesey, Espiner, & Donald, 1996).

Social Cognitive Effects of Exercise

The social–cognitive effects of physical activity may also play a key role in the prevention of depression. For instance, physical activity can lead to increases in self-esteem and self-efficacy, low levels of which are often associated with depression. Self-esteem refers to an individual's overall evaluation of their self-worth and self-efficacy may be defined as the degree of confidence an individual feels in accomplishing a given task. By increasing levels of self-esteem and self-efficacy through physical activity, factors that may be especially helpful in elevating the moods of adolescents and for individuals across the lifespan, physical activity may aid in the prevention of depression. Craft (2005) found that clinically depressed participants in an aerobic exercise program significantly increased coping self-efficacy compared to a control group of nonexercisers; there was also a significant negative relationship between depression and coping self-efficacy. Others have shown that those participating in both martial arts training and stationary cycling experienced significant gains in self-efficacy as well as significant decreases in depression scores after undergoing a martial arts training session, while the same participants did not report any statistically significant changes after partaking in stationary cycling (Bodin & Martinsen, 2004). While both of these studies focused on self-efficacy's mediating role in the relationship between exercise and acute depression, self-efficacy may have similar effects in preventing depression. In a correlational study, Ryan (2008) found that self-esteem and self-efficacy were both individually potent enough mechanisms to account for the antidepressant effects of physical activity in nonclinical sample of 381 undergraduate students.

Physical Effects of Exercise

Physical activity may also act to prevent depression through potential physiological effects such as an increased ability to regulate weight and sleep. The perception of being overweight during adolescence is a significant risk factor for depression in young men and women (Al Mamun et al., 2007). Therefore, physical activity may prevent the development of depression through improved weight management, which likely results in enhanced body-image. For example, a randomized controlled trial for overweight (BMI 25–39) women ($N=401$) showed that those receiving an intervention that incorporated both nutrition and PA counseling reported greater decreases in CESD scores over the 12-month study period than those in the control group (Kerr et al., 2008). A New Zealand study comparing a "nondieting" program (group-based vs. mail-delivered) to a relaxation training program for overweight women ($N=222$) lead to increased PA, weight loss, and decreased depression in all treatment groups, with the greatest changes in depression reported by the relaxation training group (Katzer et al., 2008). They did not report a correlation between changes in PA and changes in depression. This study also examined the effects of the treatment groups on other outcomes such as stress management, spiritual growth, and self-efficacy, but did not test whether these factors mediated treatment effects on depression.

It is also important to note that in studies where positive effects are observed there are demonstrated improvements in affect without noticeable increases in physical fitness (Physical Activity Guidelines Advisory Committee, 2008). Weight management benefits of physical activity may enhance body-image or a sense of self-control for individuals at risk for developing depression because of their perceived weight. Physical activity may also aid in regulating irregular sleep patterns (Lancel, Droste, Sommer, & Reul, 2003; Tanaka & Shirakawa, 2004; Youngstedt, 2005), a common symptom of depression. Physical activity likely increases the quality of sleep by depleting the body's energy, raising the body's core temperature, and breaking down body tissue; all processes that sleep has been hypothesized to restore (Youngstedt). Finally, physical activity can reduce the impact of medical illness on the development of depression (Harris et al., 2006)

Social Effects of Exercise

Another potential mediator of the relationship between physical activity and the prevention of depression may be the increased social interaction that often accompanies physical activity. Social relationships and mutual support for other people in an exercise setting may provide a significant proportion of the effect of exercise on mental health (Faulkner & Carless, 2006). The role of social interaction in physical activity may be especially important during early adolescence when adolescents have the opportunity to develop more peer relationships. Consequently, physical activity interventions for adolescents may benefit from the incorporation of group activity, as seen in team sports. The role of social relationships in physical activity may have antidepressant effects for those who are lonely or who have fewer relationships than they desire.

Affect Regulation and Coping

Acute bouts of aerobic exercise generally lead to improved affect (Reed & Ones, 2006). Specifically, just 30 min of moderate intensity exercise is associated with increased positive affect and tranquility and decrease negative affect and fatigue

(Kwan & Bryan, 2010). These effects are stronger for those beginning exercise in a more negative state, such that exercise is particularly beneficial for one's well-being when experiencing acute negative affect. While these effects tend not to be long-lasting (for some returning to baseline in as short as 15 min post-exercise), even temporary relief may be enough to disrupt the cycle of negative thoughts and feelings that over time may lead to the onset of a depressive episode. Thus, those at risk for depression might be encouraged to develop regular exercise regimens so that they might counteract transient negative moods and cope more effectively during times of increased stress. The establishment of physical activity as an affect regulation strategy may be particularly important during adolescence, when problem solving, coping and affect regulation mechanisms are especially relevant to the risk of depression (Compas, Jaser, & Benson, 2009).

Behavioral Activation

Finally, it has been suggested that physical activity may be associated with depression because it represents a form of behavioral activation, a therapeutic approach that seeks to alleviate depression by increasing people's activity associated with pleasure and mastery as well as improving problem solving, decreasing avoidance, and overcoming barriers to activation (Dimidjian et al., 2006). Depression tends to be associated with substantial periods of inactivity, characterized by depressed mood and passivity, offering little opportunities for reward or accomplishment (Martinsen, 2008). In many cases, people fail to recognize the connection between their behavior and their feelings. In this way, depression begets more depression. Physical activity—a broad term that encompasses a wide variety of activities that could be deemed pleasurable, uplifting and rewarding—is in direct opposition to these depressive tendencies. In the context of prevention, passive, sedentary behaviors that may lead to the onset of depression can be replaced with physical activity so as to reduce the downward spiral of depressed mood and inactivity. Youth can be taught to recognize what might be unhealthy behaviors with potential deleterious effects on mood, and to replace these behaviors with activities that will better support their general well-being. While it has been increasingly suggested that physical activity aids in both the prevention and treatment of depression via behavioral activation, direct evidence for this hypothesis does not yet exist. Future research should consider this as a possible mechanism.

Future Directions for Research on Physical Activity and Depression Prevention

Based on this review, there is promising but as yet inconclusive evidence in support of physical activity as an effective way to prevent depression. While a substantial amount of cross-sectional and prospective data exists, more experimental evidence is needed. In particular, longitudinal, randomized controlled trials testing a broad range of hypothesized mechanisms are needed. While certainly physical activity *promotion* should be done at the universal level and may be protective against risk for depression, research designed to understand the mechanisms by which physical activity prevents depression may be best aimed at selected and indicated approaches. For instance, a better understanding of the neurobiological mechanisms of the link between exercise, affect, and depression—such as those reflecting the experience of mastery, reward and pleasure (i.e., factors associated with behavioral activation)— would be valuable. Importantly, this knowledge may help determine for whom exercise may effectively prevent depression, and for whom it might not.

Recommendations for Practitioners Regarding the Use of Physical Activity to Prevent Depression

Questions remain regarding the dose of physical activity that might be required to prevent depression and symptoms of depression, and the domains, populations, and developmental stages in which there might be an effect. Physical activity at a level consistent with current government recommendations—at least 150 min per week of moderate intensity, or 75 min per week of vigorous intensity exercise (Haskell et al., 2007)—is likely sufficient. Yet it is possible that even light physical activity as replacement for sedentary activities, such as watching television, playing video games and sitting at the computer, may play some role in preventing symptoms. As discussed above, physical activity may serve as behavioral activation when depressive tendencies emerge, especially when performed in a social context (e.g., going out dancing with friends) or a context that offers the opportunity for mastery and/or pleasure (e.g., gardening). A practitioner (or parent or significant other) may be able to recognize the onset of depressive tendencies toward sedentary behavior, social isolation, and withdrawal from reward and encourage the substitution of physical activity.

However, there may be situations in which physical activity for depression prevention may be ineffective or potentially detrimental. For instance, exercise may be contraindicated for individuals experiencing comorbidities such as body dysmorphic disorder, body image problems, and eating disorders. Also, there are individuals for whom exercise is associated with negative affect, such as those who are overweight (Ekkekakis & Lind, 2006). Children who are overweight tend to have negative experiences with physical activity (Lagerberg, 2005). As suggested by the reference to physical activity as affect regulation, we might not expect that physical activity would lead to less depression when physical activity is unpleasant or painful.

What might ultimately be most important for prevention of depression are the social and contextual circumstances under which physical activity is performed. When physical activity is performed in environments that support the opportunity for personal choice, the need to feel competent and the need to feel a sense of belonging, an intrinsic motivation for physical activity is more likely to develop

(Ryan & Deci, 2000). Intrinsic motivation to exercise is characterized by inherent interest and pleasure with respect to exercise, and is associated with greater behavior maintenance over time and more positive psychological well-being (Deci & Ryan, 2008). Establishing healthy attitudes towards physical activity, especially in childhood and adolescence, would likely confer the best opportunity for a finite physical activity intervention to have long-term effects on depression outcomes.

Just as prevention of heart disease, diabetes, and cancer is emerging as a healthcare priority, so too is the prevention of depression. There are an increasing number of appeals for better integration of physical and mental healthcare. For example, the Institute of Medicine has recommended that a variety of mechanisms be developed to coordinate research and services across the currently fragmented system of research and delivery of services (National Research Council and Institute of Medicine, 2009). The promotion of physical activity as treatment and prevention for a number of mental and physical health problems is one way to support such integration.

References

Abu-Omar, K. (2004). Mental health and physical activity in the European Union. *Sozial-Und Praventivmedizin, 49*(5), 301–309.

Adams, T. B., Moore, M. T., & Dye, J. (2007). The relationship between physical activity and mental health in a national sample of college females. *Women and Health, 45*(1), 69–85.

Akerblad, A. C., Bengtsson, F., von Knorring, L., & Ekselius, L. (2006). Response, remission and relapse in relation to adherence in primary care treatment of depression: a 2-year outcome study. *International Clinical Psychopharmacology, 21*, 117–124.

Al Mamun, A., Cramb, S., McDermott, B. M., O'Callaghan, M., Najman, J. M., & Williams, G. M. (2007). Adolescents' perceived weight associated with depression in young adulthood: a longitudinal study. *Obesity, 15*(12), 3097–3105.

Allison, K. R., Adlaf, E. M., Irving, H. M., Hatch, J. L., Smith, T. F., Dwyer, J. J. M., et al. (2005). Relationship of vigorous physical activity to psychologic distress among adolescents. *Journal of Adolescent Health, 37*(2), 164–166.

American Psychiatric Association. (1994). *Diagnostic and statistical manual of mental disorders, DSM-IV* (4th ed.). Washington, DC: American Psychiatric Association.

Azar, D., Ball, K., Salmon, J., & Cleland, V. (2008). The association between physical activity and depressive symptoms in young women: a review. *Mental Health and Physical Activity, 1*(2), 82–88.

Bernaards, C. M., Jans, M. P., van den Heuvel, S. G., Hendriksen, I. J., Houtman, I. L., & Bongers, P. M. (2006). Can strenuous leisure time physical activity prevent psychological complaints in a working population? *Occupational and Environmental Medicine, 63*(1), 10–16.

Birkeland, M. S., Torsheim, T., & Wold, B. (2009). A longitudinal study of the relationship between leisure-time physical activity and depressed mood among adolescents. *Psychology of Sport and Exercise, 10*(1), 25–34.

Bodin, T., & Martinsen, E. W. (2004). Mood and self-efficacy during acute exercise in clinical depression. A randomized, controlled study. *Journal of Sport and Exercise Psychology, 26*(4), 623–633.

Boecker, H., Sprenger, T., Spilker, M. E., Henriksen, G., Koppenhoefer, M., Wagner, K. J., et al. (2008). The runner's high: opioidergic mechanisms in the human brain. *Cerebral Cortex, 18*(11), 2523–2531.

Brown, W. J., Ford, J. H., Burton, N. W., Marshall, A. L., & Dobson, A. J. (2005). Prospective study of physical activity and depressive symptoms in middle-aged women. *American Journal of Preventive Medicine, 29*(4), 265–272.

Burnham, T. R., & Wilcox, A. (2002). Effects of exercise on physiological and psychological variables in cancer survivors. *Medicine and Science in Sports and Exercise, 34*(12), 1863–1867.

Camacho, T. C., Roberts, R. E., Lazarus, N. B., Kaplan, G. A., & Cohen, R. D. (1991). Physical activity and depression—evidence from the Alameda County Study. *American Journal of Epidemiology, 134*(2), 220–231.

Clark, C., Haines, M. M., Head, J., Klineberg, E., Arephin, M., Viner, R., et al. (2007). Psychological symptoms and physical health and health behaviours in adolescents: a prospective 2-year study in East London. *Addiction, 102*(1), 126–135.

Compas, B. E., Jaser, S. S., & Benson, M. A. (2009). *Coping and emotion regulation: implications for understanding depression during adolescence.* New York, NY: Routledge/Taylor & Francis.

Cooper-Patrick, L., Ford, D. E., Mead, L. A., Chang, P. P., & Klag, M. J. (1997). Exercise and depression in midlife: a prospective study. *American Journal of Public Health, 87*(4), 670–673.

Courneya, K. S. (2001). Exercise interventions during cancer treatment: biopsychosocial outcomes. *Exercise Sport Science Review, 29*(2), 60–64.

Craft, L. L. (2005). Exercise and clinical depression: examining two psychological mechanisms. *Psychology of Sport and Exercise, 6*(2), 151–171.

Cuijpers, P., van Straten, A., Smit, F., Mihalopoulos, C., & Beekman, A. (2008). Preventing the onset of depressive disorders: a meta-analytic review of psychological interventions. *American Journal of Psychiatry, 165*(10), 1272–1280.

Culos-Reed, S. N., Carlson, L. E., Daroux, L. M., & Hately-Aldous, S. (2006). A pilot study of yoga for breast cancer survivors: physical and psychological benefits. *Psycho-Oncology, 15*(10), 891–897.

Daley, A. (2002). Exercise therapy and mental health in clinical populations: is exercise therapy a worthwhile intervention? *Advances in Psychiatric Treatment, 8,* 262–270.

Daley, A., Jolly, K., & MacArthur, C. (2009). The effectiveness of exercise in the management of post-natal depression: systematic review and meta-analysis. *Family Practice, 26*(2), 154–162.

De Moor, M. H. M., Boomsma, D. I., Stubbe, J. H., Willemsen, G., & de Geus, E. J. C. (2008). Testing causality in the association between regular exercise and symptoms of anxiety and depression. *Archives of General Psychiatry, 65*(8), 897–905.

Deci, E. L., & Ryan, R. M. (2008). Facilitating optimal motivation and psychological well-being across life's domains. *Canadian Psychology/Psychologie canadienne, 49*(1), 14–23.

Desha, L. N., Ziviani, J. M., Nicholson, J. M., Martin, G., & Darnell, R. E. (2007). Physical activity and depressive symptoms in American adolescents. *Journal of Sport and Exercise Psychology, 29*(4), 534–543.

Dietrich, A. (2006). Transient hypofrontality as a mechanism for the psychological effects of exercise. *Psychiatry Research, 145*(1), 79–83.

Dietrich, A., & McDaniel, W. F. (2004). Endocannabinoids and exercise. *British Journal of Sports Medicine, 38*(5), 536–541.

Dimidjian, S., Hollon, S. D., Dobson, K. S., Schmaling, K. B., Kohlenberg, R. J., Addis, M. E., et al. (2006). Randomized trial of behavioral activation, cognitive therapy, and antidepressant medication in the acute treatment of adults with major depression. *Journal of Consulting and Clinical Psychology, 74*(4), 658–670.

Dishman, R. K., Berthoud, H. R., Booth, F. W., Cotman, C. W., Edgerton, V. R., Fleshner, M. R., et al. (2006). Neurobiology of exercise. *Obesity, 14,* 345–356.

Dishman, R. K., & O'Connor, P. J. (2009). Lesson in exercise neurobiology: the case of endorphins. *Mental Health and Physical Activity, 2,* 4–9.

Downs, D. S., DiNallo, J. M., & Kirner, T. L. (2008). Determinants of pregnancy and postpartum depression: prospective influences of depressive symptoms, body image satisfaction, and exercise behavior. *Annals of Behavioral Medicine, 36*(1), 54–63.

Droste, S. K., Gesing, A., Ulbricht, S., Muller, M. B., Linthorst, A. C. E., & Reul, J. (2003). Effects of long-term voluntary exercise on the mouse hypothalamic-pituitary-adrenocortical axis. *Endocrinology, 144*(7), 3012–3023.

Dunn, A.L., Cheng, Y.L., Sinclair, E.L., Trivedi, M.H., & Kampert, J.B. (2003). Maintaining physical activity predicts fewer symptoms of depression. Society of Behavioral Medicine 24th Annual Meeting, March 21, 2003, Salt Lake City, Utah.

Dunn, A. L., & Weintraub, P. (2008). Exercise in the prevention and treatment of adolescent depression: a promising but little researched intervention. *American Journal of Lifestyle Medicine, 2*(6), 507–518.

Ekkekakis, P., & Lind, E. (2006). Exercise does not feel the same when you are overweight: the impact of self-selected and imposed intensity on affect and exertion. *International Journal of Obesity, 30*(4), 652–660.

Ernst, C., Olson, A. K., Pinel, J. P. J., Lam, R. W., & Christie, B. R. (2006). Antidepressant effects of exercise: evidence for an adult-neurogenesis hypothesis? *Journal of Psychiatry and Neuroscience, 31*(2), 84–92.

Farmer, M. E., Locke, B. Z., Moscicki, E. K., Dannenberg, A. L., Larson, D. B., & Radloff, L. S. (1988). Physical activity and depressive symptoms— the NHANES-I epidemiologic follow-up study. *American Journal of Epidemiology, 128*(6), 1340–1351.

Faulkner, G., & Carless, D. (2006). Physical activity in the process of psychiatric rehabilitation: theoretical and methodological issues. *Psychiatric Rehabilitation Journal, 29*(4), 258–266.

Field, T., Diego, M., & Sanders, C. (2001). Adolescent depression and risk factors. *Adolescence, 36*(143), 491–498.

Fulkerson, J. A., Sherwood, N. E., Perry, C. L., Neumark-Sztainer, D., & Story, M. (2004). Depressive symptoms and adolescent eating and health behaviors: a multifaceted view in a population-based sample. *Preventive Medicine, 38*(6), 865–875.

Gillham, J. E., Reivich, K. J., Freres, D. R., Chaplin, T. M., Shatte, A. J., Samuels, B., et al. (2007). School-based prevention of depressive symptoms: a randomized controlled study of the effectiveness and specificity of the Penn Resiliency Program. *Journal of Consulting and Clinical Psychology, 75*(1), 9–19.

Goodwin, R. D. (2003). Association between physical activity and mental disorders among adults in the United States. *Preventive Medicine, 36*(6), 698–703.

Haarasilta, L. M., Marttunen, M. J., Kaprio, J. A., & Aro, H. M. (2004). Correlates of depression in a representative nationwide sample of adolescents (15–19 years) and young adults (20–24 years). *The European Journal of Public Health, 14*(3), 280–285.

Harbour, V. J., Behrens, T. K., Kim, H. S., & Kitchens, C. L. (2008). Vigorous physical activity and depressive symptoms in college students. *Journal of Physical Activity and Health, 5*(4), 516–526.

Harris, A. H. S., Cronkite, R., & Moos, R. (2006). Physical activity, exercise coping, and depression in a 10-year cohort study of depressed patients. *Journal of Affective Disorders, 93*(1–3), 79–85.

Haskell, W. L., Lee, I. M., Pate, R. R., Powell, K. E., Blair, S. N., Franklin, B. A., et al. (2007). Physical activity and public health: updated recommendation for adults from the American College of Sports Medicine and the American Heart Association. *Medicine and Science in Sports and Exercise, 39*(8), 1423–1434.

Hill, M. N., & Gorzalka, B. B. (2005). Is there a role for the endocannabinoid system in the etiology and treatment of melancholic depression? *Behavioural Pharmacology, 16*(5–6), 333–352.

Jane-Llopis, E., Hosman, C., Jenkins, R., & Anderson, P. (2003). Predictors of efficacy in depression prevention programmes—meta-analysis. *British Journal of Psychiatry, 183*, 384–397.

Johnson, C. C., Murray, D. M., Elder, J. P., Jobe, J. B., Dunn, A. L., Kubik, M., et al. (2008). Depressive symptoms and physical activity in adolescent girls. *Medicine and Science in Sports and Exercise, 40*(5), 818–826.

Katzer, L., Bradshaw, A. J., Horwath, C. C., Gray, A. R., O'Brien, S., & Joyce, J. (2008). Evaluation of a "Nondieting" stress reduction program for overweight women: a randomized trial. *American Journal of Health Promotion, 22*(4), 264–274.

Kennard, B. D., Emslie, G. J., Mayes, T. L., & Hughes, J. L. (2006). Relapse and recurrence in pediatric depression. *Child and Adolescent Psychiatric Clinics of North America, 15,* 1057–1079.

Kerr, J., Patrick, K., Norman, G., Stein, M. B., Calfas, K., Zabinski, M., et al. (2008). Randomized control trial of a behavioral intervention for overweight women: impact on depressive symptoms. *Depression and Anxiety, 25*(7), 555–558.

King, A. C., Ahn, D. F., Atienza, A. A., & Kraemer, H. C. (2008). Exploring refinements in targeted behavioral medicine intervention to advance public health. *Annals of Behavioral Medicine, 35,* 251–260.

Kraemer, H. C., Stice, E., Kazdin, A., Offord, D., & Kupfer, D. (2001). How do risk factors work together? Mediators, moderators, and independent, overlapping, and proxy risk factors. *American Journal of Psychiatry, 158,* 848–856.

Kraemer, H. C., Wilson, G. T., Fairburn, C. G., & Agras, W. S. (2002). Mediators and moderators of treatment effects in randomized clinical trials. *Archives of General Psychiatry, 59,* 877–883.

Kwan, B. M., & Bryan, A. D. (2010). In-task and post-task affective response to exercise: translating exercise intentions into behaviour. *British Journal of Health Psychology, 15*(pt. 1), 115–131.

Lagerberg, D. (2005). Physical activity and mental health in schoolchildren: a complicated relationship. *Acta Paediatrica, 94*(12), 1699–1701.

Lai, S. M., Studenski, S., Richards, L., Perera, S., Reker, D., Rigler, S., et al. (2006). Therapeutic exercise and depressive symptoms after stroke. *Journal of the American Geriatrics Society, 54*(2), 240–247.

Lampinen, P., Heikkinen, R. L., & Ruoppila, I. (2000). Changes in intensity of physical exercise as predictors of depressive symptoms among older adults: an eight-year follow-up. *Preventive Medicine, 30*(5), 371–380.

Lancel, M., Droste, S. K., Sommer, S., & Reul, J. (2003). Influence of regular voluntary exercise on spontaneous and social stress-affected sleep in mice. *European Journal of Neuroscience, 17*(10), 2171–2179.

Larun, L., Nordheim, L.V., Ekeland, E., Hagen, K.B., & Heian, F. (2006). Exercise in prevention and treatment of anxiety and depression among children and young people. *Cochrane Database of Systematic Reviews,* (3): CD004691. DOI: 10.1002/14651858.CD004691.pub2.

Martinsen, E. W. (2008). Physical activity in the prevention and treatment of anxiety and depression. *Nordic Journal of Psychiatry, 62,* 25–29.

Mayberg, H. S. (1997). Limbic-cortical dysregulation: a proposed model of depression. *Journal of Neuropsychiatry and Clinical Neurosciences, 9*(3), 471–481.

McKercher, C. M., Schmidt, M. D., Sanderson, K. A., Patton, G. C., Dwyer, T., & Venn, A. J. (2009). Physical activity and depression in young adults. *American Journal of Preventive Medicine, 36*(2), 161–164.

Merry, S., McDowell, H., Hetrick, S., Bir, J., & Muller, N. (2004). Psychological and/or educational interventions for the prevention of depression in children and adolescents. *Cochrane Database System of Reviews,* (1): CD003380.

Merry, S., McDowell, H., Wild, C. J., Bir, J., & Cunliffe, R. (2004). A randomized placebo-controlled trial of a school-based depression prevention program. *Journal of the American Academy of Child and Adolescent Psychiatry, 43*(5), 538–547.

Milani, R. V., Lavie, C. J., & Cassidy, M. M. (1996). Effects of cardiac rehabilitation and exercise training programs on depression in patients after major coronary events. *American Heart Journal, 132*(4), 726–732.

Mobily, K. E., Rubenstein, L. M., Lemke, J. H., Ohara, M. W., & Wallace, R. B. (1996). Walking and depression in a cohort of older adults: the Iowa 65+ Rural Health Study. *Journal of Aging and Physical Activity, 4*(2), 119–135.

Motl, R. W., Birnbaum, A. S., Kubik, M. Y., & Dishman, R. K. (2004). Naturally occurring changes in physical activity are inversely related to depressive symptoms during early adolescence. *Psychosomatic Medicine, 66*(3), 336–342.

Motl, R. W., Konopack, J. F., McAuley, E., Elavsky, S., Jerome, G. J., & Marquez, D. X. (2005). Depressive symptoms among older adults: long-term reduction after a physical activity intervention. *Journal of Behavioral Medicine, 28*(4), 385–394.

Murphy, J. M., Nierenberg, A. A., Laird, N. M., Monson, R. R., Sobol, A. M., & Leighton, A. H. (2002). Incidence of major depression: prediction from subthreshold categories in the Stirling County Study. *Journal of Affective Disorders, 68*(2–3), 251–259.

National Research Council and Institute of Medicine. (2009). *Preventing mental, emotional, and behavioral disorders among young people: Progress and possibilities.* Washington, DC: The National Academies Press.

Neidig, J. L., Smith, B. A., & Brashers, D. E. (2003). Aerobic exercise training for depressive symptom management in adults living with HIV infection. *Journal of the Association of Nurses in AIDS Care, 14*(2), 30–40.

Norris, R., Carroll, D., & Cochrane, R. (1992). The effects of physical activity and exercise training on psychological stress and well-being in an adolescent population. *Journal of Psychosomatic Research, 36*(1), 55–65.

Office of Applied Studies. (2005). *The NSDUH report: depression among adolescents.* Rockville, MD: Substance Abuse and Mental Health Services Administration.

Paffenbarger, R. S., Lee, I. M., & Leung, R. (1994). Physical activity and personal characteristics associated with depression and suicide in American college men. *Acta Psychiatrica Scandinavica. Supplementum, 377*, 16–22.

Pakkala, I., Read, S., Leinonen, R., Hirvensalo, M., Lintunen, T., & Rantanen, T. (2008). The effects of physical activity counseling on mood among 75- to 81-year-old people: a randomized controlled trial. *Preventive Medicine, 46*(5), 412–418.

Paluska, S. A., & Schwenk, T. L. (2000). Physical activity and mental health—current concepts. *Sports Medicine, 29*(3), 167–180.

Parfitt, G., & Eston, R. G. (2005). The relationship between children's habitual activity level and psychological well-being. *Acta Paediatrica, 94*(12), 1791–1797.

Paus, T., Keshavan, M., & Giedd, J. (2008). Why do many psychiatric disorders emerge during adolescence? *National Review of Neuroscience, 9*(12), 947–957.

Payne, J. K., Held, J., Thorpe, J., & Shaw, H. (2008). Effect of exercise on biomarkers, fatigue, sleep disturbances, and depressive symptoms in older women with breast cancer receiving hormonal therapy. *Oncology Nursing Forum, 35*(4), 635–642.

Perera, B., Torabi, M. R., Jayawardana, G., & Pallethanna, N. (2006). Depressive symptoms among adolescents in Sri Lanka: prevalence and behavioral correlates. *Journal of Adolescent Health, 39*(1), 144–146.

Physical Activity Guidelines Advisory Committee. (2008). *Physical activity guidelines advisory committee report, 2008.* Washington, DC: U.S. Department of Health and Human Services.

Poudevigne, M. S., & O'Connor, P. J. (2006). A review of physical activity patterns in pregnant women and their relationship to psychological health. *Sports Medicine, 36*(1), 19–38.

Reed, J., & Ones, D. S. (2006). The effect of acute aerobic exercise on positive activated affect: a meta-analysis. *Psychology of Sport and Exercise, 7*(5), 477–514.

Ryan, M. P. (2008). The antidepressant effects of physical activity: mediating self-esteem and self-efficacy mechanisms. *Psychology and Health, 23*(3), 279–307.

Ryan, R. M., & Deci, E. L. (2000). Self-determination theory and the facilitation of intrinsic motivation, social development, and well-being. *American Psychologist, 55*(1), 65–78.

Sagatun, A., Sogaard, A. J., Bjertness, E., Selmer, R., & Heyerdahl, S. (2007). The association between weekly hours of physical activity and mental health: a three-year follow-up study of 15-16-year-old students in the city of Oslo, Norway. *BMC Public Health, 7*, 155.

Sanchez-Villegas, A., Ara, I., Guillen-Grima, F., Bes-Rastrollo, M., Varo-Cenarruzabeitia, J. J., & Martinez-Gonzalez, M. A. (2008). Physical activity, sedentary index, and mental disorders in the SUN Cohort Study. *Medicine and Science in Sports and Exercise, 40*(5), 827–834.

Sims, J., Hill, K., Davidson, S., Gunn, J., & Huang, N. (2006). Exploring the feasibility of a community-based strength training program for older people with depressive symptoms and its impact on depressive symptoms. *BMC Geriatrics, 6*, 18.

Singh, N. A., Clements, K. M., & Fiatarone, M. A. (1997). A randomized controlled trial of progressive resistance training in depressed elders. *Journals of Gerontology Series A—Biological Sciences and Medical Sciences, 52*(1), M27–M35.

Sjosten, N., & Kivela, S. L. (2006). The effects of physical exercise on depressive symptoms among the aged: a systematic review. *International Journal of Geriatric Psychiatry, 21*(5), 410–418.

Smith, P. J., Blumenthal, J. A., Babyak, M. A., Georgiades, A., Hinderliter, A., & Sherwood, A. (2007). Effects of exercise and weight loss on depressive symptoms among men and women with hypertension. *Journal of Psychosomatic Research, 63*(5), 463–469.

Steinberg, H., & Sykes, E. A. (1985). Introduction to symposium on endorphins and behavioral processes—review of the literature on endorphins and exercise. *Pharmacology Biochemistry and Behavior, 23*(5), 857–862.

Strawbridge, W. J., Deleger, S., Roberts, R. E., & Kaplan, G. A. (2002). Physical activity reduces the risk of subsequent depression for older adults. *American Journal of Epidemiology, 156*(4), 328–334.

Strine, T. W., Mokdad, A. H., Dube, S. R., Balluz, L. S., Gonzalez, O., Berry, J. T., et al. (2008). The association of depression and anxiety with obesity and unhealthy behaviors among community-dwelling US adults. *General Hospital Psychiatry, 30*(2), 127–137.

Strohle, A. (2009). Physical activity, exercise, depression and anxiety disorders. *Journal of Neural Transmission, 116*(6), 777–784.

Strohle, A., Feller, C., Strasburger, C. J., Heinz, A., & Dimeo, F. (2006). Anxiety modulation by the heart? Aerobic exercise and atrial natriuretic peptide. *Psychoneuroendocrinology, 31*(9), 1127–1130.

Strohle, A., Hofler, M., Pfister, H., Muller, A. G., Hoyer, J., Wittchen, H. U., et al. (2007). Physical activity and prevalence and incidence of mental disorders in adolescents and young adults. *Psychological Medicine, 37*(11), 1657–1666.

Tanaka, H., & Shirakawa, S. (2004). Sleep health, lifestyle and mental health in the Japanese elderly—ensuring sleep to promote a healthy brain and mind. *Journal of Psychosomatic Research, 56*(5), 465–477.

Teychenne, M., Ball, K., & Salmon, J. (2008a). Associations between physical activity and depressive symptoms in women. *International Journal of Behavioral Nutrition and Physical Activity, 5*, 27.

Teychenne, M., Ball, K., & Salmon, J. (2008b). Physical activity and likelihood of depression in adults: a review. *Preventive Medicine, 46*(5), 397–411.

Thakker-Varia, S., & Alder, J. (2009). Neuropeptides in depression: role of VGF. *Behavioural Brain Research, 197*(2), 262–278.

Tomson, L. M., Pangrazi, R. P., Friedman, G., & Hutchison, N. (2003). Childhood depressive symptoms, physical activity and health related fitness. *Journal of Sport and Exercise Psychology, 25*(4), 419–439.

van Praag, H. (2008). Neurogenesis and exercise: past and future directions. *Neuromolecular Medicine, 10*(2), 128–140.

Wise, L. A., Adams-Campbell, L. L., Palmer, J. R., & Rosenberg, L. (2006). Leisure time physical activity in relation to depressive symptoms in the Black Women's Health Study. *Annals of Behavioral Medicine, 32*(1), 68–76.

Wittert, G. A., Livesey, J. H., Espiner, E. A., & Donald, R. A. (1996). Adaptation of the hypothalamopituitary adrenal axis to chronic exercise stress in humans. *Medicine and Science in Sports and Exercise, 28*(8), 1015–1019.

Youngstedt, S. D. (2005). Effects of exercise on sleep. *Clinics in Sports Medicine, 24*(2), 355–365.

Chapter 7
Physical Activity as Treatment for Obesity

Elissa Jelalian and Amy Sato

The last two decades has seen a dramatic increase in the prevalence of overweight and obesity among all segments of the US population, including children, adolescents, and adults (Ogden, Carroll, & Flegal, 2008). While these increases have been observed across the population, ethnic minority groups have been impacted differentially (Ogden et al., 2008). Given the increased prevalence of obesity, considerable attention has been focused on models of intervention for this challenging concern. This chapter focuses on the role of physical activity in the treatment of obesity, with an emphasis on interventions with pediatric samples. In particular, we provide an overview of pediatric obesity treatment approaches, discuss the potential mechanisms through which physical activity impacts outcome, present a review of interventions that include manipulation of physical activity, and conclude with recommendations for best practices and future research directions. While our focus is on the importance of physical activity for pediatric weight control, a number of concepts are illustrated through research conducted with adults. The reader is referred to several excellent reviews for consideration of physical activity as a component of weight control interventions for adults (Donnelly et al., 2009; Jakicic, 2006).

E. Jelalian (✉)
Psychiatry and Human Behavior, Brown Medical School,
Coro West, One Hoppin Street, Providence, RI 02903, USA
e-mail: Elissa_Jelalian@brown.edu

A. Sato
Department of Psychology, Kent State University, 144 Kent Hall, Kent, OH 44242, USA
e-mail: asato2@kent.edu

A.L. Meyer and T.P. Gullotta (eds.), *Physical Activity Across the Lifespan*,
Issues in Children's and Families' Lives 12, DOI 10.1007/978-1-4614-3606-5_7,
© Springer Science+Business Media New York 2012

Physical Activity as a Significant Component of Obesity Intervention

A recent review summarizes recommended treatment options for pediatric obesity, ranging from least to most intensive (Spear et al., 2007). Physical activity is considered an essential component at each stage. The first two stages are prevention focused, with attention to several eating and behavioral recommendations, such as increased consumption of fruits and vegetables, limiting "screen time" (e.g., television viewing, computer use, video gaming, etc.) to 2 hours or less per day, ensuring daily physical activity, and addressing eating behaviors (e.g., daily breakfast). The next recommended stages are more intensive and involve "structured weight management" interventions, including a plan for balanced diet (emphasizing a decreased amount of calorie-dense food), further limiting screen time and increasing physical activity, implementing child and/or parent monitoring (e.g., of dietary intake), and performing medical screening (e.g., checking vital signs such as blood pressure). The third stage involves "comprehensive multidisciplinary intervention," which includes parental involvement (especially for younger children); ongoing assessment of diet, physical activity, and weight; structured behavioral programming (e.g., monitoring, goal setting); parent/caregiver training; and structured interventions for dietary and physical activity. This stage of intervention is typically more appropriate for children with higher BMI or children who have been unsuccessful with less intensive approaches. Finally, more intensive options are available for children who are already experiencing medical complications related to obesity and need additional help. This includes continued diet and activity counseling plus consideration of meal replacement, medication, very-low-energy diet, and surgery, and would only be delivered within a pediatric weight management center or residential setting with medical supervision. As can be readily observed from these recommended intervention approaches, increasing physical activity is a key component of weight control at each stage.

Potential Mechanisms

Much of the research examining the mechanisms through which physical activity impacts weight status has been conducted with adults. We include a review of these studies with the expectation that many of the same processes would pertain to youth as well. There are several potential mechanisms through which physical activity may impact weight status. At the simplest level, physical activity is a key factor in the energy balance equation. Weight status is impacted by energy intake (calories consumed) and energy expenditure, the latter consisting of resting metabolic rate, the thermic effect of food, and physical activity. The most immediately modifiable component of energy expenditure is physical activity, making it an obvious component of weight control interventions. Because it is challenging to accomplish a caloric deficit sufficient to result in weight loss through increasing energy expenditure alone, physical activity is commonly prescribed in combination with reduction in energy intake.

Exercise may impact weight management through a variety of psychological as well as physiological mechanisms (for a thorough review, see Baker & Brownell, 2000). Participation in physical activity has been shown to have positive effects on a number of psychological constructs including mood, self-efficacy, motivation, adherence, and stress, which may in turn impact weight control behaviors. In particular, exercise can result in improvements in mood, increased self-efficacy, decreased stress, and increased motivation. These benefits may in turn translate to increased ability or interest related to weight control. While it is difficult to separate the causal role of psychological variables from the physiological effects of exercise (Baker & Brownell, 2000), for the purposes of this review potential physiological and psychological variables are considered separately.

Physiological Mechanisms

In theory, there are several key physiological mechanisms through which physical activity potentially impacts weight regulation. Exercise may affect weight loss through at least three different physiological mechanisms, including energy expenditure, metabolic rate and the preservation of lean body mass, and appetite regulation.

Energy Expenditure

Positive energy balance occurs when nutrient intake exceeds nutrient oxidation, and prolonged positive energy balance results in obesity (Maffeis & Castellani, 2007). At the most basic level, exercise increases energy (i.e., caloric) expenditure and, when energy intake is held constant, this results in a negative energy balance with the potential for weight loss. However, this is unlikely to be a primary mechanism in weight loss or maintenance given that even vigorous physical activity produces relatively small changes in caloric expenditure (Baker & Brownell, 2000).

Metabolic Rate and Body Composition

Second, exercise may be linked to weight loss through increased resting metabolic rate (RMR) and preservation of lean body mass (LBM). Specifically, it has been hypothesized that exercise in combination with dietary restriction may lead to increased fat loss and protection of LBM, which may compensate for the expected decrease in RMR usually observed during weight loss and therefore aid in weight management by increasing total energy expenditure (Catenacci & Wyatt, 2007; Stiegler & Cunliffe, 2006). This is one of the hypotheses that have been used to explain why successful maintenance of weight loss in the long-term (e.g., >1 year) is associated with high levels of physical activity (e.g., Catenacci et al., 2008). Based on their review, Stiegler and Cunliffe (2006) concluded that a considerable number of regular exercise bouts are needed for exercise to reduce fat and increase fat free mass. Although high-intensity aerobic exercise has the potential to increase resting energy expenditure by 5–15 % in the short-term (i.e., 24–48 hours; Hunter, Weinsier, Bamman, & Larson, 1998); overall, the evidence regarding the impact of exercise on RMR is inconclusive (Stiegler & Cunliffe, 2006). One study found an increase in RMR among women who participated in a 20-week strength training program (Byrne & Wilmore, 2001); however, many studies have failed to find an effect of exercise on RMR. For example, Jennings and colleagues (2009) failed to find an effect on RMR among previously sedentary adults with type 2 diabetes who had participated in a 6-month exercise program, regardless of whether the exercise program consisted of aerobic training, resistance training, or combined aerobic and resistance exercise training.

Exercise may also have beneficial effects on fat balance through fat oxidation. The role of exercise therefore becomes important because skeletal muscle (used during exercise) is the most important regulator of fat oxidation and can positively impact on fat balance and fat mass (Maffeis & Castellani, 2007). In normal weight individuals, regular aerobic exercise increases fat oxidation during exercise and in postabsorptive conditions (Maffeis & Castellani, 2007). Importantly, the total amount of fat oxidation during and following exercise varies depending on exercise intensity and the percentage of energy fat oxidation, with maximum fat oxidation occurring at moderately-intense physical activity (<65 % $VO2_{peak}$) among adults (Achten, Gleeson, & Jeukendrup, 2002; Maffeis & Castellani, 2007).

Dietary Intake and Appetite Regulation

Another potential mechanism through which exercise may affect weight status is by influencing appetite (i.e., subjective feelings of hunger) and dietary intake. In their review of the literature Martins, Morgan, and Truby (2008) suggest that appetite control, including the coupling of energy expenditure and energy intake, is disrupted when the level of physical activity is low and that exercise may "fine tune" the physiological mechanisms that regulate appetite in two ways. First, they suggest that exercise leads to improved energy compensation, such that changes in energy intake during a meal are detected and compensated for at the following meal, thereby leading to improved appetite control in the short-term (Martins, Morgan et al., 2008). Second, they suggest that exercise improves the coupling of energy intake and energy expenditure in the long term, such that changes in energy expenditure are followed by proportional changes in energy intake, so that a constant body weight is maintained over time.

In addition, the impact of acute and chronic exercise on plasma levels of appetite-related hormones appears to be favorable in terms of appetite regulation and may lead to improved appetite control in response to exercise (Martins, Morgan et al., 2008; Martins, Robertson, & Morgan, 2008). For example, recent work suggests that the impact of exercise on plasma levels of appetite-related hormones, such as leptin and ghrelin (Martins, Morgan et al., 2008), or postingestive satiety peptides (i.e., postprandial levels of glucagon-like peptide-1, polypeptide YY, and pancreatic polypeptide; Martins, Robertson et al., 2008) may be important to appetite regulation. Associations between exercise and appetite regulation likely vary depending on factors such as dietary restraint, body weight, and gender (Martins, Morgan et al., 2008).

Psychological Mechanisms

There are several psychological mechanisms through which physical activity may be linked to weight loss, including improved overall mood, self-efficacy, body image, motivation, adherence, and stress.

Mood

Exercise has consistently been linked to improved overall well-being and mood (Baker & Brownell, 2000). Several investigations support the relationship between physical activity and mood in pediatric populations. An inverse relationship between physical activity and depressive symptoms was observed in a large-scale prospective study of adolescents (Motl, Birnbaum, Kubik, & Dishman, 2004). Crews, Lochbaum, and Landers (2004) examined the effects of a structured aerobic physical fitness program on psychological well-being in low-income Hispanic children. Children in this program reported less depression and higher self-esteem than controls who engaged in limited physical activity. Brosnahan, Steffen, Lytle, Patterson, and Boostrom (2004), in a study of over 1,800 Hispanic and non-Hispanic White adolescents, found that greater levels of physical activity were associated with fewer symptoms of sadness and depression.

Interestingly, associations between mood and anxiety may vary depending upon type of exercise and baseline mood. For example, one study found decreased state anxiety in response to 8 weeks of aerobic step exercise or resistance training, with similar reductions in state anxiety for step exercise and resistance training when baseline state anxiety was high, but only a reduction in the step aerobics group when baseline anxiety was low (Hale & Raglin, 2002). This is important with respect to weight loss because improved mood may reduce the frequency of negative affect cues (which may trigger eating or binging) and also lead individuals to have greater emotional and cognitive resources, motivation, and energy to sustain a commitment to weight-loss (Baker & Brownell, 2000).

Self-Efficacy

Enhanced self-efficacy is another potential psychological mechanism through exercise may affect obesity. Baker and Brownell (2000) note that enhanced self-efficacy may lead to greater confidence in the ability to make behavioral changes and lose weight. Important to weight control, exercise has the potential not only to increase exercise self-efficacy but may also foster general weight-loss self-efficacy, with positive effects on eating self-efficacy and dietary compliance (Baker & Brownell, 2000). Associations between physical exercise and enhanced self-efficacy have been observed in adults as well as adolescents. For example, preadolescents enrolled in an after-school physical activity program had improved exercise self-efficacy, with significant correlations between exercise self-efficacy and number of exercise sessions completed (Annesi, 2006). Among a primarily African American sample of adolescents, self-efficacy for healthful eating moderated the association between physical activity and BMI percentile, further underscoring the role of self-efficacy in connection with exercise and weight status (Gamble, Parra, & Beech, 2009).

Body Image

Improved body image in response to exercise may also potentially influence weight status (Baker & Brownell, 2000). Similar to self-efficacy and exercise, there is a relatively small amount of research in this area; however, the available evidence suggests that exercise is linked to improved perceptions about one's body. For example, among overweight and obese postmenopausal women, higher levels of cardiorespiratory fitness were associated with favorable psychosocial correlates, including body esteem (Karelis et al., 2008). Children participating in a 6-week circuit training intervention had improved body esteem at postintervention compared to controls, with greater improvement in girls compared to boys, but this difference was not maintained at follow-up (Duncan, Al-Nakeeb, & Nevill, 2009). Finally, Baker and Brownell (2000) note that exercise can lead to changes in body shape which can, in turn, positively influence self-image and potentially buffer against the discouragement that individuals with poor body image may experience in response to only modest weight losses.

Motivation

The relationship between physical activity and eating behaviors may also be explained by motivational mechanisms (Mata et al., 2009). Among overweight/obese women participating in a 1-year intervention focused on promoting physical activity and internal motivation for exercise and weight loss, higher exercise motivation predicted improved eating self-regulation above and beyond general self-determination and treatment motivation (Mata et al., 2009). In addition, the association between physical activity and eating regulation was mediated by general self-determination, treatment motivation, and intrinsic exercise motivation (Mata et al., 2009).

Stress and Coping

Finally, chronic stress has been implicated in the development of obesity by inter-acting with both energy expenditure and energy intake (De Vriendt, Moreno, & De Henauw, 2009). Generally, stressors represent a broad array of phenomenon that can trigger the stress system (i.e., Hypothalamic–Pituitary–Adrenal axis, sympathetic adrenomedullary axes) and can be psychological or social in nature (e.g., demand-ing job, relational problems, absence of social support) (De Vriendt et al., 2009; Faraday, 2006). There is some research to suggest that one of the pathways through which chronic stress may be associated with the development of obesity is through a decrease in physical activity and the resultant decrease energy expenditure (De Vriendt et al., 2009). For example, among adolescents participating in an exercise program there was a negative association between level of perceived stress and lev-els of physical activity (Norris, Carroll, & Cochrane, 1992). Although there is rela-tively little research examining the associations between perceived stress and the amount of physical activity a person obtains, it is conceivable that perceived chronic stress may interfere with participation in physical activity. For example, a person who perceives multiple environmental pressures (e.g., demanding job, commute to work, caregiver responsibilities) may feel that there is not enough time to devote to physical activity. This contextual feeling of not having enough time (e.g., due to balancing work and family demands) has been implicated in food consumption and food preparation patterns (Blake et al., 2009; Jabs & Devine, 2006) that have impli-cations for obesity risk. On the other hand, physical activity appears to be an adap-tive way to cope with stress. There is a small body of literature to suggest that physical activity may buffer the relationship between psychosocial stress and obe-sity, thereby exerting a beneficial effect (Holmes, Ekkekakis, & Eisenmann, 2010). For example, a study of adolescents and young adults ages 12–24 years found that physical activity buffered the effects of chronic stress on adiposity, suggesting that physical activity is a protective factor (Yin, Davis, Moore, & Treiber, 2005). This may be especially important for those with a propensity for stress-induced eating (Torres & Nowson, 2007). Additional research is needed to better understand how chronic psychological stress affects participation in physical activity,

In summary, there are several potential physiological and psychological mecha-nisms through which physical activity may impact weight status. Although the majority of the research in this area has focused on adult populations, emerging studies with children and adolescents suggest that these variables are germane to pediatric populations.

Evidenced Based Interventions Incorporating Physical Activity

Studies evaluating exercise as a component of pediatric weight control trials date to the 1980s. In an early study with school age children, adding aerobic exercise to diet led to greater reductions in percent overweight than diet alone in the short term (Epstein, Wing, Penner, & Kress, 1985). While some studies have not documented similar changes in weight status with the addition of physical activity (Rocchini et al., 1988), there are potential benefits in other health outcomes, such as improved fitness and cardiovascular health, as well as mental health associated with exercise (e.g., Goldfield, Raynor, & Epstein, 2002, Goldfield et al., 2007; Yeter et al., 2006). Among a sample of overweight or obese breast cancer survivors, greater levels of self reported physical activity were associated with lower levels of depressive symptoms (Yeter et al., 2006). Similarly, among overweight and obese children participating in a health promotion intervention, increases in level of physical activity were positively associated with body satisfaction and overall physical self-worth, independent of changes in BMI (Goldfield et al., 2007).

Physical activity recommendations are widely included as a significant component of weight control interventions (Oude Luttikhuis et al., 2009). A recent review addresses the efficacy of exercise as an intervention strategy for overweight children and adolescents (Atlantis, Barnes, & Singh, 2006). A summary of investigations indicates significant reductions in percent body fat associated with exercise interventions, although the majority of the studies examined combined physical activity with dietary restriction, making it difficult to evaluate the unique contribution of exercise. The review also provides some evidence to suggest that a higher dose of weekly exercise, as defined by 155–180 min/week results in better outcomes than less activity (120–150 min/week). The authors also interestingly observe that there are no studies examining the benefits of 60 min of physical activity daily on most days of the week, despite the fact that this level of exercise is prescribed by a number of expert committees. Given that exercise prescription is assumed to be important to either weight control or cardiovascular health, research questions have focused on the type, intensity, and frequency of physical activity that is most beneficial for overweight children and adolescents. We review these three categories of physical activity and then discuss decreased sedentary behavior as an alternative approach.

Type of Physical Activity

Several investigations have focused on the utility of lifestyle activity compared to programmed exercise in weight control interventions, where lifestyle activity is defined as physical activity that can be easily incorporated into a child's daily routine—e.g., walking to school instead of taking the bus, and programmed aerobic exercise is defined as planned activity for a certain period of time with the specific goal of increasing heart rate. Lifestyle and programmed aerobic exercise led to comparable reductions in weight status at the end of treatment; however, lifestyle was superior at follow-up, conducted 11 months after the start of treatment (Epstein, Wing, Koeske, Ossip, & Beck, 1982). A subsequent randomized controlled trial with school age children compared three different activity interventions combined with dietary intervention—aerobic exercise, lifestyle activity, and calisthenics (Epstein, Wing, Koeske, & Valoski, 1985). Comparable decreases in percent overweight were observed across the groups immediately following the end of treatment; however, at 5-year follow-up, the lifestyle intervention was superior to calisthenics

(Epstein, McCurley, Wing, & Valoski, 1990), and at 10-years, both lifestyle and aerobic were superior to calisthenics (Epstein, Valoski, Wing, & McCurley, 1994).

More recent investigations have examined the utility of resistance training as a weight control strategy. In a small randomized controlled trial, overweight adolescent Latino boys were assigned to twice weekly resistance training or a no-treatment control condition (Shaibi et al., 2006). Adolescents randomized to resistance training significantly increased both insulin sensitivity and body strength relative to the control condition after the 16-week intervention. There is some evidence to suggest that resistance training may be an exercise modality that serves to increase participation in physical activity in adolescent males. Boys on an ice hockey team who were randomly assigned to 4 months of resistance training versus typical team training demonstrated greater energy expenditure through spontaneous physical activity both at the end of the intervention and at 12-month follow-up (Eiholzer et al., 2009). While this was a highly selective sample and was not focused on weight control, the findings provide an interesting direction for further investigation. In particular, it would be of interest to determine whether participation in strength training serves to enhance motivation for aerobic or lifestyle activity in a sample of adolescents who are not participating in a structured sport, as this may serve as an innovative strategy to increase physical activity.

Our own research group has conducted two studies comparing the efficacy of supervised aerobic exercise to physical activity obtained in the context of peer building activities. In the first study, overweight/obese adolescents were randomized to group based cognitive behavioral weight control treatment combined with either "adventure therapy" based on Outward Bound (CBT + PEAT) or supervised aerobic exercise (CBT + EXER; Jelalian, Mehlenbeck, Lloyd-Richardson, Birmaher, & Wing, 2006). Adolescents who received both interventions demonstrated significant reductions in BMI over time, with no significant advantage to the peer activity condition. However, there was a significant difference in the percentage of adolescents maintaining a minimum 10 pound weight loss at 10-month follow-up, with 35 % in the CBT + PEAT condition and 12 % in the CBT + EXER condition. A second investigation compared the same two treatment conditions in a larger sample of adolescents. Adolescents randomized to both treatment conditions demonstrated significant reductions in BMI and z-BMI that were maintained at 12 months; however, there was no advantage associated with the peer condition (Jelalian et al., 2010). Taken together, these studies suggest that there may be a number of physical activity interventions that support weight control among adolescents. One potential direction for future research is to examine whether certain activities are better suited for particular subgroups of adolescents.

Physical Activity Intensity

An early review of the area suggested potential advantages associated with high intensity exercise on energy expenditure and weight control (Hunter et al., 1998). The proposed mechanisms included volume of work and greater resting energy expenditure for the time period following exercise. Studies conducted since then are equivocal with regard to support for this conclusion. In a cross-sectional study involving a large sample of adolescents not selected for weight status, higher amounts of vigorous, but not moderate physical activity were associated with lower percent body fat (Gutin, Yin, Humphries, & Barbeau, 2005). Findings from an intervention study are inconsistent. Adolescents between the ages of 13 and 16 years were randomized to one of three treatment conditions: lifestyle education alone, lifestyle education combined with moderate intensity physical activity, or lifestyle education and high intensity physical activity (Gutin et al., 2002). Activity sessions were offered after school 5 days a week. Participants who attended at least 2 days a week of activity in either the moderate or high intensity condition demonstrated greater decrease in visceral adipose tissue and improvement in cardiovascular fitness than those who received education alone. Differences were not observed between the moderate and high intensity conditions, potentially because it was difficult to keep adolescents in this group in the target heart rate zone.

Two recent investigations have looked more specifically at the utility of interval training as a component of weight control intervention for adolescents and adults. Adult patients with metabolic syndrome were randomized to receive either continuous moderate exercise (70 % of highest measured heart rate) or aerobic interval training (90 % of highest measured heart rate) three times per week for a period of 16 weeks (Tjonna et al., 2008). Based on data collected at the end of the 16-week study, both types of exercise resulted in modest weight losses and aerobic interval training was more effective than continuous moderate exercise at reducing risk factors for metabolic syndrome and improving parameters such as blood glucose and lipogenesis. A recent study compared multidisciplinary intervention including counseling, diet, and exercise to aerobic interval training in a sample of overweight/obese adolescents (Tjonna et al., 2009). Aerobic interval training was defined as four times 4-min intervals at 90 % of maximal heart rate, with each interval separated by 3 min of moderate exercise. Interval training occurred twice a week for a total of 3 months while the multidisciplinary program was twice a month for 12 months. Adolescents randomized to interval training demonstrated modest but significantly greater reductions in BMI and percent body fat at both 3 and 12 months, as well as greater decrease in systolic blood pressure and greater improvement in peak oxygen pulse.

Physical Activity Dose

A number of studies have compared the effects of single continuous versus accumulated shorter term bouts of physical activity on body weight and cardiovascular risk factors. A recent review of the area summarizes a total of 23 studies examining both immediate and long-term effects on a range of health parameters (Murphy, Blair, & Murtagh, 2009). With regard to short-term effects (i.e., within 48 h of exercise), the tentative conclusion from this review is that breaking activity into shorter bouts does not alter its ability to elicit modest reduction in fasting or postprandial lipemia. With regard to long-term effects, there were generally no differences between accumulated versus continuous physical activity of the same duration on improvements in cardiovascular fitness, including VO$_2$ max and blood pressure. Effects on body composition were inconsistent and it was further determined that neither continuous nor accumulated bouts of moderate intensity activity ranging from 60 to 200 min/week were sufficient to improve blood lipid levels.

Other studies have specifically examined the impact of short versus long bouts of exercise on weight status. In the only randomized controlled trial evaluating this question, sedentary obese females were randomized to prescription of several short bouts (i.e., multiple 10-min bouts of exercise per day) versus one long (i.e., continuous) bout of physical activity per day, primarily consisting of walking (Jakicic, Wing, Butler, & Robertson, 1995). Overall, exercising in multiple short bouts per day was more effective in supporting adherence to exercise prescription, and equally effective to continuous exercise in improving cardiovascular endurance and producing weight loss. There was a trend for women randomized to the short bout condition to lose more weight than those randomized to long bout, −8.9 kg versus −6.4 kg. A nonrandomized study with female college students found significant increases in VO$_2$ max, and decreases in BMI and skinfolds, regardless of whether participants exercised for three 10-min intervals, two 15-min intervals, or one 30-min interval (Schmidt, Biwer, & Kalscheuer, 2001).

Additional evidence is provided through cross-sectional studies examining the relationship between participation in bouts versus continuous physical activity and weight status. A recent investigation examined the importance of bouts of moderate-to-vigorous physical activity above and beyond total volume of activity in predicting overweight and obesity in school age children and adolescents (Mark & Janssen, 2009). Based on review of the NHANES data, these investigators found that moderate-to-vigorous physical activity accumulated in bouts predicated adiposity independent of the total volume of activity. A similar finding was reported in a study of adults, with accumulating moderate-to-vigorous physical activity in bouts less than 10 min related to lower BMI and smaller waist circumference even after controlling for potential confounding variables such as total activity (Strath, Holleman, Ronis, Swartz, & Richardson, 2008). Although in the same study, bouts of physical activity, defined as ≥10 min, were more strongly associated with lower BMI and waist circumference than were nonbouts of activity (<10 min). Taken together, research that compares short versus long bouts of physical activity suggests potential advantages to the accumulation of short bouts of physical activity, including beneficial effects on weight status, BMI, and cardiovascular health. The benefits of accumulated short bouts of physical activity have been observed among adult and child populations, and are potentially related to increased adherence with exercise recommendations.

Reduction of Sedentary Behavior

An alternative to prescribing increased physical activity is a recommendation for decreasing sedentary behavior, commonly defined as "screen time"—e.g., television viewing, computer use, video gaming, etc. There are two potential mechanisms through which decreasing sedentary behavior may be effective: (1) children may reallocate time spent in sedentary behavior to more physically rigorous activity; and/or (2) reducing screen time may result in decreased energy intake secondary to fewer opportunities for eating (e.g., watching less television may decrease amount of snacks consumed) (Epstein, Paluch, Kilanowski, & Raynor, 2004). In the first study examining the efficacy of decreasing sedentary behavior, school age children were randomly assigned to one of three behavioral weight control treatments including reinforcement for decreasing sedentary behavior, increasing physical activity, or doing both (Epstein et al., 1995). Both at the end of treatment and at 12-month follow-up, the group that was reinforced for decreasing sedentary behavior demonstrated greater reduction in percent overweight than the group reinforced for increasing physical activity. A subsequent study crossed decreasing sedentary and increasing physical activity with high versus low conditions of each of these (Epstein, Paluch, Gordy, & Dorn, 2000). Comparable reductions in percent overweight were observed in all four conditions, indicating that dose of physical activity did not impact outcome, and that children did equally well regardless of whether they were prescribed increased physical activity or decreased sedentary behavior. Finally, a recent study with young children (4–7 years) both overweight and at risk of overweight examined the use of a monitoring device to control television viewing and computer use (Epstein et al., 2008). The intervention resulted in significant decrease in sedentary behaviors, which was associated with significant reduction in z-BMI maintained through 24 months.

As noted above, reduction in sedentary behavior may impact energy balance by encouraging children to reallocate leisure time to physical activity or by reducing opportunities for eating. In a study designed to explore the mechanisms through which reducing sedentary behavior is effective, Epstein and colleagues (2004) evaluated whether weight outcomes were related to substituting physical activity for sedentary behavior or reducing calorie intake. Boys were significantly more likely than girls to substitute physical activity for sedentary behavior and there appeared to be some advantage to replacing sedentary behavior with physical activity rather than decreasing intake. Taken together, this series of studies suggests that prescribing reduction of sedentary behavior is a viable alternative to recommending increased physical activity and may be particularly effective for boys and those from lower socioeconomic backgrounds (Epstein et al., 2008).

Best Practices Related to Physical Activity and Obesity Treatment

Based on review of the existing literature, there is evidence to support physical activity as a key component of weight control interventions for both pediatric and adult populations. As a weight control strategy for treatment of an overweight/obese individual, physical activity should be prescribed in tandem with reduction of dietary intake, as the energy deficit required for weight loss is most likely accomplished through modification of both intake and expenditure. Although the prescribed amount and intensity of physical activity will likely vary depending on the person's initial level of physical fitness, recommendations for pediatric populations is for gradual increase of activity to 60 min daily for most days of the week. Of note, this recommendation is to support health in all pediatric samples and is not specific to weight loss goals. Further research is needed to more specifically examine recommended best practices with regard to the duration and intensity of physical activity required.

Whether an individual chooses to participate in aerobic activity accumulated throughout the day in several short (i.e., 10-min) bouts or in one continuous exercise session or in lifestyle activity, the benefits of physical activity appear to be fairly comparable. Therefore, what becomes important in practice is the ability of an individual to adhere to the exercise regimen over time. As reviewed earlier, this may be one advantage of lifestyle activities which can be accumulated throughout the day and easily incorporated into routines. Given the research suggesting that short bouts of accumulated activity may promote adherence, it is worthwhile considering the best "fit" for each individual. This flexible approach is underscored by research with adolescents suggesting that different forms of physical activity (e.g., activity involving peers versus supervised aerobic) may have similar results with regard to weight reduction. Given the equivocal findings regarding exercise intensity, it is not possible to identify one best practice in this regard. While there is some research to suggest that interval training may enhance the health benefits of exercise, these findings are preliminary and additional work is needed in this area. Therefore, best practice for physical activity as a component of obesity treatment requires that an individual exercise on most days of the week, but is not rigid about the exact method of accumulating activity and instead underscores the importance of adherence over time.

Finally, in tandem with the goal of increasing physical activity in the treatment of obesity, focus should be placed on reducing sedentary behaviors. In particular, reducing time spent watching television and on the computer (i.e., "screen time") may have beneficial effects. Current guidelines suggest that among youth, "screen time" should be limited to no more than 2 h per day (Spear et al., 2007).

Future Directions

Several directions are suggested for future research. First, additional work is needed to identify strategies for increasing physical activity participation among overweight youth. While a number of studies have examined factors that support and hinder participation in physical activity in children and adolescents (Sallis, Prochaska, & Taylor, 2000), very little research has been conducted to improve adherence to exercise participation in the context of weight control interventions. This is an area of particular concern for overweight/obese children and adolescents, as they tend to perceive more barriers to physical activity and have a less favorable attitude toward participation in physical activity than their normal weight peers (Deforche, De

Bourdeaudhuij, & Tanghe, 2006). Body related barriers were the most commonly identified barriers to exercise participation among overweight youth (Zabinski, Saelens, Stein, Hayden-Wade, & Wilfley, 2003), and weight criticism during physical activity has been related to more negative attitudes toward and decreased involvement in physical activity (Faith, Leone, Ayers, Heo, & Pietrobelli, 2002). This line of research suggests the need for innovative alternatives to encourage participation in physical activity, including those that address perceived criticism and teasing as well as those that offer an incremental approach to exercise involvement.

One potential approach is that of "gaming" as a strategy for increasing physical activity, particularly among adolescents. Recent research has shown that energy expenditure may be greater during more "active" wireless computer games than typically sedentary gaming, although not as great as what would be anticipated if actually participating in the sport (Graves, Stratton, Ridgers, & Cable, 2007). In a recent innovative study, energy expenditure and heart rate were measured during video gaming and treadmill walking in a small sample of 10–13 year olds, who were primarily within the normal weight range (Graf, Pratt, Hester, & Short, 2009). Energy expenditure was measured through indirect calorimetry. Results indicated that Wii games and Dance Dance Revolution resulted in increased energy expenditure compared to watching television at rest, and energy expenditure and heart rate were similar to or greater than that observed during moderate intensity walking (Graf et al., 2009). Finally, it is notable that the use of gaming to increase physical activity may have beneficial effects for adults as well as youth. For example, Lanningham-Foster and colleagues (2009) found that energy expenditure for children and adults increased significantly when playing Nintendo Wii Boxing compared to sitting, standing, or a conventional video game (Lanningham-Foster et al., 2009). To our knowledge, there have been no studies explicitly examining energy expenditure through gaming in an overweight sample of youth. This would be an interesting step toward potentially recommending active gaming as an alternative strategy for increasing physical activity.

Once established, physical activity patterns can be difficult to maintain (Wilcox, Dowda, Wegley, & Ory, 2009). Research regarding strategies to support maintenance of physical activity, including improved adherence, reduction of barriers, and development of environmental supports and effective policy is also of importance. There are fewer interventions demonstrating long-term maintenance of behavior change related to physical activity (Wilcox et al., 2009) and predictors of physical activity adoption have been found to differ from those of physical activity maintenance in adult samples (Williams et al., 2008). Interventions that are multilevel and can develop sustainable synergies between home, school policy (e.g., additional recess time, change in PE curriculum), and community (e.g., walkable community), may be particularly promising in both development of and maintenance of physical activity goals in children and adolescents (DeBate et al., 2009).

Research examining the physiological and psychological mechanisms through which physical activity impacts health and psychological outcomes could help to inform both the development and maintenance of physical activity habits among overweight populations. Identification of key mechanisms may serve to elucidate psychological, physiological, and environmental level factors that serve to both support and hinder participation in physical activity.

Finally, relatively little research has examined the impact of interventions that provide for substantive increases in vigorous physical activity. Interventions commonly prescribe increases in moderate level activity, with very few studies specifically examining the benefits of vigorous physical activity, which arguably has unique benefits particularly when outcomes of body fat and aerobic fitness are considered (Gutin, 2008). Further research regarding optimal and achievable physical activity intensity and duration has the potential to greatly enhance the efficacy of pediatric weight control interventions.

References

Achten, J., Gleeson, M., & Jeukendrup, A. E. (2002). Determination of the exercise intensity that elicits maximal fat oxidation. *Medicine and Science in Sports and Exercise, 34*, 92–97.

Annesi, J. J. (2006). Relations of physical self-concept and self-efficacy with frequency of voluntary physical activity in preadolescents: Implications for after-school care programming. *Journal of Psychosomatic Research, 61*, 515–520.

Atlantis, E., Barnes, E. H., & Singh, M. A. (2006). Efficacy of exercise for treating overweight in children and adolescents: A systematic review. *International Journal of Obesity, 30*, 1027–1040.

Baker, C. W., & Brownell, K. D. (2000). Physical activity and maintenance of weight loss: Physiological and psychological mechanisms. In B. Christopher (Ed.), *Physical activity and obesity* (pp. 311–328). Champaign, IL: Human Kinetics.

Blake, C. E., Devine, C. M., Wethington, E., Jastran, M., Farrell, T. J., & Bisogni, C. A. (2009). Employed parents' satisfaction with food-choice coping strategies. Influence of gender and structure. *Appetite, 52*, 711–719.

Brosnahan, J., Steffen, L. M., Lytle, L., Patterson, J., & Boostrom, A. (2004). The relation between physical activity and mental health among Hispanic and non-Hispanic white adolescents. *Archives of Pediatrics & Adolescent Medicine, 158*, 818–823.

Byrne, H. K., & Wilmore, J. H. (2001). The effects of a 20-week exercise training program on resting metabolic rate in previously sedentary, moderately obese women. *International Journal of Sport Nutrition and Exercise Metabolism, 11*, 15–31.

Catenacci, V. A., Ogden, L. G., Stuht, J., Phelan, S., Wing, R. R., Hill, J. O., et al. (2008). Physical activity patterns in the National Weight Control Registry. *Obesity (Silver Spring), 16*, 153–161.

Catenacci, V. A., & Wyatt, H. R. (2007). The role of physical activity in producing and maintaining weight loss. *Nature Clinical Practice. Endocrinology & Metabolism, 3*, 518–529.

Crews, D. J., Lochbaum, M. R., & Landers, D. M. (2004). Aerobic physical activity effects on psychological well-being in low-income Hispanic children. *Perceptual and Motor Skills, 98*, 319–324.

DeBate, R. D., Baldwin, J. A., Thompson, Z., Nickelson, J., Alfonso, M. L., Bryant, C. A., et al. (2009). *VERB* ™ Summer Scorecard: Findings from a multi-level community-based physical activity intervention for tweens. *American Journal of Community Psychology, 44*, 363–373.

Deforche, B. I., De Bourdeaudhuij, I. M., & Tanghe, A. P. (2006). Attitude toward physical activity in normal-weight, overweight and obese adolescents. *Journal of Adolescent Health, 38*, 560–568.

De Vriendt, T., Moreno, L. A., & De Henauw, S. (2009). Chronic stress and obesity in adolescents: Scientific evidence and methodological issues for epidemiological research. *Nutrition, Metabolism, and Cardiovascular Diseases, 19*, 511–519.

Donnelly, J. E., Blair, S. N., Jakicic, J. M., Manore, M. M., Rankin, J. W., & Smith, B. K. (2009). American College of Sports Medicine Position Stand. Appropriate physical activity intervention strategies for weight loss and prevention of weight regain for adults. *Medicine and Science in Sports and Exercise, 41*, 459–471.

Duncan, M. J., Al-Nakeeb, Y., & Nevill, A. M. (2009). Effects of a 6-week circuit training intervention on body esteem and body mass index in British primary school children. *Body Image, 6*, 216–220.

Eiholzer, U., Meinhardt, U., Petro, R., Witassek, F., Gutzwiller, F., & Gasser, T. (2009). High-intensity training increases spontaneous physical activity in children: A randomized controlled study. *Journal of Pediatrics, 156*, 242–246.

Epstein, L. H., McCurley, J., Wing, R. R., & Valoski, A. (1990). Five-year follow-up of family-based behavioral treatments for childhood obesity. *Journal of Consulting and Clinical Psychology, 58*, 661–664.

Epstein, L. H., Paluch, R. A., Gordy, C. C., & Dorn, J. (2000). Decreasing sedentary behaviors in treating pediatric obesity. *Archives of Pediatrics & Adolescent Medicine, 154*, 220–226.

Epstein, L. H., Paluch, R. A., Kilanowski, C. K., & Raynor, H. A. (2004). The effect of reinforcement or stimulus control to reduce sedentary behavior in the treatment of pediatric obesity. *Health Psychology, 23*, 371–380.

Epstein, L. H., Roemmich, J. N., Robinson, J. L., Paluch, R. A., Winiewicz, D. D., Fuerch, J. H., et al. (2008). A randomized trial of the effects of reducing television viewing and computer use on body mass index in young children. *Archives of Pediatrics & Adolescent Medicine, 162*, 239–245.

Epstein, L. H., Valoski, A., Wing, R. R., & McCurley, J. (1994). Ten-year outcomes of behavioral family-based treatment for childhood obesity. *Health Psychology, 13*, 373–383.

Epstein, L. H., Valoski, A. M., Vara, L. S., McCurley, J., Wisniewski, L., Kalarchian, M. A., et al. (1995). Effects of decreasing sedentary behavior and increasing activity on weight change in obese children. *Health Psychology, 14*, 109–115.

Epstein, L. H., Wing, R. R., Koeske, R., Ossip, D. J., & Beck, S. (1982). A comparison of lifestyle change and programmed aerobic exercise on weight and fitness changes in obese children. *Behavior Therapy, 13*, 651–665.

Epstein, L. H., Wing, R. R., Koeske, R., & Valoski, A. (1985). A comparison of lifestyle exercise, aerobic exercise and calisthenics on weight loss in obese children. *Behavior Therapy, 16*, 345–356.

Epstein, L. H., Wing, R. R., Penner, B. C., & Kress, M. J. (1985). Effect of diet and controlled exercise on weight loss in obese children. *Journal of Pediatrics, 107*, 358–361.

Faith, M. S., Leone, M. A., Ayers, T. S., Heo, M., & Pietrobelli, A. (2002). Weight criticism during physical activity, coping skills, and reported physical activity in children. *Pediatrics, 110*, e23. Retrieved May 12, 2010 from http://www.pediatrics.org/cgi/content/full/110/2/e23.

Faraday, M. M. (2006). Stress revisited: A methodological and conceptual history. In S. Yehuda & D. I. Mostofsky (Eds.), *Nutrients, stress, & medical disorders* (pp. 3–20). Totowa, New Jersey: Humana.

Gamble, H. L., Parra, G. R., & Beech, B. M. (2009). Moderators of physical activity and obesity during adolescence. *Eating Behaviors, 10*, 232–236.

Goldfield, G. S., Mallory, R., Parker, T., Cunningham, T., Legg, C., Lumb, A., et al. (2007). Effects of modifying physical activity and sedentary behavioral on psychosocial adjustment in overweight/obese children. *Journal of Pediatric Psychology, 32*, 783–793.

Goldfield, G. S., Raynor, H. A., & Epstein, L. H. (2002). Treatment of pediatric obesity. In T. A. Wadden & A. J. Stunkard (Eds.), *Handbook of obesity treatment* (pp. 232–555). New York: Guilford.

Graf, D. L., Pratt, L. V., Hester, C. N., & Short, K. R. (2009). Playing active video games increases energy expenditure in children. *Pediatrics, 124*, 534–540.

Graves, L., Stratton, G., Ridgers, N. D., & Cable, N. T. (2007). Comparison of energy expenditure in adolescents when playing new generation and sedentary computer games: Cross sectional study. *British Medical Journal, 335*, 1282–1284.

Gutin, B. (2008). Child obesity can be reduced with vigorous activity rather than restriction of energy intake. *Obesity (Silver Spring), 16*, 2193–2196.

Gutin, B., Barbeau, P., Owens, S., Lemmon, C. R., Bauman, M., Allison, J., et al. (2002). Effects of exercise intensity on cardiovascular fitness, total body composition, and visceral adiposity of obese adolescents. *American Journal of Clinical Nutrition, 75*, 818–826.

Gutin, B., Yin, Z., Humphries, M. C., & Barbeau, P. (2005). Relations of moderate and vigorous physical activity to fitness and fatness in adolescents. *American Journal of Clinical Nutrition, 81*, 746–750.

Hale, B. S., & Raglin, J. S. (2002). State anxiety responses to acute resistance training and step aerobic exercise across eight weeks of training. *The Journal of Sports Medicine and Physical Fitness, 42*, 108–112.

Holmes, M. E., Ekkekakis, P., & Eisenmann, J. C. (2010). The physical activity, stress and metabolic syndrome triangle: A guide to unfamiliar territory for the obesity researcher. *Obesity Reviews, 11*(7), 492–507. Epub Nov 5, 2009. DOI: 10.1111/j.1467-789X.2009.00680.x.

Hunter, G. R., Weinsier, R. L., Bamman, M. M., & Larson, D. E. (1998). A role for high intensity exercise on energy balance and weight control. *International Journal of Obesity and Related Metabolic Disorders, 22*, 489–493.

Jabs, J., & Devine, C. M. (2006). Time scarcity and food choices: An overview. *Appetite, 47*, 196–204.

Jakicic, J. J. (2006). Treatment and prevention of obesity: What is the role of exercise? *Nutrition Reviews, 64*, S57–S61.

Jakicic, J. M., Wing, R. R., Butler, B. A., & Robertson, R. J. (1995). Prescribing exercise in multiple short bouts versus one continuous bout: Effects on adherence, cardiorespiratory fitness, and weight loss in overweight women. *International Journal of Obesity and Related Metabolic Disorders, 19*, 893–901.

Jelalian, E., Lloyd-Richardson, E. E., Mehlenbeck, R. S., Hart, C. N., Flynn-O'Brien, K., Kaplan, J., et al. (2010). Behavioral weight control treatment with supervised exercise or peer-enhanced adventure for overweight adolescents. *The Journal of Pediatrics, 157*(6), 923–928.

Jelalian, E., Mehlenbeck, R., Lloyd-Richardson, E. E., Birmaher, V., & Wing, R. R. (2006). 'Adventure therapy' combined with cognitive-behavioral treatment for overweight adolescents. *International Journal of Obesity, 30*, 31–39.

Jennings, A. E., Alberga, A., Sigal, R. J., Jay, O., Boule, N. G., & Kenny, G. P. (2009). The effect of exercise training on resting metabolic rate in type 2 diabetes mellitus. *Medicine and Science in Sports and Exercise, 41*, 1558–1565.

Karelis, A. D., Fontaine, J., Messier, V., Messier, L., Blanchard, C., Rabasa-Lhoret, R., et al. (2008). Psychosocial correlates of cardiorespiratory fitness and muscle strength in overweight and obese post-menopausal women: A MONET study. *Journal of Sports Sciences, 26*, 935–940.

Lanningham-Foster, L., Foster, R. C., McCrady, S. K., Jensen, T. B., Mitre, N., & Levine, J. A. (2009). Activity-promoting video games and increased energy expenditure. *Journal of Pediatrics, 154*, 819–823.

Maffeis, C., & Castellani, M. (2007). Physical activity: An effective way to control weight in children? *Nutrition, Metabolism, and Cardiovascular Diseases, 17*, 394–408.

Mark, A. E., & Janssen, I. (2009). Influence of bouts of physical activity on overweight in youth. *American Journal of Preventative Medicine, 36*, 416–421.

Martins, C., Morgan, L., & Truby, H. (2008). A review of the effects of exercise on appetite regulation: An obesity perspective. *International Journal of Obesity (London), 32*, 1337–1347.

Martins, C., Robertson, M. D., & Morgan, L. M. (2008). Effects of exercise and restrained eating behaviour on appetite control. *Proceedings of the Nutritional Society, 67*, 29–41.

Mata, J., Silva, M. N., Vieira, P. N., Carraca, E. V., Andrade, A. M., Coutinho, S. R., et al. (2009). Motivational "spill-over" during weight control: Increased self-determination and exercise intrinsic motivation predict eating self-regulation. *Health Psychology, 28*, 709–716.

Motl, R. W., Birnbaum, A. S., Kubik, M. Y., & Dishman, R. K. (2004). Naturally occurring changes in physical activity are inversely related to depressive symptoms during early adolescence. *Psychosomatic Medicine, 66*, 336–342.

Murphy, M. H., Blair, S. N., & Murtagh, E. M. (2009). Accumulated versus continuous exercise for health benefit: A review of empirical studies. *Sports Medicine, 39*, 29–43.

Norris, R., Carroll, D., & Cochrane, R. (1992). The effects of physical activity and exercise training on psychological stress and well-being in an adolescent population. *Journal of Psychosomatic Research, 36*, 55–65.

Ogden, C. L., Carroll, M. D., & Flegal, K. M. (2008). High body mass index for age among US children and adolescents, 2003–2006. *Journal of the American Medical Association, 299*, 2401–2405.

Oude Luttikhuis, H., Baur, L., Jansen, H., Shrewsbury, V. A., O'Malley, C., Strolk, R. P., et al. (2009). Interventions for treating obesity in children. *Cochrane Database of Systematic Reviews*, Issue 1. Art. No.: CD001872. DOI: 10.1002/14651858.CD001872.pub2.

Rocchini, A. P., Katch, V., Anderson, J., Hinderliter, J., Becque, D., Martin, M., et al. (1988). Blood pressure in obese adolescents: Effect of weight loss. *Pediatrics, 82*, 16–23.

Sallis, J. F., Prochaska, J. J., & Taylor, W. C. (2000). A review of correlates of physical activity of children and adolescents. *Medicine and Science in Sports and Exercise, 32*, 963–975.

Schmidt, W. D., Biwer, C. J., & Kalscheuer, L. K. (2001). Effects of long versus short bout exercise on fitness and weight loss in overweight females. *Journal of the American College of Nutrition, 20*, 494–501.

Shaibi, G. Q., Cruz, M. L., Ball, G. D., Weigensberg, M. J., Salem, G. J., Crespo, N. C., et al. (2006). Effects of resistance training on insulin sensitivity in overweight Latino adolescent males. *Medicine and Science in Sports and Exercise, 38*, 1208–1215.

Spear, B. A., Barlow, S. E., Ervin, C., Ludwig, D. S., Saelens, B. E., Schetzina, K. E., et al. (2007). Recommendations for treatment of child and adolescent overweight and obesity. *Pediatrics, 120*(Suppl 4), S254–S288.

Stiegler, P., & Cunliffe, A. (2006). The role of diet and exercise for the maintenance of fat-free mass and resting metabolic rate during weight loss. *Sports Medicine, 36*, 239–262.

Strath, S. J., Holleman, R. G., Ronis, D. L., Swartz, A. M., & Richardson, C. R. (2008). Objective physical activity accumulation in bouts and nonbouts and relation to markers of obesity in US adults. *Preventing Chronic Disease, 5*(4), A131. Retrieved May 5, 2010 from http://www.cdc.gov/pcd/issues/2008/oct/07_0158.htm.

Tjonna, A. E., Lee, S. J., Rognmo, O., Stolen, T. O., Bye, A., Haram, P. M., et al. (2008). Aerobic interval training versus continuous moderate exercise as a treatment for the metabolic syndrome: A pilot study. *Circulation, 118*, 346–354.

Tjonna, A. E., Stolen, T. O., Bye, A., Volden, M., Slordahl, S. A., Odegard, R., et al. (2009). Aerobic interval training reduces cardiovascular risk factors more than a multitreatment approach in overweight adolescents. *Clinical Science (London), 116*, 317–326.

Torres, S. J., & Nowson, C. A. (2007). Relationship between stress, eating behavior, and obesity. *Nutrition, 23*, 887–894.

Wilcox, S., Dowda, M., Wegley, S., & Ory, M. G. (2009). Maintenance of change in the Active-for-Life initiative. *American Journal of Preventive Medicine, 37*, 501–504.

Williams, D. M., Lewis, B. A., Dunsiger, S., Whitely, J. A., Papandonatos, G. D., Napolitano, M. A., et al. (2008). Comparing psychosocial predictors of physical activity adoption and maintenance. *Annals of Behavioral Medicine, 36*, 186–194.

Yin, Z., Davis, C. L., Moore, J. B., & Treiber, F. A. (2005). Physical activity buffers the effects of chronic stress on adiposity in youth. *Annals of Behavioral Medicine, 29*, 29–36.

Yeter, K., Rock, C. L., Pakiz, B., Bardwell, W. A., Nichols, J. F., & Wilfley, D. E. (2006). Depressive symptoms, eating psychopathology, and physical activity in obese breast cancer survivors. *Psycho-Oncology, 15*, 453–462.

Zabinski, M. F., Saelens, B. E., Stein, R. I., Hayden-Wade, H. A., & Wilfley, D. E. (2003). Overweight children's barriers to and support for physical activity. *Obesity Research, 11*, 238–246.

Chapter 8
Physical Activity and Obesity Prevention*

Nicole Zarrett and Dawn K. Wilson

The prevalence of overweight and obesity among children and adolescents has more than tripled in the last three decades (Hedley et al., 2004; Ogden, Flegal, Carroll, & Johnson, 2002; Troiano & Flegal, 1998). The sharp rise in overweight and obesity rates among youth has prompted major public health concerns in recent years (Olshansky et al., 2005). Body mass index (BMI) between the 85th and 95th percentile for age and sex is considered at-risk for overweight, and BMI above the 95th percentile is considered overweight or obese (Centers for Disease Control and Prevention, 2001). Based on this sex-specific BMI for age criteria (see the Centers for Disease Control and Prevention growth charts for all BMI ranges), the U.S. Department of Health and Human Services (2008) reported that child and adolescent obesity had reached a national high with 17.0 % of youth considered overweight or obese. Moreover, if current trends continue, the prevalence of overweight in children and adolescents has been estimated to increase 1.6-fold to approximately 30 % by the year 2030 (Wang, Beydoun, Liang, Caballero, & Kumanyika, 2008).

Consequently, the life expectancy for today's generation of children has fallen for the first time in over a century, projected to be the first to have shorter, less healthy lives than their parents if population-level changes in obesity rates are not achieved (Levi, Vinter, St. Laurent, & Segal, 2008; Olshansky et al., 2005). Recognized as the primary health threat for young people, increased rates of obesity have led to major increases in the prevalence of type 2 diabetes mellitus, high blood pressure, and high cholesterol among US children and adolescents, and sets them on a lifetime trajectory of obesity and related disease (Berenson, 2005; Marcovecchio,

*This article was supported in part by a grant (R01 HD 045693) funded by the National Institutes of Child Health and Human Development to Dawn K. Wilson, Ph.D.

N. Zarrett (✉) • D.K. Wilson
Department of Psychology, Barnwell College, University of South Carolina,
1512 Pendleton St., Columbia, SC 29208, USA
e-mail: zarrettn@mailbox.sc.edu

A.L. Meyer and T.P. Gullotta (eds.), *Physical Activity Across the Lifespan*,
Issues in Children's and Families' Lives 12, DOI 10.1007/978-1-4614-3606-5_8,
© Springer Science+Business Media New York 2012

Mohn, & Chiarelli, 2005; Sinha et al., 2002). In addition to long-term physical health risks, overweight and obese children and adolescents face significant mental health morbidities (Schwimmer, Burwinkle, & Varni, 2003; Zametkin, Zoon, Klein, & Munson, 2004) and these are linked to potentially long-term health problems (Needham & Crosnoe, 2004; Ross, 1994). The growing economic impact of obesity is also a concern (Wang & Dietz, 2002). Thus, research with a focus on preventing obesity in youth has become a high priority.

Along with increased consumption of soft drinks (Sinha et al., 2002) and fast foods (Berenson, 2005; Sinha et al., 2002), a potentially primary cause of the increase in obesity among children and adolescents is that today's American youth are less physically active as compared to previous generations. A constellation of social changes, including extensive accessibility of computers and videogames (Schwimmer et al., 2003; Zametkin et al., 2004), increased amount of television viewing (Needham & Crosnoe, 2004), declines in required everyday PA (e.g., walking to school) (Marcovecchio et al., 2005), and reduced value for activities within important social institutions (e.g., school recess/PE classes), have also been identified as contributors to these decreases in PA.

Frequent engagement in PA has been shown to provide substantial health benefits to youth, and has been implemented as an effective strategy for preventing juvenile obesity and related disease (American Heart Association, 2001; Centers for Disease Control and Prevention, 2001). National recommendations and empirical research have suggested that children need a minimum of 60 min of moderate-to-vigorous PA (MVPA) per day.

Despite the health benefits of engaging in PA, over 50 % of youth do not meet the national guidelines for engaging in regular PA (U.S. Department of Health and Human Services, 2008) and there are significant declines in PA as youth mature; declining as much as 50 % between the ages of 6 and 16 years old (Nader, 2003; Nader, Bradley, Houts, McRitchie, & O'Brien, 2008). PA participation peaks very early in the lifespan, reaching its maximum between the ages of 10 and 13 for a majority of individuals (Weinberg & Gould, 2007). Thereafter, age-related declines in PA are observed through the remainder of adolescence and continue throughout adulthood (Gordon-Larsen, Nelson, & Popkin, 2004; Livingstone, Robson, Wallace, & McKinley, 2003; Weinberg & Gould, 2007).

Although studies have documented age-related PA declines for both boys and girls, these declines have consistently been found to be greater and to occur earlier in development for girls than boys (Janz, Dawson, & Mahoney, 2000; Nelson, Neumark-Stzainer, Hannan, Sirard, & Story, 2006). Where declines in girls' PA begin during mid-to-late childhood, boys tend to increase their vigorous PA through the transition into early adolescence, declining during mid-to-late adolescence. During middle childhood the higher rates of PA among boys than girls are due mainly to girls' greater decreases in PA during the evening hours. Morning and afternoon activities of boys and girls remain similar during these years (Janz et al., 2000; Nelson et al., 2006). Differences between males' and females' PA that emerge during the mid-to-late childhood years persist throughout adulthood (Busseri, Rose-Krasnor, Willoughby, & Chalmers, 2006; Malina, 2001; Pate, Dowda, O'Neill, & Ward, 2007).

Low levels of PA and higher rates of obesity and obesity-related diseases have been found to be especially problematic among minority and low-income youth (U.S. Department of Health and Human Services, 2008) who have less access to safe and well-resourced community and school contexts (Molnar, Gortmaker, Bull, & Buka, 2004), and less family support and greater family barriers (e.g., financial strain, erratic work schedules) to participate in PA (Casey, Ripke, & Huston, 2005; Pettit, Laird, Bates, & Dodge, 1997). The increase in adolescent obesity has been more pronounced within African American and Latino adolescents with 22 % of African Americans and 24 % of Latinos currently considered overweight (as compared to 17 % of Caucasian adolescents), and another 40 % of African American adolescents considered at-risk for overweight or obesity (Kumanyika, 2008; Ogden et al., 2006). In particular, African American females are considered at greatest risk for current and continued increases in prevalence of obesity, projected to have the highest incidence of obesity (41.1 %) by 2030, a figure 10 % above the estimated national average (Wang et al., 2008).

In response to this epidemic, several health organizations have issued nation- and statewide mandates to increase the PA of children and adolescents (Cotton, Stanton, Acs, & Lovegrove, 2006). The Healthy People 2010 initiative outlined multiple objectives to increase youth PA, including an objective that emphasized daily school participation in physical education (PE; Objectives 22-8 and 22-9) (U.S. Department of Health and Human Services, 2000). Despite these mandates, there remains considerable variation across the country and the state in both PE requirements and support for implementing effective PA programs that consistently engage youths' interest and participation in MVPA. For example, using national data Nader (2003) found that only 5.9 % of third graders participated in PE class five times per week and minimal PE class time was spent in vigorous activities (under 5 min per lesson) or MVPA (about 12 min per lesson). Moreover, findings suggest PE-based interventions and other school health initiatives have little effect on increasing the PA of youth (Baranowski, Cerin, & Baranowski, 2009). For example, McKenzie et al. (2004) evaluated a school-based physical education intervention on increasing MVPA in 25,000 middle school students (55 % minorities). The 2-year intervention resulted in a 3 min per session increase in MVPA based on observational evaluation methods of lessons. Several other investigators have also conducted school programs that have demonstrated significant moderate increases in MVPA in middle school students, although these studies did not focus on low-income or minority populations specifically (Martinez Vizcaino et al., 2008; Simon et al., 2008). Recent reviews, however, have indicated that *most* PA-based interventions have attained limited or no behavior changes, have rarely affected targeted physiological or anthropometric health outcomes, or identified common patterns of effects that distinguish the few successful from unsuccessful programs (Baranowski et al., 2009; Lemmens, Oenema, Klepp, Henriksen, & Brug, 2008; Salmon, Booth, Phongsavan, Murphy, & Timperio, 2007; Summerbell et al., 2005).

Despite declines in youth PA and the challenges faced in engaging youth in PA, researchers have found some indication of continuity in PA participation (Busseri et al., 2006; Malina, 2001; Taylor, Blair, Cummings, Wun, & Malina, 1999).

Specifically, participation in PA during the earlier years of development, as well as having PA skills and being physically fit, is predictive of PA participation in later adolescence and adulthood (Malina, 2001; Pate et al., 2007; Taylor et al., 1999). Stability of sedentary behaviors over time has also been documented. For example, boys who spent the greatest amount of time watching television, and boys and girls who spent the most time playing video games during childhood were more likely to show high rates of sedentary behaviors during adolescence (Janz et al., 2000; Janz, Burns, & Levy 2005). Therefore, the primary question for researchers, policy makers, and other youth advocates is "what is needed to encourage youths' initial and continued engagement in PA?"

Domains of Influence (Theoretical Foundations and Empirical Support for Promoting PA)

PA participation can be best understood through a dynamic systems perspective of human development (see Baltes, 1997; Bronfenbrenner, 2005; Eccles, Wigfield, & Schiefele, 1998; Lerner, 2006; Magnusson & Stattin, 2006; Overton, 2006 for examples of the conceptualization and application of this theoretical framework). Although a number of different systems models exist, all share the core belief that behavior is influenced by the synergistic relations between individuals and their multiple levels of individual and environmental subsystems over time (Bronfenbrenner, 2005; Bronfenbrenner & Morris, 2006; Sallis et al., 2006). In particular, Bronfenbrenner's (2005) Bioecological Model provides a strong macroparadigm for looking at development as resulting from a complex system of interactions between individuals and the various levels of their environment over time. This model provides a framework for understanding development of health behaviors as shaped by environmental subsystems that include the integration of intrapersonal factors, microsystemic factors (families and institutions), mesosystemic factors (interactions between family and institutions), exosystemic factors (communities, policies), and macrosystemic effects (all systems, micro-, meso-, and exo-, are related to a culture or subculture).

Bronfenbrenner's earlier work stressed the interplay within and across levels of individuals' environments as the primary influence on development, and focused less on the child's own role (e.g., biological contributions) in the developmental process. However, more recent versions of the bioecological theory emphasize that all characteristics of the individual—biological, psychological, social, and emotional—must also be considered to understand development (Bronfenbrenner & Morris, 2006). In this more recent model, the child is seen as an active, purposeful agent in the developmental process; characteristics of the whole child both affect and are affected by the interactions that occur within their various environments in a reciprocal fashion over time.

A direct implication of this proposition is that understanding adolescent health behaviors, and development more generally, requires that the network of relations between characteristics of the individual and the ecologies in which he/she develops must be studied in an integrated and temporal manner (Magnusson & Stattin, 2006). Moreover, this idea of a multilevel developmental system emphasizes the potential for change both in the individual and the contexts in which individuals develop in the service of promoting positive development. This underscores the general assumption guiding most modern developmental theories: Development occurs through a process of systemic interactions within and between the individual and the environment, over time (cf., Cairns, Elder, & Costello, 1996; Magnusson & Stattin, 1998; Mahoney & Bergman, 2002). This theoretical framework provides a guide to testing and evaluating critical elements that may be related at multiple levels of the system in understanding protective and risk factors related to the development of obesity in youth. In addition, it allows for further understanding of potential mechanisms that may lead to or prevent the development of obesity over time. Specifically, applying the Bioecological Model to individuals' motivation to engage in PA stresses the importance of examining the connected nature between individuals and the social and material influences that characterize their various daily contexts, whereby PA choices involve reciprocal processes between the contextual constraints and opportunities for participation within the family, school, community, and individuals' own motivations to participate (Bouffard et al., 2006; Elder & Conger, 2000; Mahoney, Larson, & Eccles, 2005; Zarrett, 2007; Zarrett, Peck, & von Eye, under review).

Intrapersonal Characteristics for Youth PA

Beyond general indicators of youth functioning, such as their academic achievement (e.g., Marsh & Kleitman, 2002), social competence (e.g., Mahoney, Cairns, & Farmer, 2003; Persson, Kerr, & Stattin, 2007), and overall adjustment (Busseri et al., 2006), adolescents' self-concept of ability, also referred to as "self-efficacy," and interest (value) in an activity have been identified both theoretically and empirically as the strongest predictors of youth activity participation (Ryan & Deci, 2000; Wigfield & Eccles, 2002). Multiple psychological theories (e.g., attribution theory, self-efficacy theory, expectancy-value model) suggest that youth are more motivated to select increasingly challenging tasks when they feel that they have the ability to accomplish such tasks (Bandura, 1997; Eccles & Wigfield, 2002; Ryan & Deci, 2000). In terms of PA participation, this means that if an adolescent feels highly competent in playing a soccer game in gym class then s/he will likely be motivated to continue playing soccer, and seek other more competitive venues as his or her skills developed. Research has provided ample empirical evidence that ability beliefs are related to achievement and long-term engagement in a variety of domains, even after controlling for previous achievement or ability (Eccles, Wigfield, Harold, & Blumenfeld, 1993; Eccles & Wigfield, 2002). With respect to the PA literature, strong evidence is accumulating indicating that self-efficacy for PA is a strong predictor of PA in youth (e.g., Cox, Smith, & Williams, 2008; DiLorenzo, Stucky-Ropp, Vander Wal, & Gotham, 1998; Wilson et al., 2005; Winters, Petosa,

& Charlton, 2003). For example, Wilson and her colleagues (2002) implemented an after-school-based intervention that targeted improvements in the PA self-concepts of underserved sixth grade youth (defined by both minority status and low SES). Youth in the intervention showed greater increases in PA self-concept and objectively measured PA as compared to youth in the health education-only comparison program (Wilson, Teasley, Friend, Green, & Sica, 2002).

Adolescents also enroll and persist in an activity because of their expressed value of, or interest in, the activity (Luthar, Shoum, & Brown, 2006; Scanlan, Babkes, & Scanlan, 2005). In fact, several studies have provided support for the strong relation between adolescents' self-concept of ability and values (see Harter, 1998; Jacobs, Lanza, Osgood, Eccles, & Wigfield, 2002; Wigfield & Eccles, 2002). This research has found that if an individual values the activity for which they feel competent, s/he will experience high levels of motivation to participate. For example, using a longitudinal design, Barber, Jacobson, Eccles, and Horn (1997) found that ratings of enjoyment, perceived importance, and self-concept of ability in sports during the tenth grade predicted persistence in sports 2 years later. Moreover, Jacobs et al. (2002) found that the relations between adolescents' self-concept of ability, interest, and their participation in the activity are reciprocal across time.

In summary, previous research indicates that self-efficacy, motivation, and self-concept are important factors in understanding PA engagement that should be a focus of on-going investigations for preventing the development of obesity in children. Early participation (during childhood and early adolescence), where youth build their activity-specific skill set and increased internal motivation, predicts sustained participation (Busseri et al., 2006; Jordan & Nettles, 2000; Mahoney et al., 2003) even when physical activities become competitive in high school (Quiroz, 2000; Simpkins, Ripke, Huston, & Eccles, 2005). However, these internal motivations (values and ability beliefs) often develop as a result of participation due to external motivating factors (Pearce & Larson, 2006). The influence of other people, including encouraging parents, participating friends, teachers, and coaches are common external reasons that adolescents provide for why they first enrolled in the activity (Loder & Hirsch, 2003).

Family Characteristics for Youth PA

The socialization process that occurs within families has been studied for decades and recognized for the prominent role it has in child and adolescent development (Collins, Maccoby, Steinberg, Hetherington, & Bornstein, 2000). Parents provide needed resources and encouragement to promote and sustain youth participation in PA. Parent education, occupation, and income (SES) (Bartko & Eccles, 2003), and the selection of neighborhoods and schools are often reflective of parents' SES (Parke et al., 2003) and have been associated with youth access to PA. In addition, previous research indicates that parents' PA beliefs and behaviors play an important role in children's initial engagement and continued pursuit of PA-related activities.

Specifically, this research has identified three parenting mechanisms by which parents influence their children's activity participation: role modeling (e.g., Anderson, Funk, Elliot, & Smith, 2003; Huebner & Mancini, 2003; Simpkins, Fredricks, Davis-Kean, & Eccles, 2006; Spurrier, Magarey, Golley, Curnow, & Sawyer, 2008), direct provision of activity-related experiences (including social support and encouragement) (Fredricks & Eccles, 2005; Horn, 1987; Spurrier et al., 2008), and their own beliefs about the activity (the degree to which they believe their child is competent in the activity and how much they view the activity as important) (e.g., Eccles et al., 1998; Goodnow & Collins, 1990; Jacobs, Vernon, & Eccles, 2005).

For example, parental behaviors such as mothers' frequency of walking, as well as aspects of the physical home environment (e.g., availability of outdoor play equipment), were associated with PA levels in youth (Spurrier et al., 2008). Research suggests that parents' expectations of their children's athletic ability in the elementary school years (e.g., perceived ability and future success, and the importance of child's engagement in the activity) predicted changes in their children's sports self-concepts from first grade through high school (Fredricks & Eccles, 2005).

Within the family, siblings can influence each other's development beyond that accounted for by the contributions of shared genetics and parenting (Slomkowski, Rende, Novak, Lloyd-Richardson, & Niaura, 2005). Typically, younger siblings are influenced by their older siblings who function as both role models, and providers of opportunities and experiences (Whiteman, McHale, & Crouter, 2007). However, research on the extent to which these processes operate and influence youth PA participation has been rarely measured. In a recent study, Whiteman et al. (2007) assessed the link between adolescents' perceptions of sibling influence and sibling similarities in athletic interests. Their findings showed that younger siblings shared similar activity interests as their older siblings when they viewed their older sibling as highly influential, and when the older sibling was highly interested in the PA activity (Whiteman et al., 2007). Further research is needed to identify the longitudinal nature of these relations and how younger siblings might influence their older sibling's behaviors or PA preferences.

Peers Characteristics for Youth PA

Where there is limited research on sibling influence, there has been much more research on the nature of peer influence on youth PA choices. The relation between activity participation and peers, often referred to as a "leisure culture," and its link to developmental outcomes has been well documented (Eccles, Barber, Stone, & Hunt, 2003; Kinney, 1993; Mahoney et al., 2003). Empirical research has shown that adolescents' friend groups (e.g., "crowd"), and the social identities they attach to this affiliation, are critical predictors of whether adolescents participate in PA (Eccles & Barber, 1999; Huebner & Mancini, 2003; Luthar et al., 2006).

The establishment of positive peer relationships (friendships) within a PA setting is believed to foster continued PA engagement because the setting fulfills adolescents' socio-emotional needs of belonging/relatedness. In fact, youth report "spending time with friends" as a central motivating factor for why they first chose to participate in an activity (e.g., organized sports), their enjoyment in the activity, and whether they persist or dropout of an activity (Borden, Perkins, Villarruel, & Stone, 2005; Persson et al., 2007; Smith, 1999; Weiss & Smith, 2002). In addition, social support from peers has been shown to significantly contribute to an adolescent's level of PA (Beets, Vogel, Forlaw, Pitetti, & Cardinal, 2006; Martin & McCaughtry, 2008; Springer, Kelder, & Hoelscher, 2006). For example, Duncan, Duncan, and Strycker (2005) found that support from friends was a stronger predictor of PA in children than was support from either parents or siblings among children aged 10–14. Springer and colleagues (2006) found that social encouragement from friends was the only factor among multiple family, intrapersonal, and environmental factors measured that was positively associated with vigorous PA in sixth grade girls (Springer et al., 2006). Lastly, youth with physically active friends are more physically active than those whose friends are not active (Duncan, Duncan, Strycker, & Chaumeton, 2007).

In summary, peer behavior and social support has been shown to be a strong predictor of child PA; however, much of the research has focused on white, middle class populations rather than low-income or minority youth. Given the strong cultural ties to family in minority populations, it is not clear how much parent versus peer support will be instrumental in understanding long-term engagement in PA among underserved youth.

Neighborhood/Community

Researchers have also considered the importance of the neighborhood and community supports for promoting PA (see Chap. 7 of this book for a more extensive discussion of the impact of the Built Environment on PA). Neighborhood resources, such as parks, community centers, playing fields, and positive adult mentors that implement and oversee youth activities, are a necessity for youth participation in PA during their leisure time. Within economically disadvantaged urban neighborhoods and poor, isolated rural areas, where youth have the greatest needs for PA-based supports, these types of provisions are often sparse (e.g., Duncan & Brooks-Gunn, 2000; Hirsch et al., 2000; Quinn, 1999; Rural School & Community Trust, 2005; Save the Children, 2002; Storey & Brannen, 2000). Youth from such low-income neighborhoods attend schools that also have limited economic resources and are less equipped to provide the variety and quality of curricular and extracurricular PA opportunities and resources that are typically available to youth attending schools in wealthier neighborhoods (Dunbar, 2002; Leventhal & Brooks-Gunn, 2000; Pedersen & Seidman, 2005).

Moreover, many youth have limited access to the activities that are available in their communities because of family constraints and concerns. Extracurricular activities can be costly, involving enrollment fees, uniforms, and other equipment, and require transportation which can be difficult for parents who are under financial strain and rigorous, erratic work schedules (e.g., Casey et al., 2005). Where there are youth programs and other affordable PA-based extracurricular activities provided in low-income communities, issues of safety and access often remain primary sources of deterrence to youth participation (Weir, Etelson, & Brand, 2006). Many parents limit their child's attendance in youth programs to avoid exposure to these risks (Fauth, Roth, & Brooks-Gunn, 2007; Jarrett, 1997; Molnar et al., 2004; Shann, 2001). For example, Weir et al. (2006) studied the influence of parent perceptions of neighborhood safety on child PA levels. Greater parent perceptions of neighborhood crime were negatively correlated with reported levels of child PA.

Differences in community supports, and the level in which these supports meet the needs of youth and their families, also impact individuals' orientation towards, and selection into, certain PA activities. In particular, low-income families are more likely to take advantage of activity opportunities offered by their religious institutions (e.g., church-sponsored basketball leagues) and local community centers (e.g., Boys and Girls Clubs) than those offered by other institutions (e.g., the school) because they tend to be more affordable, more readily available, and easier to access in their communities (Simpkins et al., 2005). In summary, neighborhood levels of access to safe places for youth PA are highly dependent on financial resources which may limit the ability of low-income and minority youth to engage in PA opportunities on a regular basis.

Quality of the PA Setting

In addition to availability and access for PA opportunities, the overall quality of the PA settings offered to youth within their communities is also an essential element for promoting youth participation in regular PA. To best understand youth sustained participation in PA it is important to consider the relation between the characteristics of the activity context and of the individual, or what has been termed the "person-environment fit" (Eccles et al., 1993; Erikson, 1968; Hunt, 1975; Magnusson & Stattin, 1998). From this perspective, individuals have needs that require appropriate responses from their social contexts to support healthy development. In the case of physical activities, a context where participation is highly voluntary, youth will select into or out of activities depending on whether these needs are met. Among the most basic of these needs is physical safety, and individuals' socio-emotional needs for achievement (competence), relatedness, and autonomy (Ryan & Deci, 2000). Researchers have proposed that successful activity contexts (both in terms of adolescent enrollment/retention rates and the promotion of positive development) are those which provide optimally challenging experiences, including the opportunity to acquire and practice specific social, physical, and intellectual skills that are useful in a wide variety of settings (see Wilson et al., 2008, for example).

Developmental Maturation (Chronosystem)

Incorporating information about developmental change into the person-environment fit model yields a "stage-environment fit" model that addresses how personal and social changes across *developmental time* impact the person-environment fit (Eccles & Midgley, 1989). PA contexts that are appropriate for adolescents are not necessarily appropriate for children. Instead, programs developed to cater to the needs of children and adolescents must map on to their growing maturity and expertise. Therefore, developmental period will dictate the type, duration, and intensity of the PA. For example, where 30–60 minutes of daily activity are recommended for both children and adolescence, to engage preadolescent children in PA it may be more effective for the activity to be broken down into 15-minute segments throughout the day given their shorter attention spans and physical abilities (Strong et al., 2005; U.S. Department of Agriculture (USDA), 2005). Moreover, as youth move through the middle to late adolescent years, youth contexts must provide PA opportunities that map onto their greater aerobic and anaerobic capacities (Wilmore & Costill, 1994), increasing cognitive capacities and identity concerns (Gerrard, Gibbons, & Bushman, 1996; Harter, 1999, 2003), additional autonomy needs, and their movement towards adulthood, including a focus on future plans (Eccles & Gootman, 2002; Zarrett & Eccles, 2006). Activities that are appropriate in terms of skill level and adolescent needs (e.g., opportunities for leadership) promote participation (Lauver & Little, 2005; Pearce & Larson, 2006) by optimizing adolescent learning and motivation (Rogoff, 2003; Ryan & Deci, 2000). In contrast, adolescents' negative responses to a specific PA (e.g., experiences of increased stress) have been shown to lead to decreased motivation and increased drop out rates of PA (Cumming, Smith, & Smoll, 2006; Scanlan et al., 2005).

Summary and Conclusions

In summary, the bioecological framework provides a guide for understanding the factors identified in correlational and quasi-experimental studies that are important in understanding child-related PA behavior. Interpersonal factors that have been demonstrated to be strongly associated with PA in youth include self-efficacy, motivation, and self-concept related to engaging in PA. For family, siblings, and peers, both direct role modeling and social support have been important factors that have been correlated with greater levels of PA in youth, although much of the previous literature has focused on the white, middle class rather than underserved minority youth. Finally, environmental factors related to neighborhood resources are important to consider in terms of increasing youth access and safety for engaging in PA. The developmental maturity of youth will also interact with understanding how each of these bioecological factors is associated with PA levels.

Prevention Programs That Foster Protective Factors for Promoting PA

In addition to the longitudinal quasi-experimental and cross-sectional studies reviewed above, it is important to highlight similar key bioecological factors that have been evaluated in the context of intervention studies. Although some PA-based interventions have been moderately effective for increasing youth PA, related healthy behaviors, and intrapersonal factors during the intervention phase, convincing effective long-lasting population-based prevention programs are still lacking (Doak, Visscher, Renders, & Seidell, 2006; Kahn et al., 2002; Sharma, 2006; Summerbell et al., 2005). Moreover, comprehensive PA-based interventions have typically included common behavior modification components including self-monitoring of PA, goal setting, and behavioral skills training, however, little attention has been given to establishing an activity climate that provides youth opportunities to exercise their autonomy (e.g., youth help develop program ideas or PA choices), that nurtures a sense of relatedness/belonging (e.g., teamwork and cooperation among peers; the development of friendships), or that facilitates a sense of mastery (self-efficacy/competency) and enjoyment in PA (Baranowski, Anderson, & Carmark, 1998; Gortmaker, Cheung et al., 1999; Kelder, Perry, & Klepp, 1989; Killen et al., 1988; Saunders, Ward, Felton, Dowda, & Pate, 2006). Interventions that address these important motivational facets of the individual and the activity context may enhance more intrinsic motivation, and thus, increase the likelihood of continued engagement in PA outside of the intervention setting.

For example, in a recent RCT known as the "Active by Choice Today" (ACT) trial, the efficacy of a motivational plus behavioral skill intervention was evaluated for increasing PA outside of school time. The trial involved 24 middle schools (1,560 sixth graders) in South Carolina that were randomly assigned to one of two after-school programs (motivational and behavioral skills intervention, or general health education). The intervention integrated constructs from Self-Determination and Social Cognitive Theories to enhance intrinsic motivation and behavioral skills for PA. The intervention targeted skill development for PA outside of program days and the after-school program social environment (autonomy, choice, participation, belongingness, fun, enjoyment, support) was designed to positively impact cognitive mediators (self-efficacy, perceived competence), and motivational orientation (intrinsic motivation, commitment, positive self-concept). It was hypothesized that the 17-week motivational and life skills intervention would lead to greater increases in MVPA (based on 7-day accelerometry estimates) at mid-intervention and 2 weeks post-intervention as compared to the general health education program. Results are forth coming that provide partial support for these hypotheses (Wilson et al., 2009, 2011). This trial is one of the first to implement a social environmental intervention to enhance long-term motivation for increasing PA in underserved adolescents with high fidelity and dose of implementation documented (Wilson et al., 2006, 2011).

Moreover, few interventions have focused on establishing social norms for PA or developing social supports/networks within and across the multiple contexts in which youth are embedded. Interventions that integrate environmental changes that facilitate values for PA and reduce the barriers for adopting an active lifestyle have a higher potential for changing PA habits (Wilson et al., 2008). Along with an array of after-school programs (Beets, Bieghle, Erwin, & Huberty, 2009), such as the ACT program described above, some researchers have begun to target other important contexts to promote youth healthy development.

School-Based Interventions

In recent years schools have been called on to expand their efforts to increase PA opportunities for youth and have become the focal point for interventions designed to increase PA in children and adolescents. The majority of youth attend school, and schools have both the facilities and personnel necessary to support PA. Physical education, recess, classroom-based activities, staff wellness, intramural activities, school-based athletics, parental involvement, and community collaboration can all be implemented within the school context to promote PA. Previous school-based studies aimed at preventing or treating obesity have demonstrated minimal to modest effects on increasing youth PA over time and, consequently, have failed to impact BMI trajectories (Baranowski et al., 2009; Baranowski, Cullen, Nicklas, Thompson, & Baranowski, 2002; Doak et al., 2006; Shaya, Flores, Gbarayor, & Wang, 2008). Among interventions that used curriculum change as their only strategy (Bush et al., 1989; Gortmaker, Peterson et al., 1999; Marcus, Wheeler, Cullen, & Crane, 1987; Palmer, Graham, & Elliott, 2005; Robinson, 1999; Salmon et al., 2007), the three that have shown notable effects were implemented by researchers rather than school staff. The Know Your Body Program (Marcus et al., 1987) was a successful multiple risk factor program implemented over 18 weeks for underserved children aged 9–11. However, when this program was delivered by different investigators to a different sample of children, these findings were not replicated. The Planet Health study (Gortmaker, Peterson et al., 1999) was shown to be effective at reducing TV viewing in adolescent boys and girls, and increasing fruit-vegetable consumption in girls, but did not meet their aims of increasing youth PA. Lastly, the Stanford Adolescent Heart Health program (Killen et al., 1988) showed that 30 % of the previously inactive youth became active after the 7-week intervention compared to 20 % in control schools. However, the intervention was delivered by university staff, significantly limiting program sustainability.

In light of research and theory that suggests the effectiveness of an integrative systems approach, The Centers of Disease Control and Prevention have proposed a coordinated school health model that highlights a wide range of school programs and components, beyond just PE, that can be implemented to increase PA in youth (Centers for Disease Control and Prevention, 1997; Koplan, Liverman, Kraak, & Wisham, 2007). Researchers have increasingly begun to adopt this proposed school-wide design, involving several school components in their interventions, and, at times, incorporating community and/or family involvement. Researchers have found that involving several school components (e.g., PE, health education, school nurse) in a health promotion intervention increased the likelihood that students adopted health-ier behaviors (e.g., increased fruit and vegetable (FV) intake, increased MVPA in PE) (Mukoma & Flisher, 2004; Parcel, Simons-Morton, & Kolbe, 1988; St Leger, 2004; Veugelers & Fitzgerald, 2005). In particular, intervention programs that focused on new PE strategies along with broad school-based changes have shown the most prom-ise for increasing youth MVPA during PE (McKenzie et al., 2004; Sallis et al., 2003), but still remain relatively unsuccessful in changing PA outside of school or overall (Cass & Price, 2003; McKenzie et al., 2004; Sahota et al., 2001; Sallis et al., 2003). For example, The Child and Adolescent Trial for Cardiovascular Health (CATCH), involved behaviorally based classroom curricula for Grades 3 through 5, school envi-ronment changes related to cafeteria food services, PE-based changes for increasing PA, and family-based activities. Where CATCH showed a significant difference in vigorous PA amounting to an 8-minute difference between intervention and control participants at a 3-year follow-up, there were no differences in total minutes of youth PA across light, moderate, and vigorous activities combined (Nader et al., 1999).

Findings indicate that the barriers to quality PE and coordinated school health programs include lack of engagement, support, and input of teachers and staff, the low priority that is placed on health-related curricula relative to other academic subjects, and insufficient training and resources (Barroso, McCullum-Gomez, Hoelscher, Kelder, & Murray, 2005). For example, schools which sustained the SPARK PE intervention, a school environmental- and behavioral skills-based pro-gram, were more likely than non-sustained SPARK users to have principals who supported PE programs and endorsed projects and campaigns for increasing PA promoted by the PE teachers, and parents who actively supported PE programs. Sustained SPARK programs were 4.4 times more likely to be in schools that had adequate equipment for PE and 4.7 times more likely to participate in 30 minutes of PA per day than nonusers (Dowda, Sallis, McKenzie, Rosengard, & Kohl, 2005). These findings exemplify that the establishment of a supportive environment for youth depends on the quality (e.g., teaching style, engagement, skill) of the specific agents of change (e.g., activity leaders, teachers, parents) within each environment, and setting up social norms that promote healthy choices for engaging in PA. Therefore, rather than considering the school simply as a setting for implementing a program, these findings suggest that we need to create and sustain change within a school through empowering school staff and students, and building social climate capacity that promotes PA (Bond, Glover, Godfrey, Butler, & Patton, 2001; Ward et al., 2006; Wilson et al., 2008). This will entail instilling a greater value for PA within the school and fostering motivation, self-efficacy, and intentions for increas-ing PA in school staff. To date, little research has been conducted that examines what types of methods are needed to build this local capacity.

Family-Based Interventions

Although less common than school-based interventions, there have been a few family-based PA interventions that have targeted children and adolescents (Wilson &

Kitzman-Ulrich, 2008). Many of these interventions have focused on the family system as an environment that can influence the adoption and maintenance of health behaviors including PA through some of the important mediators identified by theory and research (as discussed in the family section above), such as role modeling/coactivity, provision of resources, experiences, emotional/motivational support for engaging in healthy behaviors, and the creation of a supportive environment for sustained health behavior change (Benton, 2004; Ward-Begnoche & Speaker, 2006). However, there has been wide variation in the strategies researchers have used to engage the family environment and to foster PA in youth. For example, encouragement of parent and child coactivity, like that which was fostered in the Daughters and Mothers Exercising Together program (Ransdell, Dratt, Kennedy, O'Neill, & DeVoe, 2001), showed promise for increasing the physical health of adolescent girls (aged 11–17 years). In this program, mother–daughter pairs and triads attended physical activity and classroom sessions twice weekly. Although the program was only a 12-week pilot ($n = 20$ families), significant improvements were observed in perceived sport competence, physical condition, and strength and muscularity. Researchers assert that parent participation along with their child in the activity gives parents the opportunity to actively coach and teach their children skills and to provide performance feedback including direct positive and negative reinforcements for participating. Moreover, parents' involvement in their adolescents' activities further relays messages to their children about the relative importance of the activity, where high rates of involvement communicate high importance. In contrast, low parental involvement (less emotional, financial, or functional investment in their child's physical activities) is likely to undermine youth interest and engagement in such activities (Fredricks & Eccles, 2005; Horn, 1987).

Use of media, such as print materials, radio programs, and meetings with parents, has also been facilitated to engage parents in promoting their child's healthy behaviors (e.g., Cookson, Heath, & Bertrand, 2000; Saakslahti et al., 2004). Although some family-based interventions have been effective for promoting youth PA (Cookson et al., 2000; Nader, Sallis, Patterson, & Abramson, 1989; Ransdell et al., 2001, 2003; Saakslahti et al., 2004), many efforts have been small pilot studies with a wide variation of strategies (part of the US Girls' Health Enrichment Multisite Studies) and generalizability of the interventions still need to be tested. Moreover, concern about compliance (Sallis et al., 2003) and retention rates (Cookson et al., 2000) indicates that further research is needed to identify effective strategies for engaging the family in efforts to increase youth PA.

Multisystemic Interventions

Health promotion programs that have targeted more than one of adolescents' primary contexts (e.g., combined school and family intervention) have been shown to overcome some of the barriers identified by single target interventions (Barroso et al., 2005; Hopper, Munoz, Gruber, & MacConnie, 1996; Hopper, Munoz, Gruber, &

Nguyen, 2005; Johnson et al., 1991; Manios, Moschandreas, Hatzis, & Kafatos, 1999; McKenzie et al., 1996; Nader et al., 1989, 1999; Ward et al., 2006; Vandongen et al., 1995). Examples of family components used in these studies include family homework assignments, parent meetings and family fun nights (Davis et al., 2003; Manios et al., 1999; McKenzie et al., 1996), family group meetings held at the school (Nader et al., 1989), provision of behavioral reinforcements to families such as point systems and stickers (Hopper et al., 1996, 2005), and phone calls, newsletters, multimedia curriculum, and media displays to engage families (Hopper et al., 1996; Sallis et al., 1997). For example, the Sports, Play, and Active Recreation for Kids (SPARK) intervention (Sallis et al., 1997) was a 2-year program for fourth graders, which involved physical education lessons, PA-based homework, and monthly newsletters to parents to stimulate parent–child interaction that was successful in increasing youth MVPA during the school day (13 more hours of MVPA across the school year in comparison to youth in the control group) but did not produce any out-of-school effects. The Know Your Body intervention (Manios, Kafatos, & Mamalakis, 1998), a 6-year study with first graders in Greece, is known as one of the most successful long-term interventions for promoting continued child PA. The intervention included physical education lessons, classroom sessions, homework activities for children and their parents, and parental meetings at the school. Children in the intervention group had significantly greater increases in PA outside of school across the 6-year study compared with the control group, and these effects were maintained at the 4-year follow-up. However, the program had the strongest effects on increasing boys' PA; there were minimal differences between the groups in girls' PA.

Although some interventions that incorporated school- and family-based components have been effective for promoting increases in at least some aspects of PA among children (Luepker et al., 1996; Manios et al., 1998; Sallis et al., 1997; Story et al., 2003; Warren, Henry, Lightowler, Bradshaw, & Perwaiz, 2003), there are little-to-no studies that include school and family components in promoting adolescents' PA (see Salmon et al., 2007 review). Moreover, among child interventions that combined a school and family component, few have focused on underserved child populations (minority, low SES) or have used more objective measures of PA (e.g., accelerometer data). Most multilevel school- and family-based programs targeting underserved children have not been effective for promoting PA (Caballero et al., 2003; Coleman et al., 2005; Fitzgibbon et al., 2005; Goran & Reynolds, 2005; Gortmaker, Cheung et al., 1999; Paradis et al., 2005). However, without process evaluation it is not clear if these interventions have been ineffective because of lack of being implemented at a level that would be required to demonstrate effectiveness (Wilson et al., 2009). We found only one effective school- and family-based intervention that both focused on underserved children and that used an objective measure of PA. The Minnesota GEMS program (Story et al., 2003), an after-school obesity prevention program for African American girls aged 8–10 years, incorporated a family component that sent home weekly family packets to the parents containing healthful eating and exercise topics and recipes, and held family night events where families set activity and eating goals with their children. Follow-up phone calls by GEM staff to parents were conducted throughout the intervention to motivate and check the families' progress on the goals that they set. PA accelerometer measures and self-report showed consistently greater activity levels in the intervention as compared to the control group.

In summary, theoretical and empirical evidence indicates that an effective intervention for promoting youth PA involves the integration of various components within and between levels of the developmental system. However, despite advances made in youth PA behavior change through after-school, school-wide, family-based, and multi-contextual interventions, barriers still exist for sustaining effective health initiatives within these contexts for promoting youth continued engagement in PA.

Future Directions in Research

The utilization of a variety of research approaches, including randomized control trials (that involve a community-based participatory approach), qualitative assessments, longitudinal mediation models, and process evaluations, is essential for the advancement of PA prevention programs.

Use of Randomized Control Trials with a Community-Based Participatory Approach

The use of randomized controlled trials (RCTs) is important for the field of PA in that scientific integrity promotes evidence-based research that can advance the field in meaningful ways. However, the tight scientific rigor of RCTs can sometimes limit the engagement and willingness for community members to engage in the research process. This has led researchers to employ a community-based participatory approach that utilizes on-going input from the community for the development, implementation, and evaluation of RCTs in order to increase the long-term effectiveness of the prevention program.

RCTs are considered the gold-standard of research designs in that systematic error is minimized, and that results represent true findings (Kaptchuk, 2001).[1] Random assignment of participants reduces threats to internal validity and increases the extent to which group differences can be attributed to the intervention under study (Kazdin, 2003). Another component of well-conducted RCTs is blind assessment, which assures that treatment and outcome measures are not influenced by bias

---

[1] The CONSORT statement provides a tool for researchers to accurately describe their RCT, which in turn will improve the design and conduction of RCTs in the future (Freemantle, Mason, Haines, & Eccles, 1997; Moher, Schulz, & Altman, 2001). Several peer-reviewed medical and health-related journals require authors to follow the CONSORT statement (Freemantle et al., 1997), and data suggest that the implementation of CONSORT has improved the quality of reporting RCTs (Moher et al., 2001).

(Kaptchuk, 2001). Findings from RCTs guide clinical practice and the development of future research hypotheses, and are also critical in establishing evidence-based practice guidelines (Kao, Tyson, Blakely, & Lally, 2008). Therefore, well-conducted RCTs are essential to the research process and translation of efficacious interventions to clinical practice and public health interventions.

However, very few RCTs have focused on evaluating the long-term efficacy of interventions that specifically alter community level supports for PA. Consequently, community researchers have argued for more community-based participatory research (CBPR) approaches in order to better understand and sustain intervention effects over the long term (Israel, Schulz, Parker, & Becker, 2001). The CBPR approach often involves obtaining qualitative data from community participants about the PA barriers and facilitators that they encounter within their neighborhoods, schools, and families. These data are applied to the development/design of the RCT to increase the "fit" of the program with the needs of the community it serves. Community leaders and participants are also recruited and trained to help implement the intervention, increasing the likelihood of continued engagement and program implementation post-trial. Lastly, process evaluations are conducted with community participants throughout the trial to identify and alter less effective components of the intervention and maintain program quality. RCT trials that not only test scientific premises but also integrate community input throughout the developmental implementation and evaluation processes have a higher probability of success because community engagement is enhanced.

Several RCTs that have used a CBPR approach have focused on developing community coalitions to face and overcome barriers to PA, such as issues of safety and access to PA, within underserved neighborhoods. In particular, there has been a recent influx of CBPR interventions that involve the development and promotion of neighborhood walking trails that have been shown to be successful for increasing PA in adults (Morbidity and Mortality Weekly Report (MMWR), 1999; Wilson, Kirtland, Ainsworth, & Addy, 2004). For example, Brownson et al. (1996) examined the impact of PA-based community coalitions in rural Missouri which included developing walking clubs, aerobic classes, and fitness festivals with exercise demonstrations. Among well-organized coalitions, these activities significantly decreased sedentary behavior. In a study by Fisher and Li (2004), community residents in a metropolitan area of Portland, Oregon were recruited and randomized to participate in either a neighborhood peer-led walking group or an information only control group. Intervention participants participated in a peer-led neighborhood walk and received information materials and monthly newsletters. Neighborhoods in the control condition received health education information only. Compared to the control neighborhoods, results of the multilevel intervention showed increases in walking after 6-months of intervention (see Wilson et al., 2009 for an example RCT that utilizes a community-based participatory approach). Based on the studies reviewed above it is not clear that simply building a walking trail will promote walking without active engagement of the community residents. Further research is also needed to better understand the impact of community-based PA intervention programs on promoting PA in youth.

Identifying, Implementing, and Assessing Behavior Change Processes (Mediation Factors)

Further research that utilizes qualitative assessments, longitudinal methods, and process evaluation is also critical for identifying, implementing, and assessing the mediation factors, or process variables, within PA-based interventions. The mediating variable model (Baranowski et al., 2009) asserts that interventions change target behaviors by inducing change in mediating factors, such as the intrapersonal, social, and ecological factors discussed above. Importantly, identifying and then targeting change in key mediating factors will result in inducing relatively stable changes in target behaviors (e.g., PA), rendering interventions consistently more effective.

A recent report by Masse, Dassa, Gauvin, Giles-Corti, and Motl (2002) outlines the importance of using qualitative methods to better understand theoretical constructs that may mediate behavior change. These methods have been especially effective for identifying barriers and facilitators of PA across the lifespan and in subgroups that may be at increased risk for developing chronic disease and increased rates of mortality. A number of focus group studies have been conducted (Griffin, Wilson, Wilcox, Buck, & Ainsworth, 2008; Wilson et al., 2005) that indicate several clear barriers to PA exist especially in underserved populations (low income, minorities) and which have provided a basis for developing effective interventions by designing programs that best meet the needs and capitalizes on the strengths of the particular subgroup of the population in which the intervention targets.

Qualitative data can also serve as an important tool to examine the climate of the environment in which the intervention will be delivered (e.g., school, family). That is, the choice of the intervention's environment engages both its strengths and limitations. Therefore, identifying baseline climate, challenges, and strengths of the environment, as well as gaining valuable input/insights from the community in which the PA program targets, will greatly inform the final intervention design (Baranowski et al., 2009; Gucciardini, Cameron, Liao, Palmer, & Steward, 2007).

After mediation factors are identified and implemented within interventions, researchers must measure whether the intervention procedures are, in fact, manipulating these mediators, and whether the degree of manipulation is at effective levels to induce long-term change (referred to as "fidelity" and "dose," respectively). Through the utilization of process evaluation and longitudinal research methods, researchers will gain a greater understanding of the processes that occur within the activity setting, and how these processes help facilitate youth long-term engagement and development (Vandell, Shumow, & Posner, 2005).

The importance of process evaluations for monitoring program implementation has been highlighted in some large-scale trials (Durlak & DuPre, 2008; Griffin et al., 2009; Lillehoj, Griffin, & Spoth, 2004; Marcoux et al., 1999; McGraw et al., 2000; Saunders et al., 2006; Steckler & Linnan, 2002) and there is strong evidence that the level of implementation impacts study outcomes (Durlak & DuPre, 2008). Implementation monitoring can be done in both a formative and a summative manner. Formative evaluations can be defined as utilizing data to provide on-going monitoring and quality assessment to maximize the performance of a program (Devaney & Rossi, 1997; Helitzer & Yoon, 2002; Helitzer, Yoon, Wallerstein, & Garcia-Velarde, 2000; Viadro, Earp, & Altpeter, 1997). Summative evaluations analyze data at the conclusion of an intervention to provide a conclusive rating of the extent to which intended outcomes were achieved and whether the program was implemented as intended (Devaney & Rossi, 1997; Helitzer et al., 2000). Another summative purpose of process evaluation is to include level of implementation data in the outcome analysis (Baranowski & Stables, 2000; Shadish, Cook, & Campbell, 2002). Evaluations of implementation are especially important given that few studies have achieved full implementation in real-world settings (Shadish et al., 2002). This is also true of health promotion efforts, as researchers have noted the great variability in program implementation and policy adoption in community and school settings (Dusenbury, Brannigan, Falco, & Hansen, 2003; Lillehoj et al., 2004).

Lastly, combining theoretically driven longitudinal research that focuses on understanding mediational factors along with these other methods described above will provide detailed documentation of behavior and behavior change processes as interventions are implemented and sustained overtime.

In summary, a CBPR approach to RCTs, qualitative research, process evaluations, and longitudinal mediation models are essential for the advancement of both the health and health psychology fields in designing effective PA-based programs for obesity prevention. Although there are some limitations that scientific rigor can produce in developing effective community-based interventions, as long as RCTs are based on qualitative input, continue to integrate communities' values and beliefs throughout the developmental stage, incorporate key mediation factors in the design, and conduct rigorous process evaluations across the course of the intervention, the more likely there will be success in engaging the targeted community in the process of change and sustaining these changes overtime.

Strategies to Build Local Capacity

Given the extensive empirical support for the dynamic systems theoretical perspective, which asserts that health behaviors are shaped by individuals' interactions with their multiple environmental subsystems, researchers need to focus more on how to build local capacity across individuals' neighborhood, school, family, and peer group to increase the effectiveness of PA programs. For example, the majority of school-based health promotion interventions have focused on training teachers to implement a curriculum developed by the research team (e.g., The Planet Health project; The Stanford Adolescent Heart Health Program; Gortmaker, Peterson et al., 1999; Killen et al., 1988). This approach fails to consider some of the key mechanisms that help engage youth in the program's mission, such as the classroom climate (e.g., teaching style, engagement, skill) and the broader climate of the school (e.g., communication across principals, teachers, and staff), as well as the characteristics of the community (e.g., access to safe PA) and the family (e.g., parent encouragement for youth PA) in which youth reside. Lack of sufficient focus on facilitating communication across adolescents' contexts often results in no observable changes in youth PA outside of school hours.

PA interventions that focus on changing the overall school climate, connecting schools with community youth organizations, and involving parents and peers will be more likely to establish contextual climates that provide youth support and opportunities to exercise their autonomy in making their own positive health behavior choices (e.g., PA opportunities). This will include instilling a greater value for PA, and fostering motivation/engagement and PA-based competence within youth and the key agents within their ecologies (within their families, friends, schools, and neighborhoods), as well as finding ways to better connect youths' various contexts so that, in combination, they form a cohesive positive social norm around PA. A combination of multiple safe, nurturing, and caring environments will facilitate adolescents' initial and continued engagement by enabling youth to explore a variety of options and roles, establish positive mentor relationships, and develop personal assets (e.g., self-esteem, social skills) (Dunbar, 2002; Roffman, Suaurez-Orozco, & Rhodes, 2003).

Recommendations for Practitioners

Given the theoretical and empirical research reviewed above, for youth to achieve the recommended 60 minutes of PA per day will require change both in the individual and the contexts in which individuals develop. At the contextual level, this requires that researchers and practitioners focus on: (1) increasing access and safety for engaging in PA and (2) fostering increased social support, role modeling, and engagement of important socializers (e.g., teachers, parents, peers) across many of the contexts in which youth are embedded to help reinforce the positive PA attitudes and behaviors youth acquire in the PA setting. Individuals bring their own set of values, interests, identity needs, and previous socialization experiences to their activity choices. Therefore, different activities, each with their own set of tasks, skills, goals, and general structure, will appeal to different youth. This is critical to engagement. Therefore, there needs to be a multitude of PA opportunities available to youth to ensure that all individuals find an enjoyable activity (or activities) in which to engage. Opportunities to engage in PA in various contexts across adolescents' day will increase the likelihood that they find enough activities in which they enjoy to meet the daily recommendations.

Furthermore, researchers and practitioners must focus on fostering youth's PA self-efficacy, value, and motivations to participate in PA. This will require the establishment of an activity setting that meets individuals' needs for physical safety and socio-emotional needs for achievement (competence), relatedness, and autonomy (Ryan & Deci, 2000). For example, providing an activity climate that requires teamwork and cooperation among peers will nurture a sense of relatedness/belonging. Giving youth opportunities to develop segments of the PA curriculum or activity program, provide feedback about the curriculum/program, and even choose the activity offered that day from a selection will help nurture a greater sense of autonomy. Providing PA opportunities that are optimally challenging (difficult, but possible to achieve) and focused on mastery of skills, rather than performance and evaluation, will help facilitate youth's sense of mastery (self-efficacy/competency) and enjoyment (see Wilson et al., 2009 and Wilson et al., 2011 for details on a program that fosters these components). The provision of these novel, enjoyable, self-driven (autonomous), and satisfying (competence-related) experiences (considered intrinsic factors/motivators) sustain behavior more so than those produced by extrinsic factors such as external reward or coercion (Deci, Koestner, & Ryan, 1999; Ryan & Deci, 2000).

PA programs developed to cater to the needs of children and adolescents must also consider their growing maturity and expertise. Developmental period will dictate the type, duration, and intensity of the PA that would engage youth of different developmental stages. For example, practitioners who are working with preadolescent children should focus on providing multiple 15-minute segments of PA opportunities throughout the day given younger children's shorter attention spans and physical abilities. This may mean reorganizing the school day to include a 15-minute segment of activity at the beginning of the day, one or two 15-minute PA-based recesses, and a daily physical education class to ensure that children are meeting the national MVPA recommendations. Any intervention model that hopes to provide youth with the kinds of developmentally appropriate supports required to promote healthy development will need to attend explicitly to these human capacities, potentials, and needs and how they change over time during the course of development.

References

American Heart Association. (2001). *Exercise (physical activity) and children: AHA Scientific Position*. Dallas, TX: American Heart Association.

Anderson, J. C., Funk, J. B., Elliot, R., & Smith, P. H. (2003). Parental support and pressure and children's extracurricular activities: Relationships with amount of involvement and affective experience of participation. *Journal of Applied Developmental Psychology, 4*(2), 241–257.

Baltes, P. B. (1997). On the incomplete architecture of human ontogeny: Selection, optimization, and compensation as foundations of developmental theory. *American Psychologist, 52*, 366–380.

Bandura, A. (1997). *Self-efficacy: The exercise of control*. New York: W. H. Freeman & Co.

Baranowski, T., Anderson, C., & Carmark, C. (1998). Mediating variables framework in physical activity interventions. How are we doing? How might we do better? *American Journal of Preventive Medicine, 15*, 266–297.

Baranowski, T., Cerin, E., & Baranowski, J. (2009). Steps in the design, development, and formative evaluation of obesity prevention-related behavior change trials. *International Journal of Behavioral Nutrition and Physical Activity, 6, 6*.

Baranowski, T., Cullen, K. W., Nicklas, T., Thompson, D., & Baranowski, J. (2002). School-based obesity prevention: A blueprint for taming the epidemic. *American Journal of Health Behavior, 26*(6), 486–493.

Baranowski, T., & Stables, G. (2000). Process evaluations of the 5-a-day projects. *Health Education & Behavior, 27*, 157–166.

Barber, B. L., Jacobson, K. C., Eccles, J. S., & Horn, M. C. (1997). "I don't want to play any more": When do talented adolescents drop out of competitive athletics? Paper presented at the biennial meeting of the Society for Research on Child Development, Washington, DC.

Barroso, C. S., McCullum-Gomez, C., Hoelscher, D. M., Kelder, S. H., & Murray, N. G. (2005). Self-reported barriers to quality physical education by physical education specialists in Texas. *Journal of School Health, 75*(8), 313–319.

Bartko, T. W., & Eccles, J. S. (2003). Adolescent participation in structured and unstructured activities: A person-oriented analysis. *Journal of Youth and Adolescence, 32*(4), 233–241.

Beets, M. W., Bieghle, A., Erwin, H. E., & Huberty, J. L. (2009). After-school program impact on physical activity and fitness: A meta analysis. *American Journal of Preventive Medicine, 36*, 527–537.

Beets, M. W., Vogel, R., Forlaw, L., Pitetti, K. H., & Cardinal, B. J. (2006). Social support and youth physical activity: The role of provider and type. *American Journal of Health Behaviors, 30*, 278–289.

Benton, D. (2004). Role of parents in the determination of the food preferences of children and the development of obesity. *International Journal of Obesity and Related Metabolic Disorders, 28*(7), 858–869.

Berenson, G. S. (2005). Obesity—a critical issue in preventive cardiology: The Bogalusa Heart Study. *Preventive Cardiology, 8*, 234–241.

Bond, L., Glover, S., Godfrey, C., Butler, H., & Patton, G. (2001). Building capacity for system-level change in schools: Lessons from the Gatehouse Project. *Health Education & Behavior, 28*, 368–383.

Borden, L. M., Perkins, D. F., Villarruel, F. A., & Stone, M. R. (2005). To participate or not to participate: That is the question. In G. G. Noam (Ed.). H. B. Weiss, P. M. D. Little, and S. M. Bouffard (Issue Eds.), *New directions for youth development. No. 105: Participation in youth programs: Enrollment, attendance, and engagement* (pp. 33–50). New York, NY: Wiley.

Bronfenbrenner, U. (2005). *Making human beings human: Bioecological perspectives on human development*. Thousand Oaks, CA: Sage.

Bronfenbrenner, U., & Morris, P. (2006). The bioecological model of human development. In W. Daman and R. M. Lerner (Editors-in-Chief). R. M. Lerner (Volume Ed.), *Handbook of child psychology: Vol. 1. Theoretical models of human development* (pp. 793–828). Hoboken, NJ: Wiley.

Bouffard, S., Wimer, C., Caronongan, P., Little, P., Dearing, E., & Simpkins, S. D. (2006). Demographic differences in patterns of youth out-of-school time activity participation. *Journal of Youth Development, 1*(1). Retrieved February 8, 2010, from http://www.nae4ha.org/directory/jyd/intro.html.

Brownson, R. C., Smith, C. A., Pratt, M., Mack, N. E., Jackson-Thompson, J., Dean, C. G., et al. (1996). Preventing cardiovascular disease through community-based risk reduction: The Bootheel Heart Health Project. *American Journal of Public Health, 86*, 206–213.

Bush, P. J., Zuckerman, A. E., Theiss, P. K., Taggart, V. S., Horowitz, C., Sheridan, M. J., et al. (1989). Cardiovascular risk factor prevention in black schoolchildren: Two-year results of the "Know Your Body" program. *American Journal of Epidemiology, 129*, 466–482.

Busseri, M. A., Rose-Krasnor, L., Willoughby, T., & Chalmers, H. (2006). A longitudinal examination of breadth and intensity of youth activity involvement and successful development. *Developmental Psychology, 42*, 1313–1326.

Caballero, B., Clay, T., Davis, S. M., Ethelbah, B., Holy Rock, B., Lohman, T., et al. (2003). Pathways: A school-based, randomized controlled trial for the prevention of obesity in American Indian schoolchildren. *American Journal of Clinical Nutrition, 78*, 1030–1038.

Cairns, R. B., Elder, G. H., Jr., & Costello, E. J. (Eds.). (1996). *Developmental science*. Cambridge: Cambridge University Press.

Casey, D. M., Ripke, M. N., & Huston, A. C. (2005). Activity participation and the well-being of children and adolescents in the context of welfare reform. In J. L. Mahoney, R. W. Larson, &

J. S. Eccles (Eds.), *Organized activities as contexts of development* (pp. 65–84). Mahwah, NJ: Erlbaum.

Cass, Y., & Price, P. (2003). More fit-increasing physical activity in adolescent girls using the Health Promoting Schools framework. *Health Promotion Journal of Australia, 14*, 159–164.

Centers for Disease Control and Prevention. (1997). Guidelines for school and community programs to promote lifelong physical activity among young people. *Morbidity and Mortality Weekly Report, 46*, 1–36.

Centers for Disease Control and Prevention. (2001). *The importance of regular physical activity for children*. Atlanta, GA: Centers for Disease Control and Prevention.

Coleman, K. J., Tiller, C. L., Sanchez, J., Heath, E. M., Oumer, S., Milliken, G., et al. (2005). Prevention of the epidemic increase in child risk of overweight in low-income schools. *Archives of Pediatrics & Adolescent Medicine, 159*, 217–224.

Collins, W. A., Maccoby, E., Steinberg, L., Hetherington, E. M., & Bornstein, M. H. (2000). Contemporary research on parenting: The case for nature and nurture. *American Psychologist, 55*, 218–232.

Cookson, S., Heath, A., & Bertrand, L. (2000). The HeartSmart Family Fun Pack: An evaluation of family-based intervention for cardiovascular risk reduction in children. *Canadian Journal of Public Health, 91*, 256–259.

Cotton, A., Stanton, K. R., Acs, Z. J., & Lovegrove, M. (2006). The UB obesity report card: An overview. Retrieved January 8, 2010, from http://www.ubalt.edu/experts/obesity.

Cox, A. E., Smith, A. L., & Williams, L. (2008). Change in physical education motivation and physical activity behavior during middle school. *Journal of Adolescent Health, 43*, 506–513.

Cumming, S. P., Smith, R. E., & Smoll, F. L. (2006). Athlete-perceived coaching behaviors: Relating two measurement traditions. *Journal of Sport & Exercise Psychology, 28*, 205–213.

Davis, S. M., Clay, T., Smyth, M., Gittelsohn, J., Arviso, V., Flint-Wagner, H., et al. (2003). Pathways curriculum and family interventions to promote healthful eating and physical activity in American Indian schoolchildren. *Preventive Medicine, 37*(6 Pt 2), S24–S34.

Deci, E. L., Koestner, R., & Ryan, R. M. (1999). A meta-analytic review of experiments examining the effects of extrinsic rewards on intrinsic motivation. *Psychological Bulletin, 125*, 627–668.

Devaney, B., & Rossi, P. (1997). Thinking through evaluation design options. *Children and Youth Services Review, 19*, 587–606.

DiLorenzo, T. M., Stucky-Ropp, R. C., Vander Wal, J. S., & Gotham, H. J. (1998). Determinants of exercise among children. II. A longitudinal analysis. *Preventive Medicine, 27*, 470–477.

Doak, C. M., Visscher, T. L. S., Renders, C. M., & Seidell, J. C. (2006). The prevention of overweight and obesity in children and adolescents: A review of interventions and programmes. *Obesity Review, 7*, 111–136.

Dowda, M., Sallis, J. F., McKenzie, T. L., Rosengard, P., & Kohl, H. W. (2005). Evaluating the sustainability of SPARK physical education: A case study of translating research into practice. *Research Quarterly for Exercise and Sport, 76*(1), 11–19.

Dunbar, C. (2002). *Alternative schooling for African American youth: Does anyone know we're here?* New York: Peter Lang.

Duncan, G. J., & Brooks-Gunn, J. (2000). Family poverty, welfare reform, and child development. *Child Development, 71*(1), 188–196.

Duncan, S. C., Duncan, T. E., & Strycker, L. A. (2005). Sources and types of social support in youth physical activity. *Health Psychology, 24*, 3–10.

Duncan, S. C., Duncan, T. E., Strycker, L. A., & Chaumeton, N. R. (2007). A cohort-sequential latent growth model of physical activity from ages 12 to 17 years. *Annals of Behavioral Medicine, 33*, 80–89.

Durlak, J., & DuPre, E. (2008). Implementation matters: A review of research on the influence of implementation on program outcomes and the factors affecting implementation. *American Journal of Community Psychology, 41*, 327–350.

Dusenbury, L., Brannigan, R., Falco, M., & Hansen, W. B. (2003). A review of research of fidelity of implementation: Implications for drug abuse prevention in school settings. *Health Education Research, 18*, 237–256.

Eccles, J. S., & Barber, B. (1999). Student council, volunteering, basketball, or marching band: What kind of extracurricular participation matters? *Journal of Adolescent Research, 14*, 10–43.

Eccles, J. S., Barber, B., Stone, M., & Hunt, J. (2003). Extracurricular activities and adolescent development. *Journal of Social Issues, 59*(4), 865–889.

Eccles, J. S., & Gootman, J. A. (Eds.). (2002). *Community programs to promote youth development*. Washington, DC: National Academy Press.

Eccles, J. S., & Midgley, C. (1989). Stage/environment fit: Developmentally appropriate classrooms for early adolescents. In R. Ames & C. Ames (Eds.), *Research on motivation in education (Vol 3)* (pp. 139–181). New York: Academic.

Eccles, J. S., & Wigfield, A. (2002). Motivational beliefs, values, and goals. *Annual Review of Psychology, 53*, 109–132.

Eccles, J. S., Wigfield, A., Harold, R. D., & Blumenfeld, P. (1993). Age and gender differences in children's achievement self-perceptions during the elementary school years. *Child Development, 64*, 830–847.

Eccles, J. S., Wigfield, A., & Schiefele, U. (1998). Motivation to succeed. In W. Damon (Series Ed.). N. Eisenberg (Vol. Ed.), *Handbook of child psychology: Vol. 3, Social, emotional and personality development* (5th ed., pp. 1017–1094). New York: Wiley.

Elder, G. H., & Conger, R. (2000). *Children of the land*. Chicago, IL: University of Chicago Press.

Erikson, E. H. (1968). *Identity: Youth and crisis*. New York: Norton.

Fauth, R. C., Roth, J. L., & Brooks-Gunn, J. (2007). Does the neighborhood context alter the link between youth's after-school time activities and developmental outcomes? A multilevel analysis. *Developmental Psychology, 43*(3), 760–777.

Fisher, K. J., & Li, F. (2004). A community-based walking trial to improve neighborhood quality of life in adults: A multilevel analysis. *Annals of Behavioral Medicine, 28*, 186–194.

Fitzgibbon, M. L., Stolley, M. R., Schiffer, L., Van Horn, L., Kaufer Christoffel, K., & Dyer, A. (2005). Two-year follow-up results for Hip-Hop to Health Jr.: A randomized controlled trial for overweight prevention in preschool minority children. *Journal of Pediatrics, 146*, 618–625.

Fredricks, J. A., & Eccles, J. S. (2005). Family socialization, gender, and sport motivation and involvement. *Journal of Sport & Exercise Psychology, 27*, 3–31.

Freemantle, N., Mason, J. M., Haines, A., & Eccles, M. P. (1997). CONSORT: An important step toward evidence-based health care. *Annals of Internal Medicine, 126*, 81–83.

Gerrard, M., Gibbons, F. X., & Bushman, B. J. (1996). Relation between perceived vulnerability to HIV and precautionary sexual behavior. *Psychology Bulletin, 119*(1), 390–409.

Goodnow, J. J., & Collins, W. A. (1990). *Development according to parents: The nature, sources, and consequences of parents' ideas*. Hillsdale, NJ: Lawrence Erlbaum.

Goran, M. L., & Reynolds, K. (2005). Interactive multimedia for promoting physical activity (IMPACT) in children. *Obesity Research, 13*, 762–771.

Gordon-Larsen, P., Nelson, M. C., & Popkin, B. M. (2004). Longitudinal physical activity and sedentary behavior trends: Adolescence to adulthood. *American Journal of Preventative Medicine, 27*(4), 277–283.

Gortmaker, S. L., Cheung, L. W. Y., Peterson, K., Chomitz, G., Cradle, J. H., Dart, H., et al. (1999). Impact of a school-based interdisciplinary intervention on diet and physical activity among urban primary school children. Eat well and keep moving. *Archives of Pediatrics & Adolescent Medicine, 153*, 975–983.

Gortmaker, S. L., Peterson, K., Wiecha, J., Sobol, A. M., Dixit, S., Fox, M. K., et al. (1999). Reducing obesity via a school-based interdisciplinary intervention among youth: Planet health. *Archives of Pediatrics & Adolescent Medicine, 153*, 409–418.

Griffin, S., Wilcox, S., Ory, M., Lattimore, D., Leviton, L., Castro, C., et al. (2009). Results from Active for Life process evaluation: Program delivery and fidelity. *Health Education Research, 25*(2), 325–342.

Griffin, S. F., Wilson, D. K., Wilcox, S., Buck, J., & Ainsworth, B. E. (2008). Physical activity influences in a disadvantaged African American community and the communities' solutions. *Health Education Practice, 9*, 180–190.

Gucciardini, E., Cameron, J., Liao, C., Palmer, A., & Steward, D. (2007). Program design features that can improve participation in health education interventions. *BMC Health Research Methodology, 7*, 47.

Harter, S. (1998). The development of self-representations. In N. Eisenberg (Ed.). W. Damon (Series Ed.), *Handbook of child psychology: Vol 3. Social emotional, and personality development* (5th ed., pp. 553–617). New York: Wiley.

Harter, S. (1999). *The construction of the self: A developmental perspective.* New York: Guilford.

Harter, S. (2003). The development of self-representations during childhood and adolescence. In M. R. Leary & J. P. Tangney (Eds.), *Handbook of self and identity* (pp. 610–642). New York: Guilford.

Hedley, A. A., Ogden, C. L., Johnson, C. L., Carroll, M. D., Curtin, L. R., & Flegal, K. M. (2004). Prevalence of overweight and obesity among US children, adolescents, and adults, 1999–2002. *Journal of the American Medical Association, 291*, 2847–2850.

Helitzer, D., & Yoon, S. J. (2002). Process evaluation of the Adolescent Social Action Program (ASAP). In A. Steckler and L. Linman (Eds.), *Process evaluation for public health interventions and research* (Chap. 4, pp. 83–109). San Francisco, CA: Jossey Bass.

Helitzer, D., Yoon, S., Wallerstein, N., & Garcia-Velarde, L. D. (2000). The role of process evaluation in the training of facilitators for an adolescent health education program. *Journal of School Health, 70*(4), 141–147.

Hirsch, B. J., Roffman, J. G., Deutsch, N. L., Flynn, C. A., Loder, T. L., & Pagano, M. E. (2000). Inner-city youth development organizations: Strengthening programs for adolescent girls. *Journal of Early Adolescence, 20*(2), 210–230.

Hopper, C. A., Munoz, K. D., Gruber, M. B., & MacConnie, S. (1996). A school-based cardiovascular exercise and nutrition program with parent participation: An evaluation study. *Children's Health Care, 25*(3), 221–235.

Hopper, C. A., Munoz, K. D., Gruber, M. B., & Nguyen, K. P. (2005). The effects of a family fitness program on the physical activity and nutrition behaviors of third-grade children. *Research Quarterly for Exercise and Sport, 76*(2), 130–139.

Horn, T. S. (1987). The influence of teacher-coach behavior on the psychological development of children. In D. Gould & M. R. Weiss (Eds.), *Advances in pediatric sport sciences* (Behavioral issues, Vol. 2, pp. 121–142). Champaign, IL: Human Kinetics.

Huebner, A. J., & Mancini, J. A. (2003). Shaping structured out-of-school time use among youth: The effects of self, family, and friend systems. *Journal of Youth and Adolescence, 32*(6), 453–463.

Hunt, D. E. (1975). Person-environment interaction: A challenge found wanting before it was tried. *Review of Educational Research, 45*, 209–230.

Israel, B. A., Schulz, A. J., Parker, E. A., & Becker, A. B. (2001). Community-based participatory research: Policy recommendations for promoting a partnership approach in health research. *Education and Health, 14*, 182–197.

Jacobs, J. E., Lanza, S., Osgood, D. W., Eccles, J. S., & Wigfield, A. (2002). Changes in children's self-competence and values: Gender and domain differences across grades one through twelve. *Child Development, 73*(2), 509–527.

Jacobs, J. E., Vernon, M. K., & Eccles, J. S. (2005). Activity choices in middle childhood: The roles of gender, self-beliefs, and parents' influence. In J. L. Mahoney, R. W. Larson, & J. S. Eccles (Eds.), *Organized activities as contexts of development: Extracurricular activities, after-school and community programs* (pp. 235–254). Mahwah, NJ: Lawrence Erlbaum Associates.

Janz, K. F., Burns, T. L., & Levy, S. M. (2005). Tracking of activity and sedentary behaviors in childhood: The Iowa Bone Development Study. *American Journal of Preventative Medicine, 29*(3), 171–178.

Janz, K. F., Dawson, J. D., & Mahoney, L. T. (2000). Tracking physical fitness and physical activity from childhood to adolescence: The Muscatine Study. *Medicine & Science in Sports & Exercise, 32*(7), 1250–1257.

Jarrett, R. L. (1997). African American family and parenting strategies in impoverished neighborhoods. *Qualitative Sociology, 20*, 275–288.

Johnson, C. C., Nicklas, T. A., Arbeit, M. L., Harsha, D. W., Mott, D. S., Hunter, S. M., et al. (1991). Cardiovascular intervention for high-risk families: The Heart Smart Program. *South African Medical Journal, 84*(11), 1305–1312.

Jordan, W. J., & Nettles, S. M. (2000). How students invest their time outside of school: Effects on school-related outcomes. *Social Psychology of Education, 3*, 217–243.

Kahn, E. B., Ramsey, L. T., Brownson, R. C., Heath, G. W., Howze, E. H., Powell, K. E., et al. (2002). The effectiveness of interventions to increase physical activity: A systematic review. *American Journal of Preventive Medicine, 22*(Suppl 4), 73–107.

Kao, L. S., Tyson, J. E., Blakely, M. L., & Lally, K. P. (2008). Clinical research methodology I: Introduction to randomized trials. *Journal of the American College of Surgeons, 206*(2), 361–369.

Kaptchuk, T. J. (2001). The double-blind, randomized, placebo-controlled trial: Gold standard or golden calf? *Journal of Clinical Epidemiology, 54*(6), 541–549.

Kazdin, A. E. (2003). *Research design in clinical psychology* (4th ed.). Boston, MA: Allyn & Bacon.

Kelder, S. H., Perry, C. L., & Klepp, K. I. (1989). Community-wide youth exercise promotion: Long-term outcomes of the Minnesota Heart Health Program and the Class of 1989 study. *Journal of School Health, 63*, 218–223.

Killen, J. D., Telch, M. J., Robinson, T. N., Maccoby, N., Taylor, C. B., & Farquhar, J. W. (1988). Cardiovascular disease risk reduction for tenth graders: A multiple-factor school-based approach. *Journal of the American Medical Association, 260*, 1728–1733.

Kinney, D. A. (1993). From nerds to normals: The recovery of identity among adolescents from middle school to high schools. *Sociology of Education, 66*, 21–40.

Koplan, J. P., Liverman, C. T., Kraak, V. I., & Wisham, S. L. (2007). *Progress in preventing childhood obesity: How do we measure up?* Washington (DC): Committee on Progress in Preventing Childhood Obesity, Food and Nutrition Board, Institute of Medicine of the National Academies.

Kumanyika, S. K. (2008). Environmental influences on childhood obesity: Ethnic and cultural influences in context. *Physiology & Behavior, 94*(1), 61–70.

Lauver, S., & Little, P. M. D. (2005). Recruitment and retention strategies for out-of-school time programs. In G. G. Noam (Ed.). H. B. Weiss, P. M. D. Little, and S. M. Bouffard (Issue Eds.), *New directions for youth development. No. 105: Participation in youth programs: Enrollment, attendance, and engagement* (pp. 71–89). New York, NY: Wiley.

Lemmens, V. E., Oenema, A., Klepp, K. I., Henriksen, H. B., & Brug, J. (2008). A systematic review of the evidence regarding efficacy obesity prevention interventions among adults. *Obesity Review, 9*(5), 446–455.

Lerner, R. M. (2006). Developmental science, developmental systems, and contemporary theories of human development. In W. Damon and R. M. Lerner (Eds.), *Handbook of child psychology Vol. 1: Theoretical models of human development* (6th ed., pp. 1–17). Hoboken, NJ: Wiley.

Leventhal, T., & Brooks-Gunn, J. (2000). The neighborhoods they live in: The effects of neighborhood residence on child and adolescent outcomes. *Psychological Bulletin, 126*(2), 309–337.

Levi, J., Vinter, S., St. Laurent, R., & Segal, L. M. (2008). F as in fat: How obesity policies are failing in America. Trust for America's Health Issue Report. Retrieved November 24, 2008, from http://healthyamericans.org/reports/obesity2008/obesity2008report.pdf.

Lillehoj, C., Griffin, K., & Spoth, R. (2004). Program provider and observer ratings of school-based preventive intervention implementation: Agreement and relation to youth outcomes. *Health Education & Behavior, 31*, 242–257.

Livingstone, M. B., Robson, P. J., Wallace, J. M., & McKinley, M. C. (2003). How active are we? Levels of routine physical activity in children and adults. *Proceedings of the Nutrition Society, 62*(3), 681–701.

Loder, T. L., & Hirsch, B. J. (2003). Inner-city youth development organizations: The salience of peer ties among early adolescent girls. *Applied Developmental Science, 7*(1), 2–12.

Luepker, R. V., Perry, C. L., McKinlay, S. M., Nader, P. R., Parcel, G. S., Stone, E. J., et al. (1996). Outcome of a field trial to improve children's dietary patterns and physical activity. The Child and Adolescent Trial for Cardiovascular Health (CATCH). *Journal of the American Medical Association, 275*, 768–776.

Luthar, S. S., Shoum, K. A., & Brown, P. J. (2006). Extracurricular involvement among affluent youth: A scapegoat for "ubiquitous achievement pressures"? *Developmental Psychology, 42*(3), 583–597.

Magnusson, D., & Stattin, H. (1998). Person-context interaction theories. In W. Damon & R. M. Lerner (Eds.), *Handbook of child psychology, Vol 1: Theoretical models of human development* (5th ed., pp. 685–759). Hoboken, NJ: Wiley.

Magnusson, D., & Stattin, H. (2006). The person in the environment: Towards a general model for scientific inquiry. In W. Damon and R. M. Lerner (Eds.), *Handbook of child psychology, Vol. 1: Theoretical models of human development* (6th ed., pp. 400–464). Hoboken, NJ: Wiley.

Mahoney, J. L., & Bergman, L. R. (2002). Conceptual and methodological issues in a developmental approach to positive adaptation. *Journal of Applied Developmental Psychology, 23*, 195–217.

Mahoney, J. L., Cairns, B. D., & Farmer, T. W. (2003). Promoting interpersonal competence and educational success through extracurricular activity participation. *Journal of Educational Psychology, 95*, 409–418.

Mahoney, J., Larson, R., & Eccles, J. (Eds.). (2005). *Organized activities as contexts of development: Extracurricular activities, after-school and community programs*. Hillsdale, NJ: Lawrence Erlbaum Associates.

Malina, R. M. (2001). Physical activity and fitness: Pathways from childhood to adulthood. *American Journal of Human Biology, 13*(2), 162–172.

Manios, Y., Kafatos, A., & Mamalakis, G. (1998). The effects of a health education intervention initiated at first grade over a 3 year period: Physical activity and fitness indices. *Health Education Research, 13*, 593–606.

Manios, Y., Moschandreas, J., Hatzis, C., & Kafatos, A. (1999). Evaluation of a health and nutrition education program in primary school children of Crete over a three-year period. *Preventive Medicine, 28*, 149–159.

Marcoux, M., Sallis, J. F., McKenzie, T., Marshall, S., Armstrong, C., & Goggin, K. (1999). Process evaluation of a physical activity self-management program for children: SPARK. *Psychology and Health, 14*, 659–677.

Marcovecchio, M., Mohn, A., & Chiarelli, F. (2005). Type 2 diabetes mellitus in children and adolescents. *Journal of Endocrinological Investigation, 28*, 853–863.

Marcus, A. C., Wheeler, R. C., Cullen, J. W., & Crane, L. A. (1987). Quasi-experimental evaluation of the Los Angeles Know Your Body Program: Knowledge, beliefs, and self-reported behaviors. *Preventive Medicine, 16*, 803–815.

Marsh, H. W., & Kleitman, S. (2002). Extracurricular school activities: The good, the bad, and the nonlinear. *Educational Review, 72*, 464–514.

Martin, J. J., & McCaughtry, N. (2008). Using social cognitive theory to predict physical activity in inner-city African American school children. *Journal of Sport & Exercise Psychology, 30*, 378–391.

Martinez Vizcaino, V., Salcedo Aguilar, F., Franquelo Gutierrez, R., Torrijos Regidor, R., Morant Sanchez, A., Solera Martinez, M., et al. (2008). Assessment of an after-school physical activity program to prevent obesity among 9–10 year old children: A cluster randomized trial. *International Journal of Obesity, 32*, 12–22.

Masse, L. C., Dassa, C., Gauvin, L., Giles-Corti, B., & Motl, R. (2002). Emerging measurement and statistical methods in physical activity research. *American Journal of Preventive Medicine, 23*, 44–55.

McGraw, S. A., Sellers, D. E., Stone, E. J., Resnicow, K., Kuester, S., Fridinger, F., et al. (2000). Monitoring implementation of school programs and policies to promote healthy eating and physical activity among youth. *Preventive Medicine, 31*(2), S86–S97.

McKenzie, T. L., Nader, P. R., Strikmiller, P. K., Yang, M., Stone, E. J., Perry, C. L., et al. (1996). School physical education: Effect of the Child and Adolescent Trial for Cardiovascular Health. *Preventive Medicine, 25*, 423–431.

McKenzie, T. L., Sallis, J. F., Prochaska, J. J., Conway, T., Marshall, S., & Rosengard, P. (2004). Evaluation of a two-year middle-school physical education intervention: M-SPAN. *Medicine and Science in Sports and Exercise, 36*(94), 1382–1388.

Moher, D., Schulz, K. F., & Altman, D. G. (2001). The CONSORT statement: Revised recommendations for improving the quality of reports of parallel group randomized trials. *Medical Research Methodology, 1*(2), 1471. Retrieved March 4, 2011, from http://www.biomedcentral.com/1471-2288/1/2.

Molnar, B. E., Gortmaker, S. L., Bull, F. C., & Buka, S. L. (2004). Unsafe to play? Neighborhood disorder and lack of safety predict reduced physical activity among urban children and adolescents. *American Journal of Health Promotion, 18*(5), 378–386.

Morbidity and Mortality Weekly Report (MMWR). (1999). Neighborhood safety and the prevalence of physical inactivity—selected states. *MMWR. Morbidity and Mortality Weekly Report, 48*, 143–146.

Mukoma, W., & Flisher, A. J. (2004). Evaluations of health promoting schools: A review of nine studies. *Health Promotion International, 19*, 357–368.

Nader, P. R. (2003). National Institute of Child Health and Human Development Study of Early Child Care and Youth Development Network: Frequency and intensity of activity of third-grade children in physical education. *Archives of Pediatrics & Adolescent Medicine, 157*(2), 185–190.

Nader, P. R., Bradley, R. H., Houts, R. M., McRitchie, S. L., & O'Brien, M. (2008). Moderate-to-vigorous physical activity from ages 9 to 15 years. *Journal of the American Medical Association, 300*(3), 295–305.

Nader, P. R., Sallis, J. F., Patterson, T. L., & Abramson, I. S. (1989). A family approach to cardiovascular risk reduction: Results from the San Diego Family Health Project. *Health Education Quarterly, 16*, 229–244.

Nader, P. R., Stone, E. J., Lytle, L. A., Perry, C. L., Osganian, S. K., Kelder, S., et al. (1999). Three-year maintenance of improved diet and physical activity: The CATCH cohort. Child and Adolescent Trial for Cardiovascular Health. *Archives of Disease in Childhood, 153*, 695–704.

Needham, B., & Crosnoe, R. (2004). Overweight and depression during adolescence. *Journal of Adolescent Health, 36*, 48–55.

Nelson, M. C., Neumark-Stzainer, D., Hannan, P. J., Sirard, J. R., & Story, M. (2006). Longitudinal and secular trends in physical activity and sedentary behavior during adolescence. *Pediatrics, 118*(6), 1627–1634.

Ogden, C. L., Carroll, M. D., Curtin, L. R., McDowell, M. A., Tabak, C. J., & Flegal, K. M. (2006). Prevalence of overweight and obesity in the United States, 1999–2004. *Journal of the American Medical Association, 295*(13), 1549–1555.

Ogden, C. L., Flegal, K. M., Carroll, M. D., & Johnson, C. L. (2002). Prevalence and trends in overweight among US children and adolescents, 1999–2000. *Journal of the American Medical Association, 288*, 1728–1732.

Olshansky, S. J., Passaro, D. J., Hershow, R. C., Layden, J., Carnes, B. A., Brody, J., et al. (2005). A potential decline in life expectancy in the United States in the 21st century. *The New England Journal of Medicine, 352*(11), 1138–1145.

Overton, W. F. (2006). Developmental psychology: Philosophy, concepts, methodology. In W. Damon and R. M. Lerner (Eds.), *Handbook of child psychology, Vol. 1: Theoretical models of human development* (6th ed., pp. 18–88). Lerner, Hoboken, NJ: Wiley.

Palmer, S., Graham, G., & Elliott, E. (2005). Effects of a web-based health program on fifth grade children's physical activity knowledge, attitudes, and behavior. *American Journal of Health Education, 36*, 86–93.

Paradis, G., Levesque, L., Macauley, A. C., Cargo, M., McComber, A., Kirby, R., et al. (2005). Impact of a diabetes prevention program on body size, physical activity, and diet among Kanien'keha:ka (Mohawk) children 6 to 11 years old: 8-year results from the Kahnawake Schools Diabetes Prevention Project. *Pediatrics, 115*, 333–339.

Parcel, G. S., Simons-Morton, B. G., & Kolbe, L. J. (1988). Health promotion: Integrating organizational change and student learning strategies. *Health Education Quarterly, 15*, 436–450.

Parke, R. D., Killian, C., Dennis, J., Flyr, M., McDowell, D. J., Simpkins, S. D., et al. (2003). Managing the external environment: The parent as active agent in the system. In L. Kuczynski (Ed.), *Handbook of dynamic in parent-child relations* (pp. 247–270). Thousand Oaks, CA: Sage.

Pate, R. R., Dowda, M., O'Neill, J. R., & Ward, D. S. (2007). Change in physical activity participation among adolescent girls from 8th to 12th grade. *Journal of Physical Activity and Health, 4*(1), 3–16.

Pearce, N. J., & Larson, R. W. (2006). How teens become engaged in youth development programs: The process of motivational change in a civic activism organization. *Applied Developmental Science, 10*, 121–131.

Pedersen, S., & Seidman, E. (2005). Contexts and correlates of out-of-school activity participation among low-income urban adolescents. In J. L. Mahoney, R. W. Larson, & J. S. Eccles (Eds.), *Organized activities as contexts of development: Extracurricular activities, after-school and community programs* (pp. 85–110). Mahwah, NJ: Lawrence Erlbaum Associates.

Persson, A., Kerr, M., & Stattin, H. (2007). Staying in or moving away from structured activities: Explanations involving parents and peers. *Developmental Psychology, 43*, 197–207.

Pettit, G. S., Laird, R. D., Bates, J. E., & Dodge, K. A. (1997). Patterns of after-school care in middle childhood: Risk factors and developmental outcomes. *Merrill-Palmer Quarterly, 43*, 515–538.

Quinn, J. (1999). Where needs meet opportunity: Youth development programs for early teens. In R. Behrman (Ed.), *The future of children: When school is out* (pp. 96–116). Washington, DC: The David and Lucile Packard Foundation.

Quiroz, P. (2000). A comparison of the organizational and cultural contexts of extracurricular participation and sponsorship in two high schools. *Educational Studies, 31*, 249–275.

Ransdell, L. B., Dratt, J., Kennedy, C., O'Neill, S., & DeVoe, D. (2001). Daughters and mothers exercising together (DAMET): A 12-week pilot project designed to improve physical self-perception and increase recreational physical activity. *Women's Health, 33*, 101–116.

Ransdell, L. B., Taylor, A., Oakland, D., Schmidt, J., Moyer-Mileur, L., & Schultz, B. (2003). Daughters and mothers exercising together: Effects of home- and community-based programs. *Medicine and Science in Sports and Exercise, 35*, 286–296.

Robinson, T. N. (1999). Reducing children's television viewing to prevent obesity: A randomized control trial. *Journal of the American Medical Association, 282*, 1561–1566.

Roffman, J. G., Suaurez-Orozco, C., & Rhodes, J. (2003). Facilitating positive development in immigrant youth: The role of mentors and community organizations. In F. A. VIllarruel, D. F. Perkins, L. M. Borden, and J. G. Keith (Eds.), *Community youth development: Programs, policies, and practices* (pp. 90–117). Thousand Oaks, CA: Sage.

Rogoff, B. (2003). *The cultural nature of human development*. Oxford, UK: Oxford University Press.

Ross, C. E. (1994). Overweight and depression. *Journal of Health and Social Behavior, 33*, 63–78.

Rural School & Community Trust. (2005). Riding to school in slow motion. Retrieved January 7, 2008, from http://www.ruraledu.org/site/c.beJMIZOCIrH/b.2820295.

Ryan, R. M., & Deci, E. L. (2000). Self-determination theory and the facilitation of intrinsic motivation, social development, and well-being. *American Psychologist, 55*, 68–78.

Saakslahti, A., Numminen, P., Salo, P., Tuominen, J., Helenius, H., & Valimaki, I. (2004). Effects of a three year intervention on children's physical activity from age 4 to 7. *Pediatric Exercise Science, 16*, 167–180.

Sahota, P., Rudolf, M. C. J., Dixey, R., Hill, A. J., Barth, J. H., & Cade, J. (2001). Randomized controlled trial of primary school based intervention to reduce risk factors for obesity. *British Medical Journal, 323*, 1–5.

Sallis, J. F., Cervero, R. B., Ascher, W., Henderson, K. A., Kraft, M. K., & Kerr, J. (2006). An ecological approach to creating active living communities. *Annual Review of Public Health, 27*, 297–322.

Sallis, J., McKenzie, T., Alcaraz, J., Kolody, B., Faucette, N., & Hovell, M. F. (1997). The effects of a 2-year physical education program (SPARK) on physical activity and fitness in elementary school students. *American Journal of Public Health, 87*, 1328–1334.

Sallis, J. F., McKenzie, T. L., Conway, T. L., Elder, J. P., Prochaska, J. J., Brown, M., et al. (2003). Environmental interventions for eating and physical activity. A randomized controlled trial in middle schools. *American Journal of Preventive Medicine, 24*, 209–217.

Salmon, J., Booth, M. L., Phongsavan, P., Murphy, N., & Timperio, A. (2007). Promoting physical activity participation among children and adolescents. *Epidemiologic Reviews, 29*, 144–159.

Saunders, R. P., Ward, D., Felton, G. M., Dowda, M., & Pate, R. R. (2006). Examining the link between program implementation and behavior outcomes in a lifestyle education activity program (LEAP). *Evaluation and Program Planning, 29*, 352–364.

Save the Children. (2002). America's forgotten children: Child poverty in rural America. Retrieved January 20, 2008, from http://www.savethechildren.org/publications/.

Scanlan, T. K., Babkes, M. L., & Scanlan, L. A. (2005). Participation in sport: A developmental glimpse at emotion. In J. L. Mahoney, R. W. Larson, & J. S. Eccles (Eds.), *Organized activities as contexts of development: Extracurricular activities, after-school and community programs* (pp. 275–310). Mahwah, NJ: Lawrence Erlbaum Associates.

Schwimmer, J. B., Burwinkle, T. M., & Varni, J. W. (2003). Health-related quality of life in severely obese children and adolescents. *Journal of the American Medical Association, 289*, 1813–1819.

Shadish, W. R., Cook, T. D., & Campbell, D. T. (2002). Experimental and generalized causal inference. In W. R. Shadish, T. D. Cook & D. T. Campbell (Eds.), *Experimental and quasi-experimental designs for generalized causal inference* (pp. 1–32). Boston, MA: Houghton Mifflin Company.

Shann, M. H. (2001). Students' use of time outside of school: A case for after school programs for urban middle school youth. *The Urban Review, 33*, 339–356.

Sharma, M. (2006). School-based interventions for childhood and adolescent obesity. *Obesity Review, 7*, 261–269.

Shaya, F. T., Flores, D., Gbarayor, C. M., & Wang, J. (2008). School-based obesity interventions: A literature review. *Journal of School Health, 78*(4), 189–196.

Simon, C., Schweitzer, B., Oujaa, M., Wagner, A., Arveiler, D., Triby, E., et al. (2008). Successful overweight prevention in adolescents by increasing physical activity: A 4-year randomized controlled intervention. *International Journal of Obesity, 32*, 1489–1498.

Simpkins, S. D., Fredricks, J., Davis-Kean, P., & Eccles, J. S. (2006). Healthy minds, healthy habits: The influence of activity involvement in middle childhood. In A. C. Huston & M. N. Ripke (Eds.), *Developmental contexts in middle childhood* (pp. 283–302). New York: Cambridge University Press.

Simpkins, S. D., Ripke, M., Huston, A. C., & Eccles, J. S. (2005). Predicting participation and outcomes in out-of-school activities: Similarities and differences across social ecologies. In G. G. Noam (Ed.). H. B. Weiss, P. M. D. Little, and S. M. Bouffard (Issue Eds.). *New directions for youth development. No. 105: Participation in youth programs: Enrollment, attendance, and engagement* (pp. 51–70). New York, NY: Wiley.

Sinha, R., Fisch, G., Teague, B., Tamborlane, W. V., Banyas, B., Allen, K., et al. (2002). Prevalence of impaired glucose tolerance among children and adolescence with marked obesity. *The New England Journal of Medicine, 346*, 802–810.

Slomkowski, C., Rende, R., Novak, S., Lloyd-Richardson, E., & Niaura, R. (2005). Sibling effects on smoking in adolescence: Evidence for social influence from a genetically informed design. *Addiction, 100*, 430–438.

Smith, A. L. (1999). Perceptions of peer relationships and physical activity participation in early adolescence. *Journal of Sport & Exercise Psychology, 21*, 329–350.

Springer, A. E., Kelder, S. H., & Hoelscher, D. M. (2006). Social support, physical activity and sedentary behavior among 6th-grade girls: A cross-sectional study. *International Journal of Behavioral Nutrition and Physical Activity, 3*, 8–17.

Spurrier, N. J., Magarey, A. A., Golley, R., Curnow, F., & Sawyer, M. G. (2008). Relationships between the home environment and physical activity and dietary patterns of preschool children: A cross-sectional study. *International Journal of Behavioral Nutrition and Physical Activity, 5*, 31–42.

Steckler, A., & Linnan, L. (2002). Process evaluation for public health interventions and research: An overview. In A. Steckler & L. Linnan (Eds.), *Process evaluation for public health interventions and research* (pp. 1–21). San Francisco, CA: Jossey-Bass.

St Leger, L. (2004). What's the place of schools in promoting health? Are we too optimistic? *Health Promotion International, 19*(4), 419–427.

Storey, P., & Brannen, J. (2000). Young people and transport in rural areas. Retrieved November 2, 2007, from http://www.jrf.org.uk/knowledge/findings/socialpolicy/750.asp.

Story, M., Sherwood, N. E., Himes, J. H., Davis, M., Jacobs, D. R., Cartwright, Y., et al. (2003). An after-school obesity prevention program for African-American girls: The Minnesota GEMS pilot study. *Ethnicity & Disease, 13*, S1-54–S1-64.

Strong, W. B., Malina, R. M., Blimkie, C. J., Daniels, S. R., Dishman, R. K., Gutin, B., et al. (2005). Evidence based physical activity for school-age youth. *Journal of Pediatrics, 146*(6), 732–737.

Summerbell, C., Waters, E., Edmunds, L., Kelly, S., Brown, T., & Campbell, K. (2005). Interventions for preventing obesity in children. *Cochrane Database of Systematic Reviews, 3*, Article No.: CD001871, 1–70.

Taylor, W. C., Blair, S. N., Cummings, S. S., Wun, C. C., & Malina, R. M. (1999). Childhood and adolescent physical activity patterns and adult physical activity. *Medicine & Science in Sports & Exercise, 31*(1), 118–123.

Troiano, R. P., & Flegal, K. M. (1998). Overweight children and adolescents: Description, epidemiology, and demographics. *Pediatrics, 101*, 497–504.

U.S. Department of Agriculture (USDA). (2005). *Dietary guidelines for Americans, 2005.* Washington, DC: US Department of Health and Human Services/US Department of Agriculture.

U.S. Department of Health and Human Services. (2000). *Healthy people 2010 (conference edition in two volumes): Understanding and improving health and objectives for improving health.* Washington, DC: U.S. Department of Health and Human Services.

U.S. Department of Health and Human Services. (2008). *Physical activity guidelines advisory committee report.* Washington, DC: U.S. Department of Health and Human Services.

Vandell, D. L., Shumow, L., & Posner, J. (2005). After-school programs for low-income children: Differences in program quality. In J. L. Mahoney, R. W. Larson, & J. S. Eccles (Eds.), *Organized activities as contexts of development: Extracurricular activities, after-school and community programs* (pp. 437–456). Mahwah, NJ: Lawrence Erlbaum Associates.

Vandongen, R., Jenner, D. A., Thompson, C., Taggart, A. C., Spickett, E. E., Burke, V., et al. (1995). A controlled evaluation of a fitness and nutrition intervention program on cardiovascular health in 10- to 12-year-old children. *Preventive Medicine, 24*(1), 9–22.

Veugelers, P. J., & Fitzgerald, A. L. (2005). Effectiveness of school programs in preventing childhood obesity: A multilevel comparison. *American Journal of Public Health, 95*(3), 432–435.

Viadro, C., Earp, J., & Altpeter, M. (1997). Designing a process evaluation for a comprehensive breast cancer screening intervention: Challenges and opportunities. *Evaluation and Program Planning, 20*, 237–249.

Wang, Y., Beydoun, M. A., Liang, L., Caballero, B., & Kumanyika, S. K. (2008). Will all Americans become overweight or obese? Estimating the progression and cost of the US obesity epidemic. *Obesity, 16*(10), 2323–2330.

Wang, G., & Dietz, W. H. (2002). Economic burden of obesity in youths aged 6 to 17 years 1979–1999. *Pediatrics, 109*(5), e81. Retrieved January 7, 2008, from http://www.pediatrics.org/cgi/content/full/109/5/e81.

Ward-Begnoche, W., & Speaker, S. (2006). Overweight youth: Changing behaviors that are barriers to health. *Journal of Family Practice, 55*(11), 957–963.

Ward, D. S., Saunders, R., Felton, G. M., Williams, E., Epping, J. N., & Pate, R. R. (2006). Implementation of a school environment intervention to increase physical activity in high school girls. *Health Education Research, 21*(6), 896–910.

Warren, J. M., Henry, C. J. K., Lightowler, H. J., Bradshaw, S. M., & Perwaiz, S. (2003). Evaluation of a pilot school programme aimed at the prevention of obesity in children. *Health Promotion International, 18*, 287–296.

Weinberg, R. S., & Gould, D. (2007). Children and sport psychology. In R. S. Weinberg & D. Gould (Eds.), *Foundations of sport and exercise psychology* (pp. 514–532). Champaign, IL: Human Kinetics.

Weir, L. A., Etelson, D., & Brand, D. A. (2006). Parents' perceptions of neighborhood safety and children's physical activity. *Preventive Medicine, 43*, 212–217.

Weiss, M., & Smith, A. L. (2002). Friendship quality in youth sport: Relationship to age, gender, and motivational variables. *Journal of Sport & Exercise Psychology, 24*, 420–437.

Whiteman, S. D., McHale, S. M., & Crouter, A. C. (2007). Explaining sibling similarities: Perceptions of sibling influences. *Journal of Youth and Adolescence, 35*, 963–972.

Wigfield, A., & Eccles, J. S. (2002). Motivational beliefs, values, and goals. *Annual Review of Psychology, 53*, 109–132.

Wilmore, J. H., & Costill, D. L. (1994). Physiology of sport and exercise. In J. H. Wilmore & D. L. Costill (Eds.), *Growth development and the young athlete* (pp. 400–421). Champaign, IL: Human Kinetics.

Wilson, D. K., Evans, A. E., Williams, J., Mixon, G., Minette, C., Sirad, J., et al. (2005). A preliminary test of a student-centered program on increasing physical activity in underserved adolescents. *Annals of Behavioral Medicine, 30*, 119–124.

Wilson, D. K., Griffin, S., Saunders, R., Evans, A., Mixon, G., Wright, M., et al. (2006). Formative evaluation of a motivational intervention for increasing physical activity in youth. *Evaluation and Program Planning, 29*, 260–268.

Wilson, D. K., Griffin, S., Saunders, R., Kitzman-Ulrich, H., Meyers, D. C., & Mansard, L. (2009). Using process evaluation for program improvement in dose, fidelity and reach: The ACT Trial experience. *International Journal of Behavior Nutrition and Physical Activity, 6*, 79.

Wilson, D. K., Kirtland, K., Ainsworth, B., & Addy, C. L. (2004). Socioeconomic status and perceptions of access and safety for physical activity. *Annals of Behavioral Medicine, 28*, 20–28.

Wilson, D. K., & Kitzman-Ulrich, H. (2008). Cultural considerations in the development of pediatric weight management programs. In E. Jelalian & R. G. Steele (Eds.), *Handbook of childhood obesity* (pp. 293–312). Washington, DC: American Psychological Association.

Wilson, D. K., Kitzman-Ulrich, H., Williams, J. E., Saunders, R., Griffin, S., Pate, R., et al. (2008). An overview of the "Active by Choice Today" (ACT) trial for increasing physical activity. *Contemporary Clinical Trials, 29*, 21–31.

Wilson, D. K., Teasley, N., Friend, R., Green, S., & Sica, D. A. (2002). Motivational versus social cognitive interventions for promoting healthy diet and physical activity habits in African-American adolescents. *Annals of Behavioral Medicine, 24*, 310–319.

Wilson, D. K., Van Horn, M. L., Kitzman-Ulrich, H., Saunders, R., Pate, R., Lawman, H., et al. (2011). The results of the "Active by Choice Today" trial for increasing physical activity in underserved adolescents. *Health Psychology, 30*(4), 463–471.

Winters, E. R., Petosa, R. L., & Charlton, T. E. (2003). Using social cognitive theory to explain discretionary. 'Leisure-time' physical exercise among school students. *Journal of Adolescent Health, 32*, 436–442.

Zametkin, A. J., Zoon, C. K., Klein, H. W., & Munson, S. (2004). Psychiatric aspects of child and adolescent obesity: A review of the past ten years. *Journal of the American Academy of Child and Adolescent Psychiatry, 43*, 134–150.

Zarrett, N. R. (2007). The dynamic relation between out-of-school activities and adolescent development (Doctoral dissertation, University of Michigan, 2006). *Dissertation Abstracts International, 67*(10), 6100B.

Zarrett, N., & Eccles, J. S. (2006). The passage to adulthood: Challenges of late adolescence. In S. Piha and G. Hall (Vol. Eds.), *New directions for youth development. Preparing youth for the crossing: From adolescence to early adulthood* (Issue 111, pp. 13–28). Hoboken, NJ: Wiley Periodicals.

Zarrett, N., Peck, S. C., & von Eye, A. (under review). Do activities matter? Pathways from personal, familial, and community risk to educational achievement across the adolescent years.

Chapter 9
The Role of Physical Activity in Treatment of Substance Use Disorders

Dori W. Pekmezi, Lucas J. Carr, Brooke Barbera, and Bess H. Marcus

The term "substance use disorders" encompasses a wide-range of problems. Such a diagnosis can accurately describe individuals who regularly smoke cigarettes, as well as chronic alcoholics and/or drug addicts (American Psychiatric Association, 2000). In many cases, substance abuse and dependence are associated with negative personal, social, occupational, and/or legal consequences, which can lead individuals to seek treatment. In fact, according to facilities that report to State administrative data systems, there were nearly 1.8 million admissions for treatment of alcohol and drug abuse in 2006 (National Institute on Drug Abuse, 2009). Recently, the focus of substance use treatment has begun to shift towards promoting global health and wellness changes as part of the recovery process (Read et al., 2001). For example, health-care providers often encourage lifestyle changes (e.g., increased physical activity) to facilitate psychological and physical recovery in persons with substance use disorders (Read et al.). Physical activity is a particularly appealing treatment option as it is easily accessible, low cost, and can be pursued on one's own schedule. In this chapter, we provide an overview on substance use treatment, discuss the potential benefits of incorporating physical activity into such programs, and then examine the research literature on physical activity as an intervention for substance use disorders.

D.W. Pekmezi (✉)
Department of Health Behavior, School of Public Health, University of Alabama at Birmingham, 1665 University Blvd., 227 RPHB, Birmingham, AL 35293, USA
e-mail: dpekmezi@uab.edu

L.J. Carr
Department of Health and Human Physiology, University of Iowa,
E012 Field House, Iowa City, IA 52242, USA

Centers for Behavioral and Preventive Medicine, The Miriam Hospital and Alpert Medical School of Brown University, One Hoppin Street, Suite 500, 02903, Providence, RI, USA

B. Barbera • B.H. Marcus
Centers for Behavioral and Preventive Medicine, The Miriam Hospital and Alpert Medical School of Brown University, One Hoppin Street, Suite 500, Providence, RI 02903, USA

A.L. Meyer and T.P. Gullotta (eds.), *Physical Activity Across the Lifespan*,
Issues in Children's and Families' Lives 12, DOI 10.1007/978-1-4614-3606-5_9,
© Springer Science+Business Media New York 2012

Overview of Treatment of Substance Use Disorders

Treatment Settings

No single treatment is appropriate for all substance use disorders (National Institute on Drug Abuse, 2009) as consumption patterns, associated behaviors and thoughts, and physiological symptoms vary substantially across the classes of substances (i.e., alcohol, amphetamines, cannabis, cocaine, hallucinogens, inhalants, nicotine, opioids) (DSM-IV-TR). Thus, to serve such a diverse and variable need, the treatment of substance use disorders has been applied in a wide variety of settings and therapeutic styles.

The choice of treatment setting is usually determined by the medical and psychiatric needs of the individual (Hoffman, Halikas, Mee-Lee, & Weedman, 1991). Alternatives can be chosen based on several dimensions, including outpatient versus inpatient, group versus individual, and professional versus nonprofessional. Considerations for selecting treatment setting include acute intoxication or withdrawal potential, biomedical conditions or complications, emotional or behavioral conditions, treatment acceptance, health insurance (and comprehensiveness of coverage), relapse potential, and recovery environment (Hoffman et al. 1991). For example, some substances (e.g., alcohol and benzodiazepines) can produce such severe withdrawal symptoms (e.g., seizures) that detoxification can be life-threatening and require some level of inpatient care in either a hospital or treatment facility (Myrick & Anton, 1998). Following inpatient treatment, intermediate levels of care (e.g., halfway house) are often considered.

The next tier of care is outpatient treatment, which can vary in intensity and modality, but typically involves the patient living at home and receiving substance-specific services at a hospital, treatment facility, or community center on an individual or group basis. Groups are often popular as this setting provides opportunities for patients to receive helpful feedback from other members who may be further along in recovery. For example, peers within a smoking cessation group could share strategies to reduce cigarette consumption at high craving times (i.e., first thing in the morning, with coffee, during stressful events).

While many of the options discussed thus far involve treatment provided by trained professionals, nonprofessional options are also prevalent, such as 12-step programs. Alcoholics Anonymous (AA; http://www.aa.org/) has offered free-of-charge, supportive, peer-led group counseling since 1935 (Alcoholics Anonymous, 1972) and has an estimated 2,000,000 members. Narcotics Anonymous (NA; http://www.na.org/) was later developed for individuals who wanted to utilize the 12-step method for drug-specific dependence, and groups are available for cocaine, methamphetamines, and marijuana use (Narcotics Anonymous, 2007).

Theories of Substance Abuse Treatment

The treatment of addiction to substances is typically structured by theories on how the addictive behaviors were acquired or are maintained. While addiction can be understood in a variety of ways, the following section focuses on the three main, empirically supported approaches to the treatment of substance use disorders: cognitive-behavioral, relapse prevention, and motivational interviewing. Physical activity can be an accessible and easily integrated component within any of these theoretical approaches. Contrasted with addiction, physical activity is associated with numerous positive health benefits that can aid overall recovery across these modalities.

Cognitive-Behavioral Treatment

Cognitive-behavioral therapy regards substance dependence as learned behavior acquired through experience (Kadden et al., 1992). More specifically, alcohol and drug dependence can be understood as the result of observable antecedents and consequences to behavior. For example, an individual may experience high situational stress at work (antecedent), smoke a cigarette in response to that stress (behavior), and experience reduced tension (consequence). In this example, substance use occurs in relation to a negative situation and achieves a desired outcome. Cognitive-behavioral theory asserts that the probability of substance use behaviors occurring increases each time substance use is reinforced. By extension, treatment approaches developed from cognitive-behavioral theory have two main parts: (1) identification of needs met by substance use and/or situations that promote substance use, and (2) development of skills to cope with those situations and find alternatives to meet those needs.

Thus, treatment often involves becoming aware of triggers, such as persons, objects, and settings that have become associated with substance use through routine pairings. For example, if a client regularly drinks at a bar after work with co-workers, then these people (co-workers), places (bar), situations (after work) may constitute triggers for alcohol use. In exposure-based approaches, individuals are repeatedly exposed to these triggers but not allowed to engage in substance use (i.e., "response prevention"), thereby reducing their impact over time. Stimulus control approaches use more of a fading paradigm and aim to rid the environmental stimuli that precede substance use behavior. To fade the behavior, substance use is restricted to a highly circumscribed set of stimuli (no smoking in the house) and gradually decreased.

Other cognitive-behavioral treatment approaches such as contingency management and the Community Reinforcement Approach (CRA) are primarily focused on changing the consequences of substance use. Contingency management approaches utilize reward programs for abstinence, typically in the form of token economies (Stizter & Petry, 2006). CRA (Hunt & Azrin, 1973) is more extensive as it was developed for extremely debilitated alcoholics and focuses on improving communication skills with the participants' spouse or significant others, developing social and recreational activities not associated with alcohol, and practicing drink refusal skills, as well as job club participation for those who are unemployed.

Finally, cognitive restructuring is another important component of cognitive-behavioral treatment for substance use disorders (McCrady, 2007). This technique involves identifying maladaptive thoughts about substance use (e.g., "I will not be able to get through this party without drinking") and then challenging them. Participants are encouraged to review their self talk for distortions (e.g. "It might be possible for me to make it through this party without drinking.") and then substitute more realistic statements ("This is hard, but I can do it"). Numerous studies have indicated that cognitive-behavioral therapy (CBT) is effective in treating alcohol and drug dependence.

Relapse Prevention

The Relapse Prevention (RP) model is based on the notion that what produces initial change in behavior is not necessarily what is needed to maintain it. RP (Bandura, 1977; Marlatt & Gordon, 1985) focuses on helping participants develop coping strategies (i.e., planning ahead, seeking support, using relaxation techniques, scheduling pleasurable activities) and avoid reverting to earlier patterns of substance use in high-risk situations (Parks & Marlatt, 1999). For example, an individual whose nightly social interactions involved drinking at a local bar may brainstorm non-alcoholic activities like watching movies with a friend. Besides planning social activities that avoid drinking, individuals must also plan for interactions that involve others who continue substance use and practice declining invitations that involve substance use (Rawson, Obert, McCann, & Marinelli-Casey, 1993). Additional components of RP include anger management, normalizing cravings, and dealing with lapses (Dimeff & Marlatt, 1998). Past research has indicated that RP is not associated with higher abstinence rates, but can reduce the frequency and intensity of relapse.

Motivational Interviewing

Motivational interviewing (MI) was developed for the treatment of substance use disorders and has since been used as part of intervention for a broad range of behavioral problems (Arkowitz & Miller, 2008). Miller and Rollnick (2002) define MI as a "directive method for enhancing intrinsic motivation to change by exploring and resolving ambivalence" (Miller & Rollnick, 2002). MI is a client-centered approach, which emphasizes four main principles: expressing empathy, developing the discrepancy between a client's desired and actual behaviors, rolling with resistance, and supporting the client's self-efficacy (Miller & Rollnick, 2002). Reviews (Rubak, Sandbaek, Lauritzen, & Christensen, 2005) and past studies focused on alcohol use (Miller, Benefield, & Tonigan, 1993) have demonstrated that individuals receiving MI had better outcomes than those receiving traditional advice-giving therapies.

Physical Activity as a Component or Adjunct to Treatment

Physical activity can play a complementary role within the context of existing models and treatment approaches for addiction. Exercise can be done across all treatment settings, either alone or with others who are also practicing abstinence or reducing their substance use. Exercise options (e.g., group sports, exercise videos) are often available, if not prescribed, in inpatient treatment settings (Kremer, Malkin, & Benshoff, 1995) As a functional component within CBT or RP, exercise may be included as a potential pleasurable activity for alternative activity planning, and more generally, as a positive coping response to experiences of craving and other triggers for use. Regular participation in physical activity can elicit positive reinforcement similar to that resulting from substance use, such as increased social rewards and stress reduction (Read et al., 2001), and may be used as a "replacement" behavior by former alcohol and/or drug dependent individuals. In other words, physical activity may impact substance use behavior by increasing positive associations with nonuse within the same conditioning framework that contributed to substance use or dependence. As an adjunct to MI, physical activity, a health-promoting behavior, can increase dissonance between an individual's desired positive health outcomes and his/her actual engagement in addictive behavior.

Several health issues that are negatively impacted by substance use (e.g., sleep, cardiovascular fitness, respiratory capacity) can be improved by regular participation in physical activity (United States Department of Health and Human Services, 2008). In fact, physical activity has been linked to a variety of desirable health outcomes (e.g., cardiorespiratory fitness, musculoskeletal health, energy balance, cancer prevention). Furthermore, exercise has been shown to promote psychological well-being and is sometimes prescribed as an adjunct to treatment for psychiatric disorders, including anxiety and depression.

Lastly, physical activity has been demonstrated to decrease substance usage and self-reported cravings, particularly for cigarette smokers. While this topic is discussed later in this chapter, we briefly note that a number of studies have examined the impact of exercise on abstinence rates among nicotine-addicted individuals. With a reduction in primary addiction behaviors, these findings support the thesis of physical activity as an adjunct treatment for alcohol and drug dependence.

Potential Mechanisms Linking Substance Abuse and Physical Activity

Recent research has unearthed potentially overlapping mechanisms linking physical activity and substance use, with findings supporting a potential preventive and/or therapeutic role for physical activity on substance use disorders. Several theories have proposed psychosocial and neurobiological explanations although until recently much of this research has been unsubstantiated. Recent advances in imaging technologies such as *positron emission tomography* (PET), *magnetic resonance imaging* (MRI), and *functional MRI* (fMRI) have added to the knowledge base allowing for objective explorations into the structural and neurobiological changes in the brain common to both regular physical activity and substance abuse.

Psychosocial Factors Common to Substance Abuse and Physical Activity

Several psychosocial variables have been found to coexist with substance use disorders including depression (Coelho et al., 2000), anxiety (Norton, 2001), stress (Sinha, 2001), negative affect (Mason, Hitch, & Spoth, 2009), low self-esteem, external locus of control and inadequate coping skills (Wagner, Myers, & McIninch, 1999). Conversely, from both a primary and secondary prevention stand point, evidence supports improvements in many of these variables following increased physical activity.

The question of how physical activity acts upon these variables has yet to be answered although evidence does provide some clues. To date, the most consistent evidence of a link between physical activity and psychosocial constructs exists for self-efficacy. Specifically, there is evidence to support self-efficacy as both a predictor and mediator (Lewis, Marcus, Pate, & Dunn, 2002) of physical activity behavior. Therefore, self-efficacy will be described in more detail below.

Self-Efficacy

Correlational and intervention research have demonstrated strong associations (Bauman, Sallis, Dzewaltowski, & Owen, 2002) between increases in activity levels and improvements in self-efficacy (Gary, 2006). Craft (2005) demonstrated significant improvements in self-efficacy following 3 and 9 weeks of moderate-intensity aerobic activity compared to a non-exercise control group. Further, increased levels of self-efficacy have been associated with reduced anxiety (Bandura, 1988), reduced depressive symptomatology (Harris, Cronkite, & Moos, 2006), improved cognitive control (Bandura, 1993), and improved response to stress accompanied by lowered catecholamine production (Bandura, Taylor, Williams, Mefford, & Barchas, 1985). Finally, self-efficacy has also been found to mediate the relationship between stress and depressive symptoms (Maciejewski, Prigerson, & Mazure, 2000) adding to the potential preventive impact physical activity could have on risk of substance abuse.

Neurobiological Mechanisms

Research involving animal models and using microdialysis and high-performance liquid chromatography (HPLC) techniques coupled with advances in imaging technologies (PET, MRI, fMRI) have allowed for significant gains in the field. Imaging studies exploring structural and neurobiological changes within the brain common to both regular physical activity and substance abuse have added to the evidence base (Volkow, Fowler, Wang, & Goldstein, 2002; Volkow, Fowler, Wang, & Swanson, 2004). Studies in this area have led to several hypotheses connecting substance abuse and physical activity, most of which are anchored in the theory that drugs of abuse and physical activity are both associated with increased hedonic responses and feelings of reward. Therefore, this section focuses on two theories that have thus far received the most support: (1) the monoamine hypothesis and (2) the endorphin hypothesis.

Monoamine Hypothesis

The monoamine hypothesis is based on the premise that both drugs of abuse (e.g., cocaine, amphetamines, alcohol) and physical activity result in increased levels of monoamines, or neurotransmitters released within the reward areas of the brain (e.g., nucleus accumbens and ventral tegmental area). Much of this area of research has focused on the effects of the monoamine known as dopamine as many drugs act directly or indirectly on the mesolimbic dopaminergic pathway. Specifically, following a rewarding event such as cocaine use, neural projections are sent from the ventral tegmental area to dopamine receptors within the reward centers of the brain resulting in increased feelings of pleasure (Robinson & Berridge, 1993). Past research using animal models has also demonstrated significant increases in monoamines such as dopamine, serotonin, norepinephrine, and epinephrine with drug use (Di Chiara & Imperato, 1988). More recent research using fMRI imaging technology in humans has allowed for visual evidence of upregulated dopamine response following times of nicotine abstinence and anticipation (e.g., cravings) following smoking cues (Due, Huettel, Hall, & Rubin, 2002; McClernon, Hiott, Huettel, & Rose, 2005). Other imaging studies in humans have corroborated such findings (Volkow et al., 2002, 2004).

With repeated drug exposure, however, it is thought that a learned response to the substance is established (Jay, 2003) linking the act of drug use to the environment and setting associated with drug use. Eventually as tolerance to the substance is built, there is decreased dopamine release following substance use. However, there is an increased release of dopamine in response to exposure to familiar environmental stimuli associated with substance abuse (e.g., conditioned place preference) (Keitz, Martin-Soelch, & Leenders, 2003; Schultz, 1998). Thus, dopamine's role in drug addiction seems to be less linked to mediating the hedonic effects of addictive drugs as was once thought and may be more linked to the initial drug-seeking behavior through transfer of incentive salience to reward-related stimuli (Berridge, 2007), modulation of reward-related synaptic plasticity and learning (Schultz, 1998), and in overcoming effort-related response costs (Salamone, Correa, Mingote, & Weber, 2003).

Evidence of monoamine responses following physical activity has also been reported. Animal studies have explored the association between monoamines and physical activity and found consistent increases in noradrenaline (Dunn, Reigle, Youngstedt, Armstrong, & Dishman, 1996; Kurosawa, Okada, Sato, & Uchida,

1993; Sarbadhikari & Saha, 2006), serotonin (Gerin, Teilhac, Smith, & Privat, 2008; Kurosawa et al., 1993; Xu, Liu, & Wang, 2008), and dopamine (Bailey, Davis, & Ahlborn, 1992; Blomstrand, Perrett, Parry-Billings, & Newsholme, 1989; Meeusen, Piacentini, & De Meirleir, 2001; Meeusen et al., 1997) following acute bouts of exercise. Moreover, research involving rat models has found running upregulates dynorphin mRNA (Werme, Thoren, Olson, & Brene, 2000), which is known to be regulated by dopamine.

Human research exploring monoamine release in response to exercise is sparse although emerging. Few imaging studies have been conducted exploring the effects of exercise on neurobiological activity in the human brain. In one such study, Wang et al. (2000) reported no changes in synaptic dopamine concentrations using PET imaging. However, in a more recent fMRI study, Janse Van Rensburg, Taylor, Hodgson, & Benattayallah (2009) reported significant activation in areas associated with reward, motivation, and visio-spatial attention following smoking cues in non-exercising controls while hypo-activation of such areas was observed in an exercising group. Further these findings were corroborated by significant reductions in self-reported cravings during and following acute bouts of exercise (Janse Van Rensburg et al. 2009). These results suggest a decreased affinity for smoking following exercise. While extremely promising, further research is warranted to confirm such findings.

Endorphin Hypothesis

The complexity of the mechanisms associated with drug abuse and physical activity is illustrated in the overlap that seems to occur between the dopamine reward system and the closely associated endorphin system. The endorphin hypothesis, as it relates to physical activity, is often referred to as the "runner's high" and is founded on the principal that intense physical activity is associated with a feeling of euphoria accompanied by analgesia. Evidence for this theory is supported by a release of endogenous opioids known as endorphins following vigorous activity (Morgan, 1985).

Interestingly, studies using rat models have demonstrated significant and prolonged increases in beta-endorphins of up to 2 days following 5–6 weeks of spontaneous running (e.g., 3.5 km/24 h) (Hoffmann, Terenius, & Thoren, 1990). Endogenous opioid peptides bind to opioid receptors with high affinity for β-endorphins (Mansour, Fox, Akil, & Watson, 1995). Importantly, Werme et al. examined the regulation of mRNA of three endogenous opioid ligands (dynorphin, enkephalin, and neuropeptide substance P), following the administration of both chronic exercise and cocaine or morphine. The authors found that both cocaine administration and chronic exercise upregulated mRNA of dynorphin in Lewis strain rats. Further, when the rats were administered naloxone, a potent opioid receptor antagonist, the exercise-mediated increase in dynorphin mRNA was reversed (Werme et al., 2000). Exercise-induced increases in dynorphin have since been replicated (Chen, Zhao, Yue, & Wang, 2007) and are thought by some to be a possible antidote to cocaine.

Until recently, most of the evidence supporting a runner's high in humans was limited to self-reported improvements in mood following exercise (Janal, Colt, Clark, & Glusman, 1984), reversal of self-reported improvements in mood following administration of opioid receptor antagonists such as naloxone (Janal et al. 1984) and evidence supporting an indirect increase in endorphin levels of plasma and cerebral spinal fluid (Carr et al., 1981; Hoffmann et al., 1990; Wildmann, Kruger, Schmole, Niemann, & Matthaei, 1986). Recent advances, however, in brain imaging technologies, have provided objective evidence of increased endorphins following exercise in humans. Notably, Boecker et al. (2008) recently conducted a study in which ten endurance athletes completed PET scans and the Visual Analog Mood Scale (Aitken, 1969) at rest and following 2 h of endurance running. Significant increases in endorphin receptor binding in the prefrontal and limbic brain regions following the 2 h of running were observed. Specifically, ligand binding activity was significantly correlated with perceived ratings of euphoria suggesting exercise-induced increases in endorphin release and subsequent improvements in mood (Boecker et al. 2008).

Other Potential Hypotheses

Other potential hypotheses linking substance abuse to physical activity have been proposed. There is evidence that *brain-derived neurotrophic factor* (BDNF), a neurotrophin that supports the survival of existing neurons and encourages growth and differentiation of new neurons and synapses, could play a role in the prevention and treatment of substance abuse based on its ties with exercise, stress, and depressive symptoms. Specifically, while research using rat models has shown that stress decreases expression of BDNF (Murakami, Imbe, Morikawa, Kubo, & Senba, 2005), marked increases in BDNF mRNA expression coupled with improved cognitive function and decreased depressive symptoms have been demonstrated following regular exercise (Neeper, Gomez-Pinilla, Choi, & Cotman, 1995; Russo-Neustadt, Beard, Huang, & Cotman, 2000). The cognitive advances associated with increased BDNF are likely the result of increased brain plasticity as BDNF supports the health of glutamatergic neurons within the brain. It has also recently been hypothesized that the beneficial effects of exercise on stress may be due to exercise-induced activation of BDNF (Sarbadhikari & Saha, 2006).

Review of Evidence Based Interventions Incorporating Physical Activity

Now that we have provided an overview of substance use treatment and discussed potential mechanisms linking physical activity and substance abuse, the next section reviews the intervention research examining the efficacy of physical activity for the treatment of substance use disorders. Most of the studies examining exercise for the treatment for substance use come from the smoking cessation literature, as few studies have been conducted examining exercise's role in the treatment of substance use disorders related to alcohol and, to an even lesser extent, illicit drugs.

Smoking Cessation

For many years, exercise has been routinely recommended as an aid to smoking cessation (Ashelman, 2000; Hurt et al., 1992; Marcus, Hampl, & Fisher, 2004; QUIT, 1994; United States Department of Health and Human Services, 2008; Woodhouse & Rigg, 1990). The research literature in this area has been growing and is now quite extensive, even including a Cochrane review on the topic (Ussher, Taylor, & Faulkner, 2008).

Vigorous Exercise for Smoking Cessation

Several studies have examined the efficacy of vigorous exercise for smoking cessation. While several early studies did not support the effectiveness of vigorous exercise for smoking cessation, these findings were likely impacted by methodological flaws (i.e., small sample size) (Hill, 1985; Russell, Epstein, Johnston, Block, & Blair, 1988; Taylor, Houston-Miller, Haskell, & Debusk, 1988), poor exercise adherence, inadequate duration of exercise training (Russell et al., 1988), no formal smoking cessation treatment (Taylor et al., 1988), very brief programs (Hill, 1985), and an absence of a comparison group to control for contact time (Hill, 1985). For example, in one study (Hill, 1985), participants ($n=36$) received smoking cessation group counseling (1–1½ h sessions twice a week for 5 weeks) and were randomly assigned to either ten 30-min aerobic exercise classes or control condition. There were no significant group differences in abstinence rates immediately or 1 and 6 months after treatment. However, findings may have been due to differences in contact time between the two groups. Another study (Russell et al. 1988) involved all participants ($n=42$ women) receiving smoking cessation behavioral treatment (four 1-h sessions over a week) and then being randomly assigned to one of three maintenance programs (physical activity, smoking information, or contact control). While the physical activity program involved one supervised and two unsupervised walk/jog sessions per week, results did not indicate any improvements in fitness. Thus, the lack of significant group differences in smoking cessation at the end of treatment and at 3 and 18 months post-intervention was not surprising. Finally, results from a randomized controlled trial ($n=68$ male patients after acute myocardial infarction) conducted by Taylor et al. (1988) indicated that advice to stop smoking followed by medically supervised exercise training with frequent follow-ups reduced self-reported cigarette consumption ($p<0.03$, at 28 weeks), but did not significantly improve rates of smoking cessation or cessation maintenance.

Once again, findings were likely impacted by methodological issues, such as the lack of a formal smoking cessation program.

Recent studies of vigorous-intensity exercise for smoking cessation with more rigorous designs have shown promising results. For example, after two pilot studies (Marcus et al., 1991, 1995), Marcus and colleagues conducted a large-scale randomized controlled trial (Marcus et al., 1999) with 281 healthy sedentary female smokers. Participants were randomly assigned to receive 12 cognitive-behavioral smoking cessation group sessions (on nicotine fading, stimulus control, coping with cravings and high-risk situations, stress management, weight management, and relapse prevention) along with either an exercise or wellness contact control program. Exercise participants attended three supervised vigorous-intensity exercise sessions per week, consisting of a 5-min warm-up, 30–40 min of aerobic activity, and a 5-min cooldown period with stretching. Findings indicated that the exercise condition produced significant improvements in fitness (estimated VO2 peak, 25 ± 6–28 ± 6 ml/kg/min, $p < 0.01$), less weight gain (3.05 kg vs. 5.40 kg, $p = 0.03$), and higher rates of continuous abstinence at the end of treatment (19.4 % vs. 10.2 %, $p = 0.03$) and at 3 (16.4 % vs. 8.2 %, $p = 0.03$) and 12 months (11.9 % vs. 5.4 %, $p = 0.05$) than the control condition. Thus, this study demonstrated that vigorous-intensity exercise can facilitate smoking cessation with women when combined with a cognitive-behavioral smoking cessation program. Unfortunately, many individuals, particularly sedentary smokers, may find engaging in physical activity at such a high intensity uncomfortable and/or unappealing. Exercise at a moderate-intensity level may be more acceptable and enjoyable. Additionally, moderate-intensity exercise has benefits such as requiring less medical supervision and resulting in fewer injuries than vigorous intensity exercise (American College of Sports Medicine, 2006).

Moderate-Intensity Exercise for Smoking Cessation

In terms of moderate-intensity exercise's potential for facilitating smoking cessation, past research has demonstrated that short bouts of moderate-intensity exercise can help reduce tobacco withdrawal and urges to smoke (Daniel, Cropley, Ussher, & West, 2004; Ussher, Nunziata, Cropley, & West, 2001). Intervention studies are also available, but findings are mixed. For example, Hill, Rigdon, and Johnson (1993) examined different combinations of behavioral treatment (twelve 90-min sessions) and moderate-intensity exercise (3-month walking program) by randomly assigning participants ($n = 82$) to four groups (behavioral treatment alone, behavioral treatment plus nicotine gum, behavioral treatment plus moderate-intensity exercise, and moderate-intensity exercise only). At 12 months the percent quit across groups was respectively 31.8, 36.4, 27.8, and 10.0% indicating behavioral training facilitated cessation over the physical exercise only condition.

In a similar study, 205 recovering alcoholics were randomly assigned (Martin et al., 1997) to the following conditions: (1) standard treatment (American Lung

Association quit program plus nicotine anonymous meetings), (2) behavioral counseling (8 h-long group sessions) plus physical exercise (four weekly supervised moderate-intensity exercise sessions lasting 15–45 min with three similar exercise sessions at home), or (3) behavioral counseling plus nicotine gum. At the end of treatment, results indicated that behavioral counseling plus moderate-intensity exercise was more effective than behavioral counseling plus nicotine gum or the standard treatment. However, findings suggest that the benefits of participating in the exercise group were not maintained over time, outside of the context of an active intervention, as group differences were not significant at 6 or 12 months.

Kinnunen et al. (2008) examined the efficacy of a 19-week exercise intervention as an adjunct to nicotine gum, relative to contact control and standard care control conditions, in 182 sedentary female smokers aged 18–55 years. Exercise participants attended 40-min exercise sessions (5 min warm-up, 30 min of moderate intensity aerobic exercise, then 5 min cool-down) at a hospital cardiac rehabilitation center under the supervision of an exercise physiologist. Sessions focused on walked or running on the treadmill and occurred twice per week for first 5 weeks and then once per week for the remaining 14 weeks. Results indicated higher abstinence rates in the exercise and contact control conditions, compared to the standard care condition, at end of treatment (24.2 % and 23.2 % vs. 14.7 %, respectively) and 12 months (9.8 and 12.5 % vs. 5.9 %, respectively), with no significant advantage for exercise over the contact control condition. However, findings may have been impacted by the low rate of adherence to exercise in this study.

Next, Ussher et al. (2003) offered participants ($n=299$) a 7-week individualized smoking cessation program including nicotine replacement therapy plus either exercise counseling or health education advice. Exercise participants received 5 min of cognitive-behavioral exercise counseling focused on goal-setting, relapse prevention planning, and self-monitoring, along with 2 min of additional support per week for 7 weeks. Interestingly, while there were no group differences in smoking cessation or weight gain, the exercise group reported increased exercise and significantly less tension, anxiety and stress during the first week of smoking abstinence, less irritability during 2 weeks of abstinence ($p=0.03$), and less restlessness during 3 weeks of abstinence ($p=0.04$). Thus, results suggest that adding brief exercise counseling to a smoking cessation program had a beneficial effect on psychological symptoms among smokers trying to quit, even if it did not directly impact smoking abstinence or related weight gain. Findings may have been influenced by the slightly lower attendance rates at quit day among the exercise group, as abstinence rates were significantly higher for the exercise group versus the control up to the first 2 weeks of abstinence (when analyses were repeated including only participants present at quit day).

Finally, in another large randomized controlled trial conducted by Marcus and colleagues (2005), sedentary female smokers ($n=217$) were randomly assigned to an 8-week cognitive-behavioral smoking cessation program, along with either a moderate-intensity exercise program or wellness contact control condition. The exercise participants were required to attend a supervised, 1 h-long exercise session each week and participate in four additional 30-min (or longer) sessions either at home or onsite. While both groups were equally likely to have quit smoking at the end of treatment and 12 months, results indicated that the exercise group was more likely to report smoking cessation at the 3-month follow-up (11.9 % vs. 4.6 %, $p<0.05$), compared with the control group. Additionally exercise participants who reported high adherence to the exercise prescription were significantly more likely to be abstinent at the end of treatment than those reporting lower exercise adherence. As findings on studies examining moderate-intensity physical activity for smoking cessation are mixed, more research is needed to determine its efficacy, as well as the relative efficacy of vigorous-intensity versus moderate-intensity exercise, for smoking cessation.

Alcohol

There has been a call for increased attention to the role of exercise in treatment of alcohol use disorders. Past research has shown that brief bouts of moderate-intensity exercise can provide short-term relief from alcohol urges (Ussher, Sampuran, Doshi, West, & Drummond, 2004). In addition, there is preliminary data which indicate that exercise-based interventions would be well-received by those early in recovery from alcohol use disorders (Read et al., 2001). In fact, over 54 % ($n=57$) of that sample reported being very/extremely interested in participating in an exercise program as part of treatment. Another 21 % ($n=22$) indicated slight or moderate interest, with most participants preferring physical activities such as walking (66 %), weight lifting (66 %), and cycling (59 %). Despite data indicating acceptability and feasibility of such a treatment approach, there have been few actual intervention studies conducted in this area and the ones available have included small samples.

For example, Brown et al. (2009) pilot-tested a 12-week moderate-intensity aerobic exercise program among alcohol-dependent patients in recovery ($n=19$). This program involved supervised moderate-intensity aerobic group exercise sessions once a week with encouragement to exercise independently each day and weekly group behavioral training on topics such as American College of Sports Medicine guidelines, benefits of exercise for alcohol recovery, goal-setting, identifying and overcoming barriers, time management, and social support. Participants were provided with monetary incentives for attending group sessions and self-monitoring. Results indicated significant improvements in fitness and body mass index, as well as percentage of days abstinent and drinks per drinking day at the end of treatment and at 3 months post-intervention.

Other studies have examined the impact of more vigorous-intensity physical activity on drinking behavior and recovery. For example, Murphy, Pagano, and Marlatt (1986) randomly assigned 60 heavy-drinking male college students to the following 8-week treatment conditions: exercise (running), meditation, or no-treatment control group. Results indicated significantly reduced alcohol consumption among the exercise participants relative to the no-treatment control condition. Another study (Sinyor, Brown, Rostant, & Seraganian, 1982) compared alcoholics ($n=58$) who participated in daily fitness classes during a 6-week inpatient substance abuse treatment to patients at the same treatment center who only partially participated in the fitness program and those at another local treatment center without fitness programs. Fitness classes lasted approximately an hour and included stretching, light calisthenics, 12 min of walking/running, and then strength training (e.g., sit-ups, push-ups). Full participation in the fitness program was associated with significantly increased fitness and reduced body fat percentage, as well as improved abstinence rates 3 months posttreatment. Thus, promising findings were seen in the few studies examining the direct impact of exercise upon drinking behavior and recovery.

There have been several exercise interventions for drinking that targeted related (and potentially mediating) psychosocial variables (e.g., anxiety, depression). For example, Weber (1984) compared routine therapy alone to routine therapy plus 4 months of endurance training among 26 alcoholic patients. Results indicated stronger positive effects on stress and state anxiety for the exercise group and comparable decreases in trait anxiety in both groups. In a similar study, Gary and Guthrie (1972) found that jogging a mile per day for 20 days during inpatient treatment resulted in improved cardiovascular fitness, self-esteem, and sleep, relative to a control condition, in 20 volunteer participants. And, adult alcoholics who walked/jogged 3 days per week ($n=26$) during a 28-day inpatient treatment program reported significantly greater improvements in anxiety (both state and trait) and depression, but not self-concept or aerobic capacity, relative to control participants ($n=27$) (Palmer, Vacc, & Epstein 1988). Frankel and Murphy (1974) encouraged participants ($n=214$ male alcoholics) to exercise 5 days per week for 12 weeks and found improved fitness and MMPI scores, with the greatest change observed in decreases in anxiety and depression. Finally, one study demonstrated that participation in Sudarshana Kriya Yoga after detoxification can produce significantly greater reductions in depression and stress hormone levels (plasma cortisol, ACTH) after 2 weeks, relative to a control condition, in an alcohol-dependent sample ($n=60$) (Vedamurthachar et al., 2006). Thus, while the role of exercise in the treatment of alcohol use disorders needs further investigation, there is preliminary evidence in support of its feasibility, acceptability, and efficacy.

Illicit Drugs

Compared to the available data on smoking cessation and alcohol use disorders, there is little information on exercise as an adjunct to treatment of substance use disorders related to illicit drugs. In a correlational study, Weinstock, Barry, and Petry (2008) examined the relationship between completion of exercise-related activities and substance abuse treatment outcomes in a sample of 187 participants undergoing intensive outpatient treatment with contingency management. Almost 25 % of the sample completed at least one exercise-related activity during the 12 weeks of treatment. Results indicated that participants who engaged in exercise-related activities ($n=45$) achieved longer durations of abstinence during treatment than individuals who did not complete an exercise-related activity ($n=142$). In another study, 74 adolescents (Collingwood, Reynolds, Kohl, Smith, & Sloan, 1991) in either a school-based prevention program, community counseling agency substance abuse program, or chemical dependency inpatient hospital-based program received eight to nine, 90-min structured fitness classes emphasizing group exercise and instruction on topics such as goal-setting, stretching, strength training, and safety. Participants were encouraged to exercise independently on at least two other occasions each week. This physical activity program resulted in significant fitness gains, according to 1 mile run, 1 min sit-up, 1 min push-up, and flexibility tests. In addition, participants who decreased their one mile run time also reported significant improvements related to patterns of substance use (e.g., reduced percentage of multiple substance users) at post-test. Overall, while there is not enough research to support strong conclusions about physical activity and illicit drug use, findings from these studies suggest that exercise may be beneficial for individuals undergoing treatment for substance use disorders related to illicit drugs.

Best Practice Recommendations

A review of the research literature indicated that exercise may serve as a useful adjunct for acute treatment of substance use disorders and also prevent subsequent relapse. Exercise can be integrated into most substance use interventions with ease and offers many other health benefits to substance users with few disadvantages. Past studies have demonstrated numerous potential mechanisms for the relationship between physical activity and substance use, with recent technological advances adding a great deal of insight.

Intervention research has also been conducted in this area. In fact, physical activity has received strong support as a treatment for substance use disorders from the field of smoking cessation. There have been fewer studies conducted in the area of alcohol use disorders, but data are promising. The efficacy of physical activity for treatment of substance use disorders related to illicit drugs has been relatively unexplored at this point. While more research is needed, the evidence base is strong enough to recommend that, to facilitate recovery and maintain abstinence, individuals with substance use disorders engage in physical activity as part of treatment.

However, short-term increases in physical activity are not likely to have a substantial impact on substance use. Regular exercise habits and lifestyle changes are probably more conducive to remaining abstinent. Thus, issues related to exercise adherence must be considered. For example, individuals with substance use disorders may be more likely to participate in an exercise program if it is offered in a convenient, community-based setting. Thus, in an ongoing study, Marcus and colleagues are delivering the Commit to Quit program (vigorous-intensity exercise classes plus cognitive-behavioral treatment for smoking cessation) through neighborhood YMCA's building on some promising pilot work (Whiteley et al., 2007). Past research also suggests that individuals may be more likely to adhere to and receive greater psychological benefit (Byrne & Byrne, 1993) from a moderate-intensity exercise program (Sallis et al., 1986). In fact, walking, the most frequently reported type of exercise, is considered moderate intensity (Manson et al., 1999; Stofan, DiPietro, Davis, Kohl, & Blair, 1998). Sustaining exercise behavior change over time in individuals in recovery from substance use disorders may also require encouraging them to find ways to make physical activity more enjoyable and develop social networks that support exercise participation, with an emphasis on strategies that can be continued without heavy involvement from professionals. For example, researchers and/or clinicians could help individuals in recovery establish local walking groups and sports leagues that hold regular softball/kickball/soccer games. Furthermore, there are environmental changes that could function to promote behavior change for both physical activity and abstinence from substance use. For example, increased community presence (and perhaps even police surveillance, if necessary) in local parks could potentially reduce the amount of criminal activity occurring in these areas and thus make utilizing this space for physical activity more appealing, while also supporting abstinence from substance use by reducing the availability of illegal drugs and discouraging drug trafficking in these nearby areas. In sum, individuals who are trying to abstain from substance use are most likely to benefit from realistic (i.e., moderate intensity, enjoyable, sustainable) exercise recommendations and interventions which focus on promoting more active, healthy lifestyles.

Future Directions

There are still many gaps in this research literature. While the data from the smoking cessation field provides support for exercise for substance use treatment, the specific efficacy of physical activity for substance use disorders related to illicit drugs has yet to be examined. In addition, studies with larger samples are needed to determine the efficacy and necessary dose–response of physical activity for treatment of alcohol use disorders. Questions remain regarding what intensity levels (e.g., moderate vs. vigorous) and types (e.g., cardiovascular, strength training) of physical activity will be most beneficial for individuals in substance use treatment. Future directions should also include recruiting more diverse samples and targeting the populations most at risk for substance use disorders. And finally, future researchers should consider developing and testing strategies to help participants maintain exercise gains once the actual intervention has ended, as the focus in this research area needs to shift towards producing enduring changes in activity levels.

References

Aitken, R. C. (1969). Measurement of feelings using visual analogue scales. *Proceedings of the Royal Society of Medicine, 62*(10), 989–993.
Alcoholics Anonymous. (1972). A brief guide to alcoholics anonymous. http://www.aa.org/. Accessed 25 July 2009.

American College of Sports Medicine. (2006). *ACSM's guidelines for exercise testing and prescription* (7th ed.). Philadelphia, PA: Lippincott Williams & Wilkins.

American Psychiatric Association. (2000). *Diagnostic and statistical manual of mental disorders, 4th ed., text revision (DSM-IV-TR)*. Washington, DC: American Psychiatric Association.

Arkowitz, H., & Miller, W. R. (2008). Learning, applying, and extending motivational interviewing. In H. Arkowitz, H. Westra, W. R. Miller, & S. Rollnick (Eds.), *Motivational interviewing in the treatment of psychological problems* (pp. 1–25). New York: Guilford Publications.

Ashelman, M. W. (2000). *Stop smoking naturally*. Lincoln, IL: Keats Publishing Inc.

Bailey, S. P., Davis, J. M., & Ahlborn, E. N. (1992). Effect of increased brain serotonergic activity on endurance performance in the rat. *Acta Physiologica Scandinavica, 145*(1), 75–76.

Bandura, A. (1977). *Social learning theory*. New York: General Learning Press.

Bandura, A. (1988). Self-efficacy conception of anxiety. *Anxiety, Stress and Coping: An International Journal, 1*(2), 77–98.

Bandura, A. (1993). Perceived self-efficacy in cognitive-development and functioning. *Educational Psychologist, 28*(2), 117–148.

Bandura, A., Taylor, C. B., Williams, S. L., Mefford, I. N., & Barchas, J. D. (1985). Catecholamine secretion as a function of perceived coping self-efficacy. *Journal of Consulting and Clinical Psychology, 53*(3), 406–414.

Bauman, A. E., Sallis, J. F., Dzewaltowski, D. A., & Owen, N. (2002). Toward a better understanding of the influences on physical activity: The role of determinants, correlates, causal variables, mediators, moderators, and confounders. *American Journal of Preventive Medicine, 23*(2 Suppl), 5–14.

Berridge, K. C. (2007). The debate over dopamine's role in reward: The case for incentive salience. *Psychopharmacology, 191*(3), 391–431.

Blomstrand, E., Perrett, D., Parry-Billings, M., & Newsholme, E. A. (1989). Effect of sustained exercise on plasma amino acid concentrations and on 5-hydroxytryptamine metabolism in six different brain regions in the rat. *Acta Physiologica Scandinavica, 136*(3), 473–481.

Boecker, H., Sprenger, T., Spilker, M. E., Henriksen, G., Koppenhoefer, M., Wagner, K. J., et al. (2008). The runner's high: Opioidergic mechanisms in the human brain. *Cerebral Cortex, 18*(11), 2523–2531.

Brown, R. A., Abrantes, A. M., Read, J. P., Marcus, B. H., Jakicic, J., Strong, D. R., et al. (2009). Aerobic exercise for alcohol recovery: Rationale, program description, and preliminary findings. *Behavior Modification, 33*(2), 220–249.

Byrne, A., & Byrne, D. G. (1993). The effect of exercise on depression, anxiety and other mood states: A review. *Journal of Psychosomatic Research, 37*(6), 565–574.

Carr, D. B., Bullen, B. A., Skrinar, G. S., Arnold, M. A., Rosenblatt, M., Beitins, I. Z., et al. (1981). Physical conditioning facilitates the exercise-induced secretion of beta-endorphin and beta-lipotropin in women. *The New England Journal of Medicine, 305*(10), 560–563.

Chen, J. X., Zhao, X., Yue, G. X., & Wang, Z. F. (2007). Influence of acute and chronic treadmill exercise on rat plasma lactate and brain NPY, L-ENK, DYN A1-13. *Cellular and Molecular Neurobiology, 27*(1), 1–10.

Coelho, R., Rangel, R., Ramos, E., Martins, A., Prata, J., & Barros, H. (2000). Depression and the severity of substance abuse. *Psychopathology, 33*(3), 103–109.

Collingwood, T. R., Reynolds, R., Kohl, H. W., Smith, W., & Sloan, S. (1991). Physical fitness effects on substance abuse risk factors and use patterns. *Journal of Drug Education, 21*(1), 73–84.

Craft, L. L. (2005). Exercise and clinical depression: Examining two psychological mechanisms. *Psychology of Sport and Exercise, 6*(2), 151–171.

Daniel, J., Cropley, M., Ussher, M., & West, R. (2004). Acute effects of a short bout of moderate versus light intensity exercise versus inactivity on tobacco withdrawal symptoms in sedentary smokers. *Psychopharmacology, 174*(3), 320–326.

Di Chiara, G., & Imperato, A. (1988). Drugs abused by humans preferentially increase synaptic dopamine concentrations in the mesolimbic system of freely moving rats. *Proceedings of the National Academy of Sciences, 85*(14), 5274–5278.

Dimeff, L. A., & Marlatt, G. A. (1998). Preventing relapse and maintaining change in addictive behaviors. *Clinical Psychology: Science and Practice, 5*(4), 513–525.

Due, D. L., Huettel, S. A., Hall, W. G., & Rubin, D. C. (2002). Activation in mesolimbic and visuospatial neural circuits elicited by smoking cues: Evidence from functional magnetic resonance imaging. *The American Journal of Psychiatry, 159*(6), 954–960.

Dunn, A. L., Reigle, T. G., Youngstedt, S. D., Armstrong, R. B., & Dishman, R. K. (1996). Brain norepinephrine and metabolites after treadmill training and wheel running in rats. *Medicine and Science in Sports and Exercise, 28*(2), 204–209.

Frankel, A., & Murphy, J. (1974). Physical fitness and personality in alcoholism. Canonical analysis of measures before and after treatment. *Quarterly Journal of Studies on Alcohol, 35*(4 Pt A), 1272–1278.

Gary, R. (2006). Exercise self-efficacy in older women with diastolic heart failure: Results of a walking program and education intervention. *Journal of Gerontological Nursing, 32*(7), 31–39. quiz 40–31.

Gary, V., & Guthrie, D. (1972). The effect of jogging on physical fitness and self-concept in hospitalized alcoholics. *Quarterly Journal of Studies on Alcohol, 33*(4), 1073–1078.

Gerin, C., Teilhac, J. R., Smith, K., & Privat, A. (2008). Motor activity induces release of serotonin in the dorsal horn of the rat lumbar spinal cord. *Neuroscience Letters, 436*(2), 91–95.

Harris, A. H., Cronkite, R., & Moos, R. (2006). Physical activity, exercise coping, and depression in a 10-year cohort study of depressed patients. *Journal of Affective Disorders, 93*(1–3), 79–85.

Hill, J. S. (1985). Effect of a program of aerobic exercise on the smoking behaviour of a group of adult volunteers. *Canadian Journal of Public Health, 76*(3), 183–186.

Hill, R., Rigdon, M., & Johnson, S. (1993). Behavioral smoking cessation treatment for older chronic smokers. *Behavior Therapy, 24*(2), 321–329.

Hoffman, N. G., Halikas, J. A., Mee-Lee, D., & Weedman, R. D. (1991). *Patient placement criteria for the treatment of psychoactive substance use disorders.* Washington, D.C.: American Society of Addiction Medicine.

Hoffmann, P., Terenius, L., & Thoren, P. (1990). Cerebrospinal fluid immunoreactive beta-endorphin concentration is increased by voluntary exercise in the spontaneously hypertensive rat. *Regulatory Peptides, 28*(2), 233–239.

Hunt, G. M., & Azrin, N. H. (1973). A community-reinforcement approach to alcoholism. *Behaviour Research and Therapy, 11*(1), 91–104.

Hurt, R. D., Dale, L. C., Offord, K. P., Bruce, B. K., McClain, F. L., & Eberman, K. M. (1992). Inpatient treatment of severe nicotine dependence. *Mayo Clinic Proceedings, 67*(9), 823–828.

Janal, M. N., Colt, E. W., Clark, W. C., & Glusman, M. (1984). Pain sensitivity, mood and plasma endocrine levels in man following long-distance running: Effects of naloxone. *Pain, 19*(1), 13–25.

Janse Van Rensburg, K., Taylor, A., Hodgson, T., & Benattayallah, A. (2009). Acute exercise modulates cigarette cravings and brain activation in response to smoking-related images: An fMRI Study. *Psychopharmacology, 203*(3), 589–598.

Jay, T. M. (2003). Dopamine: A potential substrate for synaptic plasticity and memory mechanisms. *Progress in Neurobiology, 69*(6), 375–390.

Kadden, R. M., Carroll, K., Donovan, D., Cooney, N., Monti, P., Abrams, D., et al. (1992). *Cognitive-behavioral coping skills therapy manual: A clinical research guide for therapists treating individuals with alcohol abuse and dependence. Project MATCH monograph series, vol 4* (DHHS Publication No. (ADM)92-1895). Rockville, MD: National Institute on Alcohol Abuse and Alcoholism.

Keitz, M., Martin-Soelch, C., & Leenders, K. L. (2003). Reward processing in the brain: A prerequisite for movement preparation? *Neural Plasticity, 10*(1–2), 121–128.

Kinnunen, T., Leeman, R. F., Korhonen, T., Quiles, Z. N., Terwal, D. M., Garvey, A. J., et al. (2008). Exercise as an adjunct to nicotine gum in treating tobacco dependence among women. *Nicotine and Tobacco Research, 10*(4), 689–703.

Kremer, D., Malkin, M. J., & Benshoff, J. J. (1995). Physical activity programs offered in substance abuse treatment facilities. *Journal of Substance Abuse Treatment, 12*(5), 327–333.

Kurosawa, M., Okada, K., Sato, A., & Uchida, S. (1993). Extracellular release of acetylcholine, noradrenaline and serotonin increases in the cerebral cortex during walking in conscious rats. *Neuroscience Letters, 161*(1), 73–76.

Lewis, B. A., Marcus, B. H., Pate, R. R., & Dunn, A. L. (2002). Psychosocial mediators of physical activity behavior among adults and children. *American Journal of Preventive Medicine, 23*(2 Suppl), 26–35.

Maciejewski, P. K., Prigerson, H. G., & Mazure, C. M. (2000). Self-efficacy as a mediator between stressful life events and depressive symptoms. Differences based on history of prior depression. *British Journal of Psychiatry, 176,* 373–378.

Manson, J. E., Hu, F. B., Rich-Edwards, J. W., Colditz, G. A., Stampfer, M. J., Willett, W. C., et al. (1999). A prospective study of walking as compared with vigorous exercise in the prevention of coronary heart disease in women. *The New England Journal of Medicine, 341*(9), 650–658.

Mansour, A., Fox, C. A., Akil, H., & Watson, S. J. (1995). Opioid-receptor mRNA expression in the rat CNS: Anatomical and functional implications. *Trends in Neuroscience, 18*(1), 22–29.

Marcus, B. H., Albrecht, A. E., King, T. K., Parisi, A. F., Pinto, B. M., Roberts, M., et al. (1999). The efficacy of exercise as an aid for smoking cessation in women: A randomized controlled trial. *Archives of Internal Medicine, 159*(11), 1229–1234.

Marcus, B. H., Albrecht, A. E., Niaura, R. S., Abrams, D. B., & Thompson, P. D. (1991). Usefulness of physical exercise for maintaining smoking cessation in women. *The American Journal of Cardiology, 68*(4), 406–407.

Marcus, B. H., Albrecht, A. E., Niaura, R. S., Taylor, E. R., Simkin, L. R., Feder, S. I., et al. (1995). Exercise enhances the maintenance of smoking cessation in women. *Addictive Behaviors, 20*(1), 87–92.

Marcus, B. H., Hampl, J. S., & Fisher, E. B. (2004). *How to quit smoking without gaining weight.* New York: Simon and Schuster.

Marcus, B. H., Lewis, B. A., Hogan, J., King, T. K., Albrecht, A. E., Bock, B., et al. (2005). The efficacy of moderate-intensity exercise as an aid for smoking cessation in women: A randomized controlled trial. *Nicotine and Tobacco Research, 7*(6), 871–880.

Marlatt, G. A., & Gordon, J. R. (1985). *Relapse prevention: Maintenance strategies in the treatment of addictive behaviors.* New York: Guilford Press.

Martin, J. E., Calfas, K. J., Patten, C. A., Polarek, M., Hofstetter, C. R., Noto, J., et al. (1997). Prospective evaluation of three smoking interventions in 205 recovering alcoholics: One-year results of Project SCRAP-Tobacco. *Journal of Consulting and Clinical Psychology, 65*(1), 190–194.

Mason, W. A., Hitch, J. E., & Spoth, R. L. (2009). Longitudinal relations among negative affect, substance use, and peer deviance during the transition from middle to late adolescence. *Substance Use and Misuse, 44*(8), 1142–1159.

McClernon, F. J., Hiott, F. B., Huettel, S. A., & Rose, J. E. (2005). Abstinence-induced changes in self-report craving correlate with event-related FMRI responses to smoking cues. *Neuropsychopharmacology, 30*(10), 1940–1947.

McCrady, B. S. (2007). Alcohol use disorders. In D. H. Barlow (Ed.), *Clinical handbook of psychological disorders* (3rd ed., pp. 376–433). New York: Guilford.

Meeusen, R., Piacentini, M. F., & De Meirleir, K. (2001). Brain microdialysis in exercise research. *Sports Medicine, 31*(14), 965–983.

Meeusen, R., Smolders, I., Sarre, S., de Meirleir, K., Keizer, H., Serneels, M., et al. (1997). Endurance training effects on neurotransmitter release in rat striatum: An in vivo microdialysis study. *Acta Physiologica Scandinavica, 159*(4), 335–341.

Miller, W. R., Benefield, R. G., & Tonigan, J. S. (1993). Enhancing motivation for change in problem drinking: A controlled comparison of two therapist styles. *Journal of Consulting and Clinical Psychology, 61*(3), 455–461.

Miller, W. R., & Rollnick, S. (2002). *Motivational interviewing: Preparing people for change* (2nd ed.). New York, NY: Guilford.

Morgan, W. P. (1985). Affective beneficence of vigorous physical activity. *Medicine and Science in Sports and Exercise, 17*(1), 94–100.

Murakami, S., Imbe, H., Morikawa, Y., Kubo, C., & Senba, E. (2005). Chronic stress, as well as acute stress, reduces BDNF mRNA expression in the rat hippocampus but less robustly. *Neuroscience Research, 53*(2), 129–139.

Murphy, T. J., Pagano, R. R., & Marlatt, G. A. (1986). Lifestyle modification with heavy alcohol drinkers: Effects of aerobic exercise and meditation. *Addictive Behaviors, 11*(2), 175–186.

Myrick, H., & Anton, R. F. (1998). Treatment of alcohol withdrawal. *Alcohol Health and Research World, 22*(1), 38–43.

Narcotics Anonymous. (2007). Facts about NA. http://www.na.org/. Accessed 25 July 2009.

National Institute on Drug Abuse. (2009). NIDA InfoFacts: Treatment statistics. http://www.drugabuse.gov/infofacts/treatmenttrends.html. Accessed 12 Mar 2010.

Neeper, S. A., Gomez-Pinilla, F., Choi, J., & Cotman, C. (1995). Exercise and brain neurotrophins. *Nature, 373*(6510), 109.

Norton, G. R. (2001). Substance use/abuse and anxiety sensitivity – What are the relationships? *Addictive Behaviors, 26*(6), 935–946.

Palmer, J., Vacc, N., & Epstein, J. (1988). Adult inpatient alcoholics: Physical exercise as a treatment intervention. *Journal of Studies on Alcohol, 49*(5), 418–421.

Parks, G. A., & Marlatt, G. A. (1999). Relapse prevention therapy for substance-abusing offenders: A cognitive-behavioral approach in what works. In E. L. Lantham (Ed.), *Strategic solutions: The international community corrections association examines substance abuse* (pp. 161–233). Washington, DC: American Correctional Association.

QUIT. (1994). *Helping smokers to quit: A handbook for the practice nurse, health visitor and midwife*. London, UK: Department of Health.

Rawson, R. A., Obert, J. L., McCann, M. J., & Marinelli-Casey, P. (1993). Relapse prevention strategies in outpatient substance abuse treatment. *Psychology of Addictive Behaviors, 7*, 85–95.

Read, J. P., Brown, R. A., Marcus, B. H., Kahler, C. W., Ramsey, S. E., Dubreuil, M. E., et al. (2001). Exercise attitudes and behaviors among persons in treatment for alcohol use disorders. *Journal of Substance Abuse Treatment, 21*(4), 199–206.

Robinson, T. E., & Berridge, K. C. (1993). The neural basis of drug craving: An incentive-sensitization theory of addiction. *Brain Research. Brain Research Reviews, 18*(3), 247–291.

Rubak, S., Sandbaek, A., Lauritzen, T., & Christensen, B. (2005). Motivational interviewing: A systematic review and meta-analysis. *British Journal of General Practice, 55*(513), 305–312.

Russell, P. O., Epstein, L. H., Johnston, J. J., Block, D. R., & Blair, E. (1988). The effects of physical activity as maintenance for smoking cessation. *Addictive Behaviors, 13*(2), 215–218.

Russo-Neustadt, A. A., Beard, R. C., Huang, Y. M., & Cotman, C. W. (2000). Physical activity and antidepressant treatment potentiate the expression of specific brain-derived neurotrophic factor transcripts in the rat hippocampus. *Neuroscience, 101*(2), 305–312.

Salamone, J. D., Correa, M., Mingote, S., & Weber, S. M. (2003). Nucleus accumbens dopamine and the regulation of effort in food-seeking behavior: Implications for studies of natural motivation, psychiatry, and drug abuse. *Journal of Pharmacology and Experimental Therapeutics, 305*(1), 1–8.

Sallis, J. F., Haskell, W. L., Fortmann, S. P., Vranizan, K. M., Taylor, C. B., & Solomon, D. S. (1986). Predictors of adoption and maintenance of physical activity in a community sample. *Preventive Medicine, 15*(4), 331–341.

Sarbadhikari, S. N., & Saha, A. K. (2006). Moderate exercise and chronic stress produce counteractive effects on different areas of the brain by acting through various neurotransmitter receptor subtypes: A hypothesis. *Theoretical Biology and Medical Modelling, 3*, 33.

Schultz, W. (1998). Predictive reward signal of dopamine neurons. *Journal of Neurophysiology, 80*(1), 1–27.

Sinha, R. (2001). How does stress increase risk of drug abuse and relapse? *Psychopharmacology, 158*(4), 343–359.

Sinyor, D., Brown, T., Rostant, L., & Seraganian, P. (1982). The role of a physical fitness program in the treatment of alcoholism. *Journal of Studies on Alcohol, 43*(3), 380–386.

Stizter, M., & Petry, N. (2006). Contingency management for treatment of substance abuse. *Annual Review of Clinical Psychology, 2*, 411–434.

Stofan, J. R., DiPietro, L., Davis, D., Kohl, H. W., III, & Blair, S. N. (1998). Physical activity patterns associated with cardiorespiratory fitness and reduced mortality: The Aerobics Center Longitudinal Study. *American Journal of Public Health, 88*(12), 1807–1813.

Taylor, C. B., Houston-Miller, N., Haskell, W. L., & Debusk, R. F. (1988). Smoking cessation after acute myocardial infarction: The effects of exercise training. *Addictive Behaviors, 13*(4), 331–335.

United States Department of Health and Human Services. (2008). Physical activity guidelines advisory committee report to the secretary of health and human services. http://www.health. gov/PAGuidelines/committeereport.aspx. Accessed 16 Nov 2008.

Ussher, M., Nunziata, P., Cropley, M., & West, R. (2001). Effect of a short bout of exercise on tobacco withdrawal symptoms and desire to smoke. *Psychopharmacology, 158*(1), 66–72.

Ussher, M., Sampuran, A. K., Doshi, R., West, R., & Drummond, D. C. (2004). Acute effect of a brief bout of exercise on alcohol urges. *Addiction, 99*(12), 1542–1547.

Ussher, M. H., Taylor, A., & Faulkner, G. (2008). Exercise interventions for smoking cessation. *Cochrane Database of Systematic Reviews* 4, CD002295.

Ussher, M., West, R., McEwen, A., Taylor, A., & Steptoe, A. (2003). Efficacy of exercise counselling as an aid for smoking cessation: A randomized controlled trial. *Addiction, 98*(4), 523–532.

Vedamurthachar, A., Janakiramaiah, N., Hegde, J. M., Shetty, T. K., Subbakrishna, D. K., Sureshbabu, S. V., et al. (2006). Antidepressant efficacy and hormonal effects of Sudarshana Kriya Yoga (SKY) in alcohol dependent individuals. *Journal of Affective Disorders, 94*(1–3), 249–253.

Volkow, N. D., Fowler, J. S., Wang, G. J., & Goldstein, R. Z. (2002). Role of dopamine, the frontal cortex and memory circuits in drug addiction: Insight from imaging studies. *Neurobiology of Learning and Memory, 78*(3), 610–624.

Volkow, N. D., Fowler, J. S., Wang, G. J., & Swanson, J. M. (2004). Dopamine in drug abuse and addiction: Results from imaging studies and treatment implications. *Molecular Psychiatry, 9*(6), 557–569.

Wagner, E. F., Myers, M. G., & McIninch, J. L. (1999). Stress-coping and temptation-coping as predictors of adolescent substance use. *Addictive Behaviors, 24*(6), 769–779.

Wang, G. J., Volkow, N. D., Fowler, J. S., Franceschi, D., Logan, J., Pappas, N. R., et al. (2000). PET studies of the effects of aerobic exercise on human striatal dopamine release. *Journal of Nuclear Medicine, 41*(8), 1352–1356.

Weber, A. (1984). Running as treatment option: An experimental trial in stationary alcoholics. *Suchtgefahren, 30*, 160–167.

Weinstock, J., Barry, D., & Petry, N. M. (2008). Exercise-related activities are associated with positive outcome in contingency management treatment for substance use disorders. *Addictive Behaviors, 33*(8), 1072–1075.

Werme, M., Thoren, P., Olson, L., & Brene, S. (2000). Running and cocaine both upregulate dynorphin mRNA in medial caudate putamen. *European Journal of Neuroscience, 12*(8), 2967–2974.

Whiteley, J. A., Napolitano, M. A., Lewis, B. A., Williams, D. M., Albrecht, A., Neighbors, C. J., et al. (2007). Commit to Quit in the YMCAs: Translating an evidence-based quit smoking program for women into a community setting. *Nicotine and Tobacco Research, 9*(11), 1227–1235.

Wildmann, J., Kruger, A., Schmole, M., Niemann, J., & Matthaei, H. (1986). Increase of circulating beta-endorphin-like immunoreactivity correlates with the change in feeling of pleasantness after running. *Life Sciences, 38*(11), 997–1003.

Woodhouse, K., & Rigg, E. (1990). *Quit & Get Fit: A guide to running a six week course.* London, UK: HEA.

Xu, C. X., Liu, H. T., & Wang, J. (2008). Changes of 5-hydroxytryptamine and tryptophan hydroxylase expression in the ventral horn of spinal cord. *Neuroscience Bulletin, 24*(1), 29–33.

Chapter 10
Physical Activity for the Prevention of Child and Adolescent Drug Abuse

Aleta L. Meyer, Augusto Diana, and Elizabeth Robertson

Data on the relationship between physical activity and the use of alcohol, tobacco, and other drugs warrant a closer look before automatically presuming that physical activity has the potential to reduce risk for drug abuse. For example, recent analyses from the Monitoring the Future Study (MTF) between substance use and physical activity (either exercise in general or athletic team participation specifically) among US middle and high school youth from 1992 to 2009 indicates varying patterns of use by type of physical activity (Terry-McElrath, O'Malley, & Johnson, 2011). Exercise in general (reported level of participation in sports, athletics, or exercising) was associated with lower prevalence of middle and high school alcohol use, binge drinking, cigarette use, smokeless tobacco use, marijuana use, and steroid use; in contrast, athletic team participation (extent of participating in school athletic teams) was associated with lower rates of marijuana and cigarette use in middle school and higher rates of alcohol use, binge drinking, and steroid use in high school. Clearly, based on this information from the MTF data, physical activity is not the "silver

Disclaimer: The views and opinions expressed in this manuscript are those of the authors and should not be construed necessarily to represent the views of the NIDA, NIH, HHS or the US government.

A.L. Meyer (✉)
Office of Planning, Research, and Evaluation,
Administration for Children and Families, 370 L'Enfant Plaza Promenade,
SW, Washington, DC 20447, USA
e-mail: aleta.meyer@acf.hhs.gov

A. Diana
Division of Epidemiology, Services and Prevention Research, Prevention Research Branch,
National Institute on Drug Abuse (NIDA), 6001 Executive Blvd., Room 5163,
MSC 9589, Bethesda, MD 20892-9589, USA

E. Robertson
Division of Epidemiology, Services, and Prevention Research,
National Institute on Drug Abuse,
6001 Executive Blvd., Bethesda, MD 20852, USA

A.L. Meyer and T.P. Gullotta (eds.), *Physical Activity Across the Lifespan*,
Issues in Children's and Families' Lives 12, DOI 10.1007/978-1-4614-3606-5_10,
© Springer Science+Business Media New York 2012

bullet" of drug abuse prevention. However, there are many possible explanations for these relationships, and those explanations could lead to different approaches to prevention. While the MTF measurement questions around physical activity specify some distinctions in type of physical activity, those questions leave out many of the important dimensions and nuances described in Chap. 1 of this volume, which is focused on definitions of physical activity. Thus, assuming the relationships found in the MTF study relate solely to organized sports participation, without looking at the specifics such as characteristics of the sport itself and the motivation of the individual for participating, may lead to erroneous conclusions about causality and misguided direction for prevention. A more holistic view of physical activity offers the potential of elucidating multiple etiologic pathways and more targeted approaches for drug abuse prevention interventions.

A number of cross-sectional studies document associations between subgroups of individuals involved in physical activity and their use of substances; these studies help to define the complex relationship between these variables. For example, in one study that compared subgroups of adolescents by type of sport, participation in club and group sports had a significant lower negative correlation with alcohol use, whereas participation in individual-based sports did not (Vilhjalmsson & Thorlindsson, 1992). Other studies have examined single sex subsamples. Yusko, Buckman, White, and Pandina (2008) found that women's sports team athletes were significantly less likely to be substance users than female non-athletes. Similarly, the most active and fit females in a sample of college athletes had lower rates of smoking initiation than female non-athletes, independent of the sports season (Yusko et al.). These studies, and others like them, point to the many nuances in the relationships between substance use and physical activity. Cross-sectional studies help to clarify associations between variables, but do not give definitive answers as to why particular subgroups are more prone to use particular substances than other groups. For those answers well constructed experimental studies are needed.

The information in this chapter underscores the fact that the study of physical activity as drug abuse prevention is in its infancy. In fact there is little information regarding the efficacy of physical activity as an approach for drug abuse prevention in the research literature. However, over the past 20 years of prevention research using rigorous experimental designs, much has been learned about a wide range of other approaches that may be useful in making the case that physical activity is an approach worth investing time and effort in exploring (National Institute on Drug Abuse, 2003). For example, we have learned that interactive, psycho-social-educational approaches can be effective and that information-only, motivational testimonials, and scare tactics are not effective (Tobler, 2000). One can infer from this information that a physical activity approach comprised of motivational speeches or testimonials by professional athletes who have learned difficult lessons about drug use through personal experiences will not be effective. Alternately, interactive physical activity approaches that use a psychosocial educational approach and incorporate appropriate anti-drug information may be very effective.

The recent Institute of Medicine report on preventing mental, emotional, and behavioral disorders among young people states that "Mental health and physical health are inseparable" (National Research Council and Institute of Medicine, 2009, p. 17). This statement acknowledges the reciprocal relationship between physical health and mental health across the lifespan. Drug use initiation is a problem behavior that can lead to drug abuse and dependence, a chronic relapsing disease, which is closely associated with many other mental health disorders. The acknowledgement that physical health is tied to the risk factors for developing both mental health and drug abuse disorders opens the door to pursuing the possibility that improving physical health through physical activity may also be a promising approach for the prevention of drug use and other mental and emotional problem behaviors.

Theoretical Foundations and Empirical Support for Physical Activity as Drug Use Prevention

The assertion that mental and physical health are inseparable is consistent with the "whole child" view (e.g., Zigler & Trickett, 1978), a holistic approach which focuses on all areas of child and family development (e.g., cognitive, physical, and social-emotional development and contextual influences). Drawing on research built on this foundation, this chapter takes the viewpoint that youth are "whole people." Theory and empirical work that support moving in this direction include physical activity as a method to promote social-cognitive and emotional development, physical activity as an intervention modality, and physical activity as a social context for development. In the following sections a theoretical rationale, empirical support, and concrete examples of how physical activity might prevent drug use are presented.

Physical Activity to Promote Social-Cognitive and Emotional Development

Much of the progress of the drug abuse prevention field can be attributed to its strong grounding in life-course development and other ecological theories that support research on behavior change (e.g., Kellam, Koretz, & Moscicki, 1999). In the past, theories of behavior change presumed that observed behavior changes either signaled or were a reflection of internal biological changes. Advances in technologies to test internal change have confirmed this assumption and many of the assumptions of specific theories. For example, Riggs and Greenberg (2009) describe evidence that demonstrates a consistent association between neurocognitive deficits in self-regulation and early initiation of drug use. These data provide some understanding of how neurocognition is related to social-emotional competence (Riggs, Jahromi, Razza, Dillworth-Bart, & Mueller, 2006). Further, they may offer an avenue for considering whether physical activity influences risk for drug abuse.

The next section expands on this proposed link between neurocognitive development and drug abuse risk by describing possible mechanisms through which various forms of physical activity may enhance the development of self-regulation and potentially reduce drug abuse risk.

A recent observation concerning early childhood is the parallel and interdependent development of cognitive and perceptual-motor skills (Diamond, 2007). Stated simply, the mastery of bodily movements is manifested in physical changes in the brain that represent increased complexity and efficiency of neural pathways. The evidence on the relationship between motor skills and cognition suggests that participation in physical activities that involve the practice, repetition, and mastery of specific movements, such as tossing a ball or learning a particular dance step or a yoga pose may facilitate cognitive development. In fact, some psychologists hypothesize that intellectual and perceptual-motor skills are acquired in fundamentally similar ways (e.g., learning stages, training effects, the crucial role of coordination of component subskills) and that brain sites serving these processes are not as distinct as once thought, leading to the conclusion that mental operations are supported by perceptual-motor activities (Rosenbaum, Carlson, & Gilmore, 2001). Based on this research on the relationship between perceptual-motor skills and cognitive development, Rosenbaum suggests that the study of motor control is fundamental to understanding the ways in which cognition is expressed through behavior (Rosenbaum, 2005). If this is the case, interventions that involve movement and physical activity may be particularly effective for promoting behavior change over time and across domains through their dual impact on motor control and cognitive processes. For example, Diamond (2008) presents a compelling argument that participating in dance, through practice and performance, can improve children's lives, discipline, and cognitive skills.

An important dimension to consider in the relationship between cognitive and perceptual-motor skills is regulation of emotional arousal. For example, when a child learns to toss a ball, he or she may experience a combination of feelings including excitement, frustration, and fun. These feelings can serve to motivate and/or inhibit learning, depending on how well the child is able to regulate them. The process of emotional self-regulation during early childhood has been described as the ability, when aroused, to balance cognitive and emotion systems in an integrated whole (Diamond, 2007). The development of the capacity to self-regulate has been found to be important for developmental tasks such as school readiness (Blair & Diamond, 2008) and is a key resilience process to protect against later drug abuse risk (Dishion & Connell, 2006). Thus, the engagement of both the body and mind in physical activities that require the mastery or coordination of specific movements may facilitate the development of self-regulation and decision-making. Moreover, physical activities that include social aspects such as teamwork, competition, and affiliation to a group have the potential to rouse higher levels of emotion and hence require greater self-regulation. Additionally, situations that actively elicit emotion may generate memories of learning and lived experiences that are more readily accessed during social-cognitive problem-solving than memories that are not linked to an emotion (Lemerise & Arsenio, 2000).

As one transitions from childhood to adolescence, self-regulation in the form of coping with chronic and extended challenges becomes increasingly salient (Molden & Dweck, 2006). These challenges include the transition from primary to secondary school settings, the onset of puberty, the increasing significance of peer groups, the desire to establish one's own identity, pressures to perform at higher levels, and the need to learn from one's own mistakes. Many physical activities, especially being a member of a sports or performance team, may help an adolescent to learn skills and appropriate behaviors for dealing with challenges in a somewhat protected environment. For example, if a coach manages a team experience well (e.g., praises effort, teaches specific skills, refrains from humiliating players, focuses on improvement rather than winning at all costs), a child could learn the usefulness of self-discipline through daily practice, the value of trying a new strategy in the face of failure, and the benefits of pro-social problem-solving with one's peers. Researchers such as Cicchetti and Tucker (1994) argue that an individual's efforts to change his/her own behavior has enduring effects on development; the accumulation of such experiences can facilitate the development of social competence and protect against drug abuse risk.

Physical Activity as Intervention Method for Prevention

Kellam et al. (1999) discuss the importance of distinguishing between developmental theory and intervention theory when designing preventive interventions. Developmental theories, such as those that describe the development of self-regulation, describe the "putative causal elements and processes that then become potential targets" of intervention; an intervention theory describes the "process by which the intervention works" to affect positive change (Kellam et al., p. 472). Ideally, intervention design involves pairing developmental theory with intervention or change theory in a way that facilitates the targeted developmental process and the creation of an intervention approach. Tobler's (2000) finding in her meta-analysis that drug abuse prevention programs are more effective when they are interactive than when they are didactic, is an example of the mapping of intervention theory onto developmental theory. That is, a developmental task of early adolescence is greater involvement with peers; interventions for youth in this age group can capitalize on both the need for affiliation and the use of interactive techniques to maximize the effectiveness of interventions. Most successful preventive interventions are designed with both a specific developmental theory in mind and its intentional pairing with an intervention or change theory. However, physical activity has rarely been incorporated as either a necessary element of physical and emotional development or as a potential modality for change. Next we explore possibilities for considering physical activity as a method for enacting intervention theory by pairing the developmental theory on self-regulation with the intervention theories of social learning and experiential education.

Using Physical Activity to Enact Social Learning Intervention Theory

A social learning theory approach to intervention involves the processes of observation, practice, reinforcement, direct instruction, and modeling with facilitation by valued adults and peers (Bandura, 1977). Numerous effective preventive interventions have been based all or in part on the social learning approach (e.g., Adolescent Training and Learning to Avoid Steroids (ATLAS) (Goldberg et al., 2000); Life Skills Training Program (Botvin, 1996), Skills, Opportunity and Recognition (SOAR) (Hawkins, Catalano, Kosterman, Abbott, & Hill, 1999; Lonczak, Abbott, Hawkins, Kosterman, & Catalano, 2002). A physical activity preventive intervention based on social learning theory would involve the processes mentioned above in the context of valued feedback from others, with the added benefit of opportunities to learn from the natural consequences of the activity itself. The pairing of social learning theory with self-regulation theory for early adolescents through a physical activity intervention such as basketball offers opportunities for modeling (e.g., coach who models self-regulation when refereeing a game), reinforcement (e.g., being cheered on by teammates for good defense), and direct instruction and practice (e.g., demonstrating and practicing techniques for calming oneself when shooting a free throw). Organized physical activities provide many "teachable moments" such as these. Promising research is capitalizing on this through using basketball and martial arts with African American adolescent boys to promote anger management (Stevenson, 2008); similar approaches might be taken for promoting self-regulation to prevent drug abuse risk.

Using Physical Activity to Enact Experiential Education Intervention Theory

Experiential education intervention theory is based on the conceptualization of experience as (1) the sensory impact of the immediate event and (2) reflection on information from that event that allows one to make predictions about future events (Dewey, 1938). Thus, for a physical activity to qualify as an experiential education intervention modality, it must involve both the fully embodied experience of the activity and intentional reflection upon the relationship of that experience to future activities. For example, an experiential education intervention for the development of enhancement of self-regulation awareness for newly employed young adults could involve an outdoor solo trek where there is attention to the emotional experiences of the trek itself, paired with a reflective writing activities designed to promote the identification of how skills and attitudes around coping with the emotional and physical challenges encountered in the solo adventure inform coping with the stressors in one's first adult job. Processes that promote the transfer of this type of learning have been described as requiring preplanning, intentional pairings between the current learning environment and future environments, multiple opportunities for practice, natural consequences, internalized learning, involvement of significant others in the learning process, and follow-up experiences (Priest & Gass, 2005). Well-established examples of the experiential learning field, such as Outward Bound (established by Kurt Hahn) and the American Camping Association (established by Laura Mattoon), were developed around the intentional use of experience in the outdoors to enhance human development (Yerkes, 1999). While meta-analyses on outcomes of therapeutically oriented adventure programs with delinquent youth has indicated promise (Lipsey, 2009) and research comparing juvenile re-arrest rates of participants in adventure-based behavior management programs to treatment as usual has shown positive outcomes for the adventure-based behavior management approach (Gillis, Gass, & Russell, 2008), research to test to role of experiential mechanisms within such intervention approaches has not yet been conducted. Research that has focused on mechanisms of learning transfer for experiential approaches has focused on transfer to educational settings (e.g., Sibthorp, Furman, Paisley, Schumann, & Gookin, 2011; Sibthorp, Paisley, Furman, & Gookin, 2008). Up to this point, while there has been interest in research to understand the impact of experiential approaches such as summer camp on positive youth development outcomes (Bialeschki, Henderson, & James, 2007; Sibthorp, 2010), the prevention of drug abuse and other health risk behaviors has not been a focus.

Using Physical Activity to Enhance the Impact of Effective Drug Abuse Prevention

Self-regulation, or the lack thereof, has been associated with both positive and negative development. The preceding paragraphs make arguments for the ability of physical activity experiences to build or enhance self-regulatory processes. Associations between emotional reactivity and drug use and abuse have also been well documented. Given these overlapping associations, physical activity as an intervention modality might also be thought of as a way to strengthen or reinforce the impact of an existing evidence-based drug abuse prevention program. Important drug abuse prevention intervention components such as social norms for non-initiation of use, skills for refusing drug offers, and attitudes and intentions toward non-use could easily be incorporated into organized physical activities and elements of physical activity could easily be integrated into many existing efficacious and prevention programs. For example, in an elementary school using an effective classroom-based drug use prevention program, the components intended to build self-regulation and problem-solving through norms and refusal skills building could be adapted for use by physical education instructors during classroom activities, thereby reinforcing the original program. In this scenario, the physical activity intervention component is not the main approach, rather it creates the experiences that can be remembered and reflected upon to promote and retain learning.

Physical Activity as a Social Context for Development

Some have argued that within the Bronfenbrenner ecological framework (Bronfenbrenner, 1977), the sports context can be viewed as an important proximal social context for child and adolescent development, similar to the school context. For example, Danish, Petitpas, and Hale (1990) make the case that formal sports can be a context for enhancing or inhibiting development. However, they also posit that unless adults intentionally design formal sport activities to promote personal and social competence, these activities are unlikely to do so, given the highly competitive nature of professional sports in American culture. Lerner's conceptual model of developmental contextualism (Lerner & Castellino 2002), postulates a "goodness-of-fit" paradigm that involves reciprocal interactions between a child and his/her chosen context over-time. In this model, social contexts that optimize children's developmental potential have protective qualities that can be maximized over time, creating a "goodness of fit." This model could be applied to a broad range of settings where physical activities might occur, for example extracurricular sports, vigorous free play during recess, or taking one's dog for a daily walk. Using this model, prevention interventions could be designed to match individuals to activity types and settings that meet a wide range of needs and/or preferences. This targeted approach could enhance and build protective factors against drug abuse risk (e.g., poor impulse control; lack of parental monitoring; school disengagement) for individuals by need or preference.

In addition to promoting competencies, settings where physical activity occurs and the activities themselves could promote social identities that are congruent with healthy behaviors (Oyserman, Fryberg, & Yoder, 2007). Social identity involves identification with individuals and groups and with the behaviors those people participate in (e.g., people like me do x, y, and z; people like me do not do a, b, or c) (Haslam & Reicher, 2006). The identity-based motivation and health theoretical model Oyserman et al. suggests that if health promotion is not perceived as part of your in-group identity, then you are more likely to engage in unhealthy lifestyle behaviors than healthy behaviors. When Oyserman et al. tested this theoretical model on diverse samples of college students and adults, they found that indeed individuals who defined unhealthy behavior as part of their in-group identity were less likely to believe that engaging in healthy behavior would lead to positive outcomes such as improved quality and added years of life. Following from this theoretical perspective, perhaps social contexts that promote healthy behaviors and norms for in-group members can help to establish social identities where engaging in healthy behaviors and avoiding unhealthy behaviors, such as drug abuse, is consistent with one's identity.

In summary, this section described theoretical and empirical support for how physical activity might promote cognitive and emotional development, serve as an effective intervention modality, and/or function as protective social context for development. While all of these are possible avenues by which physical activity could prevent drug abuse, experimental studies are needed to test whether or not they actually operate in these ways. The following section summarizes existing research on physical activity to prevent drug abuse.

Research on Physical Activity Programs to Prevent Drug Abuse

There is a dearth of research on physical activity as an approach to prevent drug abuse; here we provide three programs of research worth examining for lessons learned. The first area focuses on the use of leisure time as a way to address drug use prevention (Caldwell, 2008). The second area focuses on common factors that exist between drug abuse risk and obesity risk (Pentz, 2008). The third area involves research on the impact of a physical activity intervention on alcohol use (Correia, Carey, Simons, & Borsari, 2003).

Research on Leisure Time Approaches to Drug Abuse Prevention

Timewise and Healthwise are leisure time-oriented expansions of the Life Skills Training middle-school drug abuse prevention curriculum (Botvin, 1996). Timewise and Healthwise are grounded in developmental neuroscience, psychosocial development, and self-determination theory (Sharp, Caldwell, Coffman, Wegner, & Flisher, 2011). Developmental neuroscience explains adolescent sensation seeking and quest for novelty, positing that rapid changes in the emotional and regulatory controls of the brain drive adolescents to seek out novelty, heightened sensations, and immediate rewards (Dahl, 2004; Steinberg, 2008). This sensation-seeking behavior may make adolescents susceptible to risk-taking behaviors like substance use if they are not having new experiences. Drawing from psychosocial development theory (Erickson, 1968), Timewise and Healthwise focus in on the role of identity formation as the primary task of adolescence. Youth often explore their identities in leisure contexts, which are free of the constraints of other more formal settings (like school and work). Timewise and Healthwise seek to exploit these adolescent tendencies by encouraging youth to engage in activity that may minimize risk factors such as boredom/loneliness, lack of motivation, and sedentary lifestyles. Self-determination theory (Ryan & Deci, 2000) is brought to bear as it helps explain individual motivation, seeing it along a continuum from internal or intrinsic rewards, such as satisfaction, to external or extrinsic rewards, including praise and acknowledgements of accomplishments by others.

Timewise is comprised of six core lessons in seventh grade, with additional boosters in eighth and ninth grades (Caldwell, Baldwin, Walls, & Smith, 2004). The curriculum includes lessons on helping youth understand their use of leisure time and on tracking and managing their daily leisure activity. In the advanced skills-building booster components, youth participants work on decision-making, risk-taking, stress management, friendships and mindfulness in their daily lives. A study of Timewise in rural Pennsylvania drew data from a pretest and posttest of a randomized control trial among students in nine rural schools (Caldwell et al., 2004). The sample was comprised of roughly half boys and half girls, 95% Caucasian, and about one-third were eligible for free or reduced lunches. Results at 5 months post-intervention showed higher posttest levels of interest in the intentional use of leisure time among girls in the Timewise group compared with those in the control group youth who exhibited more lack of motivation. In addition, Timewise boys showed significant increases in intrinsic motivation at posttest compared to control group boys. Corresponding to these positive leisure outcomes, adolescent use of alcohol increased at a significantly lower rate for Timewise than youth in the control group, and Timewise boys reported less use of cannabis and reduced inhalant use.

The Healthwise program builds on the Timewise logic and implements leisure-based activity among youth in nine schools in a peri-urban setting near Cape Town, South Africa (Caldwell, Patrick, Smith, Palen, & Wegner, 2010). Healthwise consists of 12 core lessons in eighth grade and boosters in ninth grade. The curriculum aims to reduce targeted risk behaviors, substance use, sexual risk behavior and their comorbidity, by increasing the influence of protective factors. The primary protective areas built by Healthwise are positive and meaningful leisure, risk avoidance, relationship-building, stress reduction, and meaningful information about sexual health and substance misuse. An added dimension of the Healthwise curriculum which relates to the cultural context of the program setting is promotion of community integration. This social component could yield important scientific knowledge appropriate for translation back to the US through program adaptations. For example, the community integration component seems highly compatible with the typical American community focus on recreational physical activity programming, including team sports and games, whereby a group identity can form, even when a team is not victorious, that may have potential as a protective factor.

The research on the Healthwise curriculum consisted of an effectiveness trial in nine high schools, using a pretest–posttest matched design, where schools were matched and assigned (Caldwell, Bradley, & Coffman, 2009). Data were collected in waves on three cohorts of students at approximately 6-month intervals. Early findings suggest that the leisure education intervention has effects in the promised direction on hypothesized leisure activity-related mediators and for substance abuse outcomes (Caldwell et al.). With regard to the mediators, compared to students in the comparison schools, students in the intervention schools showed increases in intrinsic motivation and decreases in a motivation over time (Caldwell et al., 2010).

Additional analyses of studies on Healthwise and Timewise are underway. One analysis found that the more consistent the sports/physical activity involvement by girls, the lower the odds of marijuana use (Tibbits, Caldwell, & Smith, 2009); results were less clear for boys. A second analysis found that the strongest predictors of substance use behaviors at baseline and over time were (1) leisure boredom, which increased the likelihood of using alcohol, cigarettes, and marijuana, and (2) healthy leisure and greater parental control, which mitigated the risk for substance use (Sharp et al., 2011). A third analysis of the HealthWise curriculum found that girls in schools with high fidelity of implementation experienced significant positive shifts in motivation directly following the physical activity component of the curriculum (Palen et al., 2009).

Research on the Healthwise and Timewise programs provide important insights into the potential value of leisure, a multi-faceted and somewhat distinct construct in the physical activity literature, on youth and drug abuse prevention. The findings also suggest preliminary support for a positive impact on sensation seeking and identity formation constructs embedded in the developmental neuroscience and psychosocial development perspectives. This work strongly suggests that attention to positive use of leisure time, devoted to proactive activities, can generate positive benefits for participants.

Research on Common Factors Between Drug Abuse Risk and Obesity Risk Approach

The second approach uses emotional self-regulation theory as its foundation with several identified risk and protective factors and their neurocognitive basis to examine the co-occurrence of substance use and obesity and then adapt an existing efficacious substance abuse prevention program to address the joint problems (Pentz, 2008). The common risk areas are poor executive function, sensation seeking, emotional dysregulation, stress/arousal, low impulse control, and peer and family influences. Pentz argues that the association between substance use and obesity risks presents the opportunity for the expansion and adaptation of evidence-based programs (EBP) for drug abuse prevention by incorporating physical activity as a focal area. Using the existing EBPs PATHS (Greenberg & Kusche, 1998) and STAR Midwestern Prevention Project (Pentz et al., 1998) programs as the basis, Pentz and colleagues (Sakuma, Riggs, & Pentz, 2012) incorporated a physical activity dimension to create the Pathways obesity prevention program. The added dimensions include recognizing sedentary vs. active lifestyles, exercise availability, and physical activity modeling by adult and peer models.

Pathways consists of 15 sessions with youth in fourth grade, ten additional sessions upon entering fifth grade, and five sessions in sixth grade (Riggs, Chou, Spruijt-Metz, & Pentz 2010a). Parent–child activities are implemented at the same time as the direct intervention with the children; these home-based activities are designed to promote homework completion (all three grades), emotional regulation and impulse control (fourth grade), and impulse control, executive function and behavior change (fifth and sixth grade). Four distinct hypotheses were tested through this research study, of which three identified physical activity as the primary intervention strategy. These hypotheses tested whether increases in physical activity promoted pro-social environment-seeking and alternative leisure time use by the children, and in turn, whether these changes led to increased dopamine and dopamine receptors. Pilot data from the study support these hypotheses (Riggs et al.). Specifically, higher levels of physical activity were associated with greater emotional control, more working memory and minimized behavioral disinhibition. In addition, higher levels of physical activity were also associated with less likelihood of tobacco use initiation (Riggs, Spruijt-Metz, Sakuma, Chou, & Pentz, 2010b). Thus this intervention shows promise for addressing the joint risk and protective factors associated with obesity and drug abuse.

Research on Physical Activity Intervention to Address Alcohol Abuse

The third example of physical activity as a possible substance abuse intervention strategy is a study of college students exposed to drug-free reinforcement techniques to minimize the likelihood of binge drinking (Correia et al., 2003). The study involved a comparison of an exercise intervention, a meditation intervention, and a no treatment control group; individuals in the exercise condition met three times per week as a group for 8 weeks in a structured and supervised running program. The meditation condition met three times weekly for 8 weeks; and the no treatment control group was comprised of comparable subjects who were only contacted for measurement sessions. Results indicated that compared to the other two groups, the exercise group not only showed an increase in physical fitness but also had the greatest reductions in alcohol consumption during the 8-week intervention and 6-week follow-up (Correia et al.).

As mentioned at the outset of this section, there is very little research linking physical activity directly to substance abuse prevention. The three approaches provided here offer promise that this area is one worthy of additional study. The three examples approaches address very different approaches and in each case, the greater the involvement in activity the lower the risk for and use of drugs. Given the limited amount of research in the area, these findings are promising and suggestive, providing impetus for additional research.

Suggestions for Practitioners Interested in Physical Activity Approaches to Drug Use Prevention

As the research on drug use prevention has developed, many lessons have been learned about what works and what does not. Whether traditional drug abuse prevention approaches and approaches that use physical activity have these lessons in common remains to be seen. However, there are some principles of prevention that are very relevant to this emerging area (National Institute on Drug Abuse, 2003). For example, as mentioned before, research has shown that interactive, psychosocial-educational approaches can be effective whereas information-only, motivational testimonials, and scare tactics approaches are ineffective (Tobler, 2000). This suggests that physical activity approaches that use a psychosocial educational approach and incorporate appropriate anti-drug information may be very effective. In the section that follows, we continue this type of reflection regarding what has been learned about effective drug use prevention and how it may apply to efforts that utilize physical activity.

Two relatively accessible approaches for blending drug use prevention with physical activity are to (1) augment existing drug use prevention efforts with physical activity or (2) build effective drug use prevention into existing physical activity venues. For both of these strategies, another relevant principle of prevention is that prevention programs should intervene in the developmental contexts proximal to the targeted children and adolescents. This principle suggests that combined drug use/physical activity prevention interventions should occur in the primary context of the individual and be developmentally appropriate for the age of the child. For example, because the family context is most important for young children, early childhood interventions should be family-based and can incorporate activities such as rough and tumble play; simple physical exercise games such as Simon Says; and access to safe, open spaces for running, jumping, skipping, and free play. Similarly, because the school context becomes increasingly important in the elementary school years, physical activity approaches that augment existing school-based drug use prevention should maximize opportunities (e.g., recess, physical education classes) and activities (e.g., dramatizing stories and measuring an acre) during the school day. In early adolescence, as youth get involved with extracurricular activities, drug abuse prevention programs for this developmental stage often include problem-solving and coping skills that could be adapted for use by coaches and other extracurricular instructors to reinforce the original program. Another research-based principle is that intervening in multiple contexts over time (e.g., the family, childcare settings, the schools, and after-school programs) with compatible, developmentally appropriate content can result in more powerful effects in promoting positive behavior and preventing drug use initiation than intervening in a single context. Therefore, developmentally appropriate, multi-contextual drug abuse/physical activity prevention interventions timed across the lifespan could be a viable approach for positively affecting public health.

As stated above, a second approach is to add effective principles of drug use prevention into real world settings that involve physical activity (e.g., childcare settings, after-school programs, summer programs, sports). Many youth-based contexts provide structured physical activities that could, but do not, incorporate a drug abuse prevention component. Moreover, these youth serving venues offer unique opportunities to reach difficult to access, vulnerable populations. If these settings actively incorporated developmentally appropriate drug use prevention into their daily activities, a large segment of the youth population would receive effective drug use prevention.

With both of these approaches that blend physical activity with effective drug use prevention, attention needs to be paid to the characteristics and supervision needs of the prevention specialist/staff who provides the programming and the supervision they would need to facilitate this blending. For example, because the use of "teachable moments" utilizes opportunities for illustrating the role that prevention skills play in real-life situations, individuals who merge these type of activities need to demonstrate their ability to actively draw these metaphors in the moment, rather than assuming children and youth will automatically see and understand the applicability of prevention skills to real-life situations. Thus, tools are needed to identify staff who are able to recognize those "moments" and spontaneously merge prevention and physical activities in real-time. Research has also demonstrated that across the course of child and adolescent development, contexts that offer warmth, support, appropriate developmental expectations, and rewards for appropriate behavior are the most successful in allowing youth to reach their full potential. For this reason, close attention should be paid to the ways in which physical activity is promoted by the facilitator. For example, is he or she using an encouraging or a competitive approach to engage or compel participation? How is he or she assessing the fit between the approach taken and the responsiveness of participants? In other words, as with all prevention and intervention efforts, there should be a strong focus on making sure to do no harm (Rhule, 2005).

Implementation considerations such as these are extremely important with preventive interventions in general and most likely will continue to be important with drug use preventive interventions that include physical activity. Implementation and dissemination research demonstrates that the competence of the facilitator/practitioner and the characteristics of the context effect implementation quality. Context impacts the feasibility, acceptability, and effectiveness of intervention strategies, often in ways that are unrelated to the intervention itself. Features such as the organization, financing, management, and staffing of contexts in which interventions take place (e.g., playground, schools, after-school programs, recreation centers, youth organizations) can influence what is implemented, who implements it, how it is implemented, and for how long it is implemented.

One final lesson from the current research on physical activity and drug abuse prevention is that practitioners should intentionally guide youth in structuring their free time. The finding that forms the basis of this lesson suggests that practitioners who help youth identify structured, proactive activities during leisure time help to promote benefits and prevent risks for youth. In sum, knowledge of the principles of prevention and lessons learned from research on physical activity can help practitioners and program providers to select and implement strategies that are developmentally appropriate, offered through contexts proximal to the target populations, including vulnerable youth, over the course of development by practitioners who promote interaction, recognize teachable moments, and approach youth with warmth and consistency.

Future Directions for Research on Physical Activity and Drug Abuse Prevention

Over the past few decades, significant progress has been made in understanding effective approaches to prevention of drug abuse in part due to the careful attention to basic developmental, biological, psychological and social processes associated with the initiation of drug use and the progression to abuse and dependence. However, the research on the relationship between physical activity and drug abuse is scant in general and specifically with regard to prevention. The life-course developmental perspective supports the position that individual and environmental factors interact to increase or reduce vulnerability to drug use with vulnerability occurring at many points along the life course and peaking at critical life transitions.

To address this complexity, intervention research has tested strategies designed to alter specified modifiable mediators in order to determine which are most related to and effective in reducing drug use initiation and escalation, with multiple audiences, and under varied conditions. As noted previously, successful drug use prevention programs have utilized a number of theories of development for intervening in drug use trajectories and for elucidating predictive mediators, or risk and protective factors, amenable to change. Because theoretical grounding of prevention programs is an essential feature of their success, further progress in prevention research relies on a stronger understanding of the internal mechanisms and processes at work when hypothesized intervention effects are realized. Moreover, further analyses of data collected during intervention trials are needed to develop a greater understanding of how and the extent to which these experiments support the theories on which they are based, as well as elucidate new theoretical approaches or meta-theories.

In this chapter, much of the theoretical focus has been on how physical activity in combination with effective drug abuse prevention approaches might promote self-regulation. However, there are many more intrapersonal, interpersonal, and environmental processes related to drug use risk and protection that could be identified as targets of a drug abuse prevention program in combination with physical activity. These processes include, but are not limited to, work and play as key social activities; sensation seeking; stress and coping; aggressive behavior; differential learning styles; family constellation, eating behaviors, and use of food as reward; and features of the built environment such as side walks and open spaces for recreation. Thus there are multiple possible new research avenues on which to build an understanding of how physical activity could prevent drug use that require empirical studies to test existing and novel theoretical frameworks. However, not all factors with empirical links to drug abuse and physical activity fit well into a theoretical basis. Rather, some empirical findings, especially those related to physiological and brain function are a-theoretical, nevertheless these data provide information important to the formation and testing of intervention strategies and may eventually support existing or be integrated into new theoretical frameworks.

A comprehensive approach to physical activity embedded within drug abuse prevention interventions would involve the entirety of physical development in context. Specifically, those aspects of physical development related to: nutrition and food habits; age and comparative physical maturation; psychological aspects of the physical self (e.g., body image, confidence in physical abilities); changing physicality over time (e.g., pubertal changes, weight gain or loss); physical abilities (e.g., grace, athleticism); social aspects of physical development (e.g., expectations based on size and appearance, feedback from significant adults and peers on physical appearance and abilities); and to local norms and resources for personal transport (e.g., mass transit, automobiles, foot travel). Some data on physical development have established relationships with drug use and abuse; notable examples relate to rumination about body image, bulimia, depressive symptoms and substance use among adolescent girls (Nolen-Hoeksema, Stice, Wade, & Bohon, 2007). However, little is known about factors such as the effect of the intrapersonal and interpersonal perceptions of physical development as risk or protective factors for drug abuse or about the role of physical activity as a mediator; even less is known about how to modify these risk factors through behavior change interventions. To advance the field of prevention, novel interventions must build on basic science findings from diverse fields to understand the pathways between physical development and activity and the rejection of or initiation of drug use.

Moreover, related to intervention theory, the actual content of interventions has been shown to influence effectiveness. For example, interactive activities and meaningful skill practices have been shown to be effective (Nichols, Graber, Brooks-Gunn, & Botvin, 2006). Therefore it is important to gain an understanding of what and how content influences intervention success. It is possible that processes posited by intervention theories such as social learning and experiential education may be as important as the developmentally based content of the intervention in accounting for beneficial changes in behaviors when they occur. However, little research has attempted to explicate how content, development, and other characteristics of the target population and content interact in creating the processes and mechanisms that contribute to intervention efficacy and effectiveness. For example, the internal processes involved through repeated physical activity or multiple exposures to anti-drug messages in multiple school venues including physical education classes may effect the expression of attitudes and intentions toward drug use through changes in cognitive processes, as well as supporting group social norms. Understanding how interventions work, for whom, and under what conditions are basic prevention research questions that could be addressed from the vantage point of physical activity.

The blending of established extracurricular and community activities that involve physical activity with effective substance use prevention programming represents another area ripe for research. The addition of an effective drug abuse intervention, as an adjunct to standard operations that include physical activity, adds to the complexity of planning and conducting a rigorous research study. However, accessing these contexts with the cooperation and collaboration of practitioners within the settings can greatly assist in the successful integration and implementation of developmentally appropriate drug abuse prevention content and activities as well as the research to support its efficacy and effectiveness. Understanding these venues, partnering with the providers, and selecting research questions that assist these venues in reaching their goals could aid in the overall process. Initial questions may include the feasibility, acceptability, and efficacy of intervention, while later questions may address issues such as fidelity and dosage, and then on to issues of financing and sustainability of the intervention.

Many research opportunities are available for those interested in physical activity research in the context of drug abuse prevention (NDA 2011). Given there are so many opportunities for research, the challenge is to narrow the scope to a manageable set of questions. The type of prevention research proposed (e.g., feasibility, efficacy, effectiveness, systems research) could offer some guidance for narrowing the scope; however, the more exciting aspects would relate to some of the most difficult questions regarding the integration of drug abuse and physical activity interventions—looking at *both* developmental and intervention theories within one research project.

References

Bandura, A. (1977). *Social learning theory*. Oxford, England: Prentice Hall.

Bialeschki, D., Henderson, K., & James, P. (2007). Camp experiences and developmental outcomes for youth. *Child and Adolescent Psychiatric and Clinical Nursing, 16*, 769–788.

Blair, C., & Diamond, A. (2008). Biological processes in prevention and intervention: The promotion of self-regulation as a means of preventing school failure. *Development and Psychopathology, 20*(3), 899–911.

Botvin, G. (1996). *Life skills training: promoting health and personal development*. Princeton, NJ: Princeton Health Press.

Bronfenbrenner, U. (1977). Toward an experimental ecology of human development. *American Psychologist, 32*(7), 513–531.

Caldwell, L. (2008). Adolescents and healthy leisure contexts: The Healthwise and Timewise interventions. Presented on 8 June 2008, Bethesda, MD: National Institute on Drug Abuse. http://grants.nih.gov/grants/guide/pa-files/PA-11-311.html. Accessed 15 Sept 2011.

Caldwell, L., Baldwin, C., Walls, T., & Smith, E. (2004). Preliminary effects of a leisure education program to promote healthy use of free time among middle school adolescents. *Journal of Leisure Research, 36*(3), 310–335.

Caldwell, L., Bradley, S., & Coffman, D. (2009). A person-centered approach to individualizing a school-based universal prevention intervention. *American Journal of Alcohol and Drug Dependence, 35*(4), 214–219.

Caldwell, L., Patrick, M., Smith, E., Palen, L., & Wegner, L. (2010). Influencing adolescent leisure motivation: Intervention effects of Healthwise South Africa. *Journal of Leisure Research, 42*(2), 203–220.

Cicchetti, D., & Tucker, D. (1994). Development and self-regulatory structures of the mind. *Development and Psychopathology, 6*, 533–549.

Correia, C., Carey, K., Simons, J., & Borsari, B. (2003). Relationship between binge drinking and substance-free reinforcement in a sample of college students: A preliminary investigation. *Addiction Behavior, 28*, 361–368.

Dahl, R. (2004). Adolescent brain development: A period of vulnerabilities and opportunities. *Annals of New York Academies of Science, 1021*, 1–22.

Danish, S., Petitpas, A., & Hale, B. (1990). Sport as a context for developing competence. In T. Gullotta, G. Adams, & R. Montemayer (Eds.), *Developing social competence in adolescence* (pp. 169–194). Newbury Park, CA: Sage Publications.

Dewey, J. (1938). *Experience and education*. New York: Collier.

Diamond, A. (2007). Interrelated and interdependent. *Developmental Science*. doi:dx.doi.org, 10, 152–158.

Diamond, A. (2008). Improving children's lives, discipline, and cognitive skills through dance. Presented on 8 June 2008, Bethesda, MD: National Institute on Drug Abuse. Retrieved 9/15/11 http://www.seiservices.com/NIDA/1014032/Final%20Presentations/NIDA%20PA%20June%206/Adele%20Diamond.pdf.

Dishion, T., & Connell, A. (2006). Adolescents' resilience as a self-regulatory process: Promising themes for linking intervention with developmental science. *Annals of the New York Academy of Science, 1094*, 125–138.

Erickson, E. (1968). *Identity: Youth and crisis*. New York: Norton.

Gillis, H., Gass, M., & Russell, K. (2008). The effectiveness of Project Adventure's behavior management programs for male offenders in residential treatment. *Residential Treatment for Children and Youth, 25*(3), 227–247.

Goldberg, L., MacKinnon, D., Elliot, D., Moe, D., Clarke, G., & Cheong, J. (2000). The adolescents training and learning to avoid steroids program: Preventing drug use and promoting health behaviors. *Archives of Pediatrics and Adolescent Medicine, 154*(4), 332–338.

Greenberg, M., & Kusche, C. (1998). Preventive interventions for school-age deaf children: The PATHS curriculum. *Journal of Deaf Studies and Deaf Education, 3*(1), 49–63.

Haslam, S., & Reicher, S. (2006). Stressing the group: Social identity and the unfolding dynamics of responses to stress. *Journal of Applied Psychology, 91*, 1037–1052.

Hawkins, J., Catalano, R., Kosterman, R., Abbott, R., & Hill, K. (1999). Preventing adolescent health-risk behaviors by strengthening protection during childhood. *Archives of Pediatric and Adolescent Medicine, 153*, 226–234.

Kellam, S., Koretz, D., & Moscicki, E. (1999). Core elements of developmental epidemiologically based prevention research. *American Journal of Community Psychology, 27*(4), 463–482.

Lemerise, E., & Arsenio, W. (2000). An integrated model of emotion processes and cognition in social information processing. *Child Development, 71*(1), 107–118.

Lerner, R., & Castellino, D. (2002). Contemporary developmental theory and adolescence: Developmental systems and applied developmental science. *Journal of Adolescent Health, 31*(Suppl6), 122–135.

Lipsey, M. (2009). The primary factors that characterize effective interventions with juvenile offenders: A meta-analytic overview. *Victims and Offenders, 4*, 124–147.

Lonczak, H., Abbott, R., Hawkins, J., Kosterman, R., & Catalano, R. (2002). Effects of the Seattle Social Development Project on sexual behavior, pregnancy, birth, and sexually transmitted disease outcomes at age 21 years. *Archives of Pediatric and Adolescent Medicine, 156*, 438–447.

Molden, D., & Dweck, C. (2006). Finding "meaning" in psychology: A lay theories approach to self-regulation, social perception, and social development. *American Psychologist, 61*(3), 192–203.

National Institute on Drug Abuse. (2003). Preventing drug use among children and adolescents: A research-based guide for parents, educators, and community leaders. Washington, DC: U.S. Department of Health and Human Services. http://www.nida.nih.gov/pdf/prevention/RedBook. pdf. Accessed 20 Oct 2011.

National Institute on Drug Abuse. (2011). Drug abuse prevention intervention research funding opportunity announcement (RO1). http://grants.nih.gov/grants/guide/pa-files/PA-11-311.html. Accessed 20 Oct 2011.

National Research Council and Institute of Medicine. (2009). Preventing mental, emotional, and behavioral disorders among young people: Progress and possibilities. Committee on the Prevention of Mental Disorders and Substance Abuse among Children, Youth, and Young Adults: Research Advances and Promising Interventions. In M. E. O'Connell, T. Boat, & K. E. Warner (Eds.). Board on Children, Youth, and Families, Division of Behavioral and Social Sciences and Education. Washington, DC: The National Academies Press. "Introduction" pp. 1–32. p. 17 specifically.

Nichols, T., Graber, J., Brooks-Gunn, J., & Botvin, G. (2006). Ways to say no: Refusal skill strategies among urban adolescents. *American Journal of Health Behavior, 30*(3), 227–236.

Nolen-Hoeksema, S., Stice, E., Wade, E., & Bohon, C. (2007). Reciprocal relations between rumination and bulimic, substance abuse, and depressive symptoms in adolescent females. *Journal of Abnormal Psychology, 116*, 198–207.

Oyserman, D., Fryberg, S., & Yoder, N. (2007). Identity-based motivation and health. *Journal of Personality and Social Psychology, 93*(6), 1011–1027.

Palen, L., Patrick, M., Gleeson, S., Caldwell, L., Smith, E., & Wegner, L. (2009). Leisure constraints for adolescents in Cape Town, South Africa: A qualitative study. *Leisure Sciences, 32*, 434–452.

Pentz, M. (2008). Translating drug use prevention to obesity prevention. Presented on "Can Physical Activity and Exercise Prevent Drug Abuse? Promoting a Full Range of Science to Inform Prevention." Presented on 8 June 2008, Bethesda, MD: National Institute on Drug Abuse. http://www.seiservices.com/NIDA/1014032/Final%20Presentations/NIDA%20PA%20 June%205/Pentz%20NIDA%20PA%20conference.pdf. Accessed 15 Sept 2011.

Pentz, M., Dwyer, J., Mackinnon, D., Flay, B., Hansen, W., Wang, E., et al. (1998). A multicommunity trial for primary prevention of adolescent drug abuse. *Journal of the American Medical Association, 261*(2), 3259–3266.

Priest, S., & Gass, M. (2005). *Effective leadership in adventure programming*. Champaign, IL: Human Kinetics.

Rhule, D. (2005). Take care to do no harm: Harmful interventions for youth problem behavior. *Professional Psychology: Research and Practice, 36*(6), 618–625.

Riggs, N., Chou, C. P., Spruijt-Metz, D., & Pentz, M. A. (2010a). Executive cognitive function as a correlate and predictor of child food intake and physical activity. *Child Neuropsychology, 16*(3), 279–292.

Riggs, N., & Greenberg, M. (2009). Neurocognition as a moderator and mediator in adolescent substance misuse prevention. *The American Journal of Drug and Alcohol Abuse, 35*(4), 209–213.

Riggs, N., Jahromi, L., Razza, R., Dillworth-Bart, J., & Mueller, U. (2006). Executive function and the promotion of social-emotional competence. *Journal of Applied Developmental Psychology, 27*, 300–309.

Riggs, N. R., Spruijt-Metz, D., Sakuma, K. L., Chou, C. P., & Pentz, M. A. (2010b). Executive cognitive function and food intake in children. *Journal of Nutrition Education and Behavior, 42*(6), 398–403.

Rosenbaum, D. (2005). The Cinderella of psychology: The neglect of motor control in the science of mental life and behavior. *American Psychologist, 60*(4), 308–317.

Rosenbaum, D., Carlson, R., & Gilmore, R. (2001). Acquisition of intellectual and perceptual-motor skills. *Annual Review of Psychology, 52*, 453–470.

Ryan, R., & Deci, E. (2000). Self-determination theory and the facilitation of intrinsic motivation, social development and well-being. *American Psychologist, 55*, 68–78.

Sakuma, K., Riggs, N., & Pentz, M. (2012). Translating evidence based violence and drug use prevention to obesity prevention: Development and construction of the pathways program. *Health Education Research, 27*(92), 343–358.

Sharp, E., Caldwell, L., Coffman, D., Wegner, L., & Flisher, A. (2011). Predicting substance use behavior among South African adolescents: The role of leisure experience across time. *International Journal of Behavioral Development, 35*(4), 343–351.

Sharp, E., Coffman, D., Caldwell, L., Smith, E., Wegner, L., Vergnani, T., et al. (2011). Predicting substance use behavior among South African adolescents: The role of leisure experiences across time. *International Journal of Behavioral Development, 35*(4), 343–351.

Sibthorp, J. (2010). Positioning outdoor and adventure programs within positive youth development. *Journal of Experiential Education, 33*(2), vi–ix.

Sibthorp, J., Furman, N., Paisley, K., Schumann, S., & Gookin, J. (2011). Mechanisms of learning transfer in adventure education: Qualitative results from the NOLS transfer survey. *Journal of Experiential Education, 34*(2), 109–126.

Sibthorp, J., Paisley, K., Furman, N., & Gookin, J. (2008). Long-term impacts attributed to participation in adventure education: Preliminary findings from NOLS. *Research in Outdoor Education, 9*, 86–102.

Steinberg, L. (2008). A social neuroscience perspective on adolescent risk-taking. *Developmental Review, 28*, 78–106.

Stevenson, H. (2008 science meeting). A potential enhancement for substance use prevention: Promoting self-control through basketball and martial arts. Presented on 8 June 2008, Bethesda, MD: National Institute on Drug Abuse. http://www.seiservices.com/NIDA/1014032/Final%20Presentations/NIDA%20PA%20June%205/Pentz%20NIDA%20PA%20conference.pdf. Accessed 15 Sept 2011.

Terry-McElrath, Y., O'Malley, P., & Johnson, L. (2011). Exercise and substance use among American youth, 1991–2009. *American Journal of Preventive Medicine, 40*(5), 530–540.

Tibbits, M., Caldwell, L., & Smith, E. (2009). The relation between profiles of leisure activity participation and substance use among South African youth. *World Leisure, 51*(3), 150–159.

Tobler, N. (2000). Lessons learned. *The Journal of Primary Prevention, 20*(4), 261–274.

Vilhjalmsson, R., & Thorlindsson, T. (1992). The integrative and physiological effects of sport participation: A study of adolescents. *The Sociological Quarterly, 33*(4), 637–647.

Yerkes, R. (1999). 1998 Kurt Hahn address: Dancing on the shores of the future. *Journal of Experiential Education, 22*(1), 20–23.

Yusko, D., Buckman, J., White, H., & Pandina, R. (2008). Alcohol, tobacco, illicit drugs, and performance enhancers: A comparison of use by college student athletes and nonathletes. *Journal of American College Health, 57*(3), 281–289.

Zigler, E., & Trickett, P. (1978). IQ, social competence, and the evaluation of early childhood intervention programs. *American Psychologist, 33*, 789–798.

Chapter 11
Individual-Level Behavior Change Strategies to Promote Physical Activity

Kyle J. Davis, Samuel Hubley, and Jenn Leiferman

Introduction

Many of us can relate to the difficulty of initiating and maintaining a regular exercise program in our daily lives. In fact, up to 60 % of people fail to maintain regular physical activity 6 months after starting an exercise program (Dishman, 1988). Despite these sobering figures, strategies drawn from modern psychological theory-based interventions can help clients initiate and maintain regular physical activity. As the effectiveness of any therapeutic technique is partly dependent on clients' motivation for change, facilitating motivation is a crucial and often overlooked aspect of initiating physical activity. Although those seeking to increase physical activity in their lives likely already possess some motivation to change their current behavior, many find it difficult to maintain regular activity as originally intended. While many have shared this experience, others are able to initiate and maintain regular physical activity throughout their lives. What accounts for this difference? We may never know the full answer to this question, but we do know that theory and techniques developed for use in psychotherapy or counseling can encourage, facilitate, and maintain a variety of behavior changes, including physical activity.

This chapter offers several strategies for helpers (i.e., health care professionals, therapists, counselors, social workers) to promote behavior change specific to increasing physical activity. The application of these strategies are drawn primarily from motivational interviewing (MI; Miller & Rollnick, 1991), and behavioral activation (BA; Jacobson, Martell, & Dimidjian, 2001), and the theoretical rationale for

K.J. Davis(✉) • S. Hubley
Department of Psychology, University of Colorado, 345 UCB,
Boulder, CO 80309, USA
e-mail: kyle.davis@colorado.edu

J. Leiferman
Department of Community and Behavioral Health, Colorado School of Public Health,
13001 E 17th Ave, C245, Aurora, CO 80045, USA

A.L. Meyer and T.P. Gullotta (eds.), *Physical Activity Across the Lifespan*,
Issues in Children's and Families' Lives 12, DOI 10.1007/978-1-4614-3606-5_11,
© Springer Science+Business Media New York 2012

employing such strategies is rooted in Self-Determination Theory (Deci & Ryan, 1985), Social Cognitive Theory (Bandura, 1986), and the Transtheoretical Model (Prochaska & Diclemente, 1983). We present the theoretical foundations of health behavior change theories, the empirical support for MI and BA, and three classes of strategies: assessment and motivation, implementing behavioral plans, and relapse prevention. Each of these three sections includes practical examples of helpers using these strategies with clients. By understanding the nuances and difficulties of initiating behavior change, helpers may find these strategies useful in helping clients make physical activity an integral part of their lives.

Theoretical Foundation and Empirical Support

Self-Determination Theory

Self-Determination Theory (SDT) posits that basic psychological needs, such as feeling competent, autonomous, and related are important factors contributing to human motivation (Ryan & Deci, 2000). According to SDT, motivation falls on a continuum between intrinsic and extrinsic motivation where intrinsic motivation refers to engaging in an activity for the inherent satisfaction of the activity itself, and extrinsic motivation refers to performing an activity to obtain a separable outcome (Ryan & Deci, 2000). Ideally, extrinsically motivated behavior becomes intrinsically motivated if a person feels competent to perform the behavior, autonomous in their actions, and that the behavior is relevant to their values. For example, some people are extrinsically motivated to cook dinner simply because they need to eat and do not cook for the sake of cooking, while others are intrinsically motivated because they may feel effective and connected to others while cooking. SDT states that the greater intrinsic motivation one has to perform a behavior, the greater likelihood that behavior will be performed (Ryan & Deci, 2000). The rationale of SDT implies that helpers can promote increases in physical activity by fostering intrinsic motivation.

Social Cognitive Theory

Social Cognitive Theory (SCT) integrates the functions of social environments and self-regulatory behaviors when adopting and maintaining new behaviors and emphasizes the theory of reciprocal determinism, a theory that describes how individuals' environments and behaviors interact and influence each other (Bandura, 1986). SCT highlights the role of self-efficacy in initiating and maintaining behavior change by emphasizing how engagement in new behavior is positively associated with the amount of confidence one feels in performing that behavior. To increase physical activity, helpers can structure activities that the participant already feels confident in by grading tasks into manageable steps so the client can develop a greater sense of self-efficacy. SCT also posits that individuals may learn new behaviors through observing behavioral models (Elder et al., 2007). Incorporating others into physical activities may help clients to both learn how others perform and maintain activity and receive increased social support.

Transtheoretical Model

The Transtheoretical Model (Prochaska & Diclemente, 1983) is a theory of behavior change developed in the context of decreasing addictive behaviors. The Transtheoretical Model highlights how behavior change progresses along a sequence of stages and that each stage is characterized by specific processes of change (Prochaska, Diclemente, & Norcross, 1992). The five stages of change include: precontemplation, contemplation, preparation, action, and maintenance. For example, consider a person trying to quit smoking cigarettes. They begin in the precontemplation stage, with no intention of quitting in the next 6 months, move to the contemplation stage when they do plan to quit in the next 6 months, and then prepare for taking action in the next month. The action stage refers to overt behavior changes to reduce smoking over the next 6 months and the maintenance phase involves relapse prevention. The Transtheoretical Model also includes ten significant processes of change: consciousness raising, self-reevaluation, self-liberation, counterconditioning, stimulus control, reinforcement management, helping relationships, dramatic relief, environmental reevaluation, and social liberation (Prochaska et al., 1992). For definitions of the stages and processes of change, please see (Glanz, Rimer, & Viswanath, 2008). While the Transtheoretical Model was developed to understand how people change addictive behaviors, it has subsequently been applied to understanding how people initiate and maintain regular physical activity (Marshall & Biddle, 2001). Helpers can use this stage model of change to assess where clients are in the process of increasing physical activity and targeting interventions accordingly.

Theories of behavior change and strategies to change behavior are closely linked. SDT, SCT, and the Transtheoretical Model provide the theoretical backbone for which MI and BA can be used to help client's change behavior. For example, MI works to facilitate intrinsic versus extrinsic motivation as posited in SDT by helping clients explore ambivalence and clarify values. As motivation will invariably waver, it is important to have well-defined goals and strategies to maintain those plans; as will become clear, these are central constructs of BA.

Empirical Evidence for Motivational Interviewing

The following two sections are meant to substantiate the use of MI and BA with clinical populations. While a full review of the MI/BA efficacy data is beyond the scope of this chapter, interested readers are encouraged to follow up on the references provided in these sections. Motivational Interviewing (MI) is a counseling style rooted in the tradition of client-centered therapy and developed as a brief intervention for problem alcohol use, where motivation is a common obstacle to behavior change (Rollnick, Miller, & Butler, 2008). MI helps clients change behavior by exploring and resolving ambivalence concerning behavior change (Miller & Rollnick, 1991). Therapists using MI work to create a warm, empathic, and supportive atmosphere where clients can safely explore reasons for and against changing their behavior (Miller & Rollnick, 1991). Since MI's inception for treating problem alcohol use, it has been adapted to increase motivation for behavior change in a variety of domains ranging from use with criminal offenders (McMurran, 2009) to voice therapy (Behrman, 2006). MI has been empirically tested as a standalone therapy for increasing physical activity in cancer survivors (Bennett, Lyons, Winters-Stone, Nail, & Scherer, 2007), people with chronic heart failure (Brodie & Inoue, 2005), in employees of a business (Butterworth, Linden, McClay, & Leo, 2006), and in primary care settings (Harland et al., 1999; Hillsdon, Thorogood, White, & Foster, 2002). Successful implementation of MI guides the client through the stages of behavior change outlined in the Transtheoretical Model, from contemplation through maintenance, and moves at a comfortable pace for the client. With promising evidence for helping clients initiate behavior change, MI is a logical choice for assessing and fostering motivation to engage in physical activity.

Empirical Evidence for Behavioral Activation

Behavioral Activation (BA) is a brief, structured psychotherapy for depression that emphasizes the role of contextual factors and behavioral patterns in the onset and maintenance of depression (Jacobson et al., 2001). BA seeks to alleviate depression by helping clients systematically reconnect with activities that elicit pleasure and mastery. Specific strategies of BA include scheduling and structuring activities, decreasing avoidance, overcoming barriers to activation, collaborative problem solving, and acting in accordance with goals rather than mood. In addition to evidence that BA is an efficacious treatment of acute depression (Dimidjian et al., 2006), it has also shown promise in the treatment of other psychological and physiological disorders such as Posttraumatic Stress Disorder (Jakupcak et al., 2006), Borderline Personality Disorder (Hopko, Sanchez, Hopko, Dvir, & Lejuez, 2003), depression in cancer patients (Hopko, Bell, Armento, Hunt, & Lejuez, 2005), and depression comorbid with obesity (Pagoto, Bodenlos, Schneider, Olendzki, & Spates, 2008). While designed for the treatment of acute depression, the techniques used in BA are amenable to the promotion of physical activity, and although they have not been tested empirically in this realm, it is a pragmatic and logical approach that meshes well with health behavior change theories. In fact, increasing physical activity is often a goal of clients undergoing treatment in BA.

Strategies to Initiate and Maintain Physical Activity

This section of the chapter provides practical techniques that health care professionals can use to help clients increase motivation, and to initiate and maintain regular physical activity in their lives. These clinical strategies are divided into *Assessment and Motivation*, *Implementing Behavioral Plans*, and *Relapse Prevention* and are used in a logical order: (1) First, helpers assess client motivation to initiate physical activity and work with clients to foster further motivation. (2) Second, helpers draw on BA techniques to increase the likelihood that clients will follow through with physical activity plans. (3) Next, helpers and clients review progress and what clients have learned about the relationship between themselves and physical activity. (4) Finally, helpers and clients make plans to overcome obstacles to maintaining regular physical activity once therapy or consultation has ended. Each section includes a theoretical overview, descriptions of specific strategies, and applied examples. We use the term helpers to describe any mental or physical health care practitioner and the term client for anyone seeking to increase physical activity. While we suspect weekly meetings between helpers and clients may be most helpful, we realize that this is unlikely in many if not most situations. Accordingly, these strategies can be applied in as little or as much time is available.

Assessment and Motivation

Most people know that physical activity is good for them. Despite this knowledge, many lack the motivation to begin regular physical activity on their own. Establishing motivation is thus the first step, and perhaps the most important, in initiating behavior change. Without motivation, most people will fail to ever begin physical activity, and the few that do may not maintain it. In order to develop motivation for change, helpers must first explore why their clients need or want to engage in physical activity. Helpers can accomplish this by utilizing a MI technique which assesses the clients' desire, ability, reason, and need (DARN; Rollnick, et al., 2008) to initiate physical activity. Assessing clients' desires, abilities, reasons, and needs to initiate physical activity provides helpers with valuable information they can use throughout treatment. A client's desire to change informs helpers of how intrinsically motivated clients are to begin physical activity. Gauging clients' abilities to engage in physical activity informs helpers of what types of activities clients feel confident in engaging and also provides insight into the level of intensity that is appropriate for clients. There are numerous evidence-based motivating factors to partake in regular physical activity such as disease prevention and control, weight management, and stress reduction. Helpers can work to aid clients in identifying factors that are motivating to each individual client. Helpers may also benefit by reminding clients of their values and why physical activity is important in their lives.

According to MI, there are five basic principles that helpers can follow in order to facilitate motivating behavior change. These principles include expressing empathy, developing discrepancy, avoiding argumentation, rolling with resistance, and sup-porting self-efficacy (Miller & Rollnick, 1991). *Expressing empathy* is a fundamen-tal component of the therapeutic process. Showing sincere care about the clients' thoughts and feelings assists helpers in joining their clients as an ally in increasing physical activity. For example, a client may reveal how embarrassed they are to start a walking program because they are less physically fit and may not be able to keep up with others in the program. In such situations, it is crucial that helpers empathize with clients and reflect how hard it may be so clients feel understood. Expressing empathy is an often overlooked step as health care providers may have a tendency to suggest what they think is best for clients without taking into consideration clients' concerns. *Developing discrepancy* in clients' thoughts concerning behavior change involves helping clients articulate how their exercise habits are different than they would like them to be and can give helpers leverage in encouraging physical activity. For example, depressed clients may say that certain activities help them feel better, but they never have time to engage in these activities. Similarly, clients may state that they do not feel like exercising, though engaging in regular physical activity is a value that they hold important. Statements like these enable helpers to point out that clients may be prioritizing other activities in their lives that do not have a positive effect on mood or are not valued activities, despite clients' desires to overcome depression or live their lives according to their values. *Avoiding argumentation* and *rolling with resistance* often go hand-in-hand. When discussing behavior change with clients, many helpers notice ambivalence about changing behavior and it is easy to fall into the trap of telling clients what is best for them. Unfortunately, this type of direct advice can actually undermine behavior change when clients are ambivalent and end up taking the side of not changing. Rather, helpers can avoid arguments and reflect back the difficulty in making changes to one's lifestyle. Encouraging such change talk can also enhance the therapeutic alliance. *Rolling with resistance* refers to not challenging or arguing with clients when they present reasons not to change. This can be accomplished by reflecting clients' reasons not to change while remain-ing empathic. For example, clients may say that they do not have time to engage in physical activity or that they do not enjoy exercising. In these situations, it is tempt-ing to point out other activities clients engage in that are not related to physical activ-ity, or to tell clients that they will like physical activity after they get used to it. In contrast, helpers can benefit from agreeing with clients about how busy their sched-ules are or agreeing with clients that physical activity is not easy and can be painful. These techniques often obviate an adversarial relationship and enable helpers to serve as allies to their clients in increasing physical activity. *Supporting self-efficacy* rewards clients for taking charge of their lives. By praising clients when they accom-plish goals, overcome obstacles, think of novel ways to increase physical activity, and take steps to be more proactive in physical activity, clients will become more confident in their ability to maintain physical activity throughout their lives.

MI posits that increased change talk and diminished resistance are directly related to behavior change. Thus, helpers seek to guide clients through their thoughts and feelings regarding increasing levels of physical activity. By affording clients the space to explore their own reasons for change as well as their reasons not to change, helpers can highlight discrepancies in how clients' resistances are keeping clients from living their desired lifestyles. Here is an example demonstrating these strategies:

HELPER: Hello Caroline, it seems like you haven't been able to be as active as you would like to be in the last 6 months. What are some reasons you have for wanting to be more active?

CAROLINE: I've been feeling pretty depressed recently and my doctor said it may help. Also, I guess I never felt as depressed when I was exercising more.

HELPER: So it seems like regular physical activity is pretty important to regulating your mood. I'm curious how it felt when you were exercising more?

CAROLINE: I just remember feeling better about myself and that I was more productive.

HELPER: Can you tell me more about being more productive?

CAROLINE: Well I would work out after work, before I got home. I would have more energy to cook and to do things around the house. I think accomplishing those types of things made me feel better about myself. Now when I get off work, I just feel really tired and pick up dinner on the way home because I don't have the energy to cook.

HELPER: Alright, so exercising more might help your mood, give you more energy and help you get more done around the house?

CAROLINE: Yeah, I mean it sounds so simple, just exercise more, but I never have the energy or time.

HELPER: From what you've told me, your life does sound very busy.

CAROLINE: Well I am busy, but I was just as busy when I was exercising in the past.

HELPER: Oh okay, so you're noticing that in the past you were busy as well but managed to find time to exercise. What do you think is different now?

CAROLINE: I guess it's the energy part. I'm just so tired when I get done at work.

HELPER: It definitely is hard to exercise when you feel like you don't have any energy.

CAROLINE: You know, I've always felt tired at the end of a work-day. It seems like I actually had more energy when I got home if I went for a walk right after work.

HELPER: I know that does seem kind of strange how exercising can make you feel like you have more energy.

CAROLINE: This all sounds nice, but I'm just not sure if I'm going to be able to actually get out there and start walking again.

HELPER: It's definitely easier said than done. From what I heard you say though, it seems like exercising would help your mood, may give you more energy and help you get more things accomplished. How important do you think those things are to you?

CAROLINE: I guess they're really important, when I'm feeling depressed I just don't really enjoy anything or get much done.

HELPER: Ah, so it sounds like exercising more really improves your life in a variety of ways.

CAROLINE: Yeah, it definitely does. I just need to start going on walks again.

The helper in this example makes use of techniques vital to MI. First, the helper assesses the client's motivation to exercise by remembering to elicit desire, ability, reasons, and needs to change from the client. The helper is also quick to express empathy when the opportunity arises. Arguments are avoided and the helper rolls with, and does not attempt to challenge, the client's resistance. The helper agrees with the client instead, but gently reminds the client of their own motivation to exercise. Finally, the helper praises the client when they generate their own ways to increase physical activity. By using MI, the helper guides the client towards realizing their own motivation to increase physical activity.

Assessment of Physical Activity

Assessment of current physical activity as well as physical capabilities is necessary to help clients set realistic goals and avoid potential failure. It would be unrealistic to assume, for example, that sedentary clients will be able to walk 2 miles three times per week. Because clients may not know their limitations or capabilities, helpers can help clients set realistic and achievable goals. In the previous example, a more realistic goal may be to start slowly by walking a half mile three times per week and eventually increase to longer distances. Helpers can base assessments on what clients have done in the past and adjust for their current physical condition. More thorough assessments may include heart rate monitors so clients' can track their heart rates. Similarly, pedometers, which are small, inexpensive, electronic step counting devices, may be used to provide helpers and clients with accurate levels of physical activity. Once baseline levels of physical activity, or steps, are established, helpers can assist clients in setting incremental, long-term goals. Pedometers are effective tools to teach behavioral skills related to self-monitoring, as they provide instant feedback on how much physical activity the client has engaged in per day.

Setting Physical Activity Goals

As a vision of a desired end state is required for any systematic effort toward behavior change, setting specific, concrete goals is a logical first step in helping clients increase physical activity. The extent to which a goal is specific and concrete depends on how precisely it is defined. For example, the goal of going to the gym more is not as precisely defined as the goal of going to the gym twice per week. Better yet is the goal of going to the gym two times per week—one 20-min session of cardio and one 20-min session of weight-training. Abstract goals ("I want to get in better shape") make behavior change difficult because progress and success in achieving an indeterminate objective is difficult, if not impossible, to achieve or measure. Helpers may find using the acronym SMART (Specific, Measureable, Achievable, Realistic, and Timely) beneficial when aiding clients in setting goals. Establishing specific, concrete goals allows clients and helpers to ensure that they are realistic and that they can be broken down and structured appropriately (see below for a discussion on structuring).

An important reason for setting physical activity goals is the sheer number and variety of activities clients can engage in to become more physically active. As activity goals may range from walking around the block to running a marathon, it is important for helpers to tailor goals to individual client needs and focus on finding activities that clients are interested in and that allow for incremental gains across the exercise program. In time, these weekly goals will hopefully develop into daily routines in the client's lifestyle.

While options to increase physical activity are numerous, it is often beneficial for helpers to encourage clients to adopt modest goals (though large, long-term goals—such as running a marathon—need not immediate dismissal). The American College of Sports Medicine and the American Heart Association (Haskell et al., 2007) recommend the following: moderate-intensity aerobic physical activity for a minimum of 30 min on 5 days per week, or vigorous-intensity aerobic physical activity for a minimum of 20 min on 3 days per week. Physical activity can be measured in terms of Metabolic Equivalent of Task (MET). One MET is equivalent to burning one kilocalorie of energy per kilogram of body weight per hour. Moderate intensity exercise may be defined as 3–5.9 METs and vigorous intensity exercise as greater than or equal to 6.0 METs (Physical Activity Guidelines Advisory Committee, 2008). Comparable amounts of physical activity are effective in the prevention and treatment of depression (Dunn, Trivedi, Kampert, Clark, & Chambliss, 2005; Physical Activity Guidelines Advisory Committee, 2008) as well as many other physical disorders. Helpers can use these findings to help clients establish realistic physical activity goals.

Finally, BA therapists often encourage clients to consider the distinction between *mood-dependent behavior* and *goal-dependent behavior*. Helpers will also likely benefit from this technique when encouraging physical activity. When faced with tasks of all kinds that are not required on a day-to-day basis (e.g., household chores, staying in touch with family, exercising) many people often wait until they *feel like it* and are thus exhibiting mood-dependent behavior. The problem with mood-dependent behavior is that, even for the mild-tempered, our moods may vary considerably from hour-to-hour, whereas our values tend to remain consistent across time. Exercising according to mood would suffice if everyone always felt like exercising, but clearly this is not the case. Success in implementing and maintaining regular physical activity is often bound by the extent to which clients can learn to recognize the pitfalls of mood-dependent exercise and replace it with a goal-dependent attitude. An example of working with a client to establish goals is provided below. The example below builds on the previous scenario in which the helper worked to establish motivation. The client ended by saying she was ready to start walking again.

HELPER: That sounds great Caroline! Do you have an idea of how far or how long you are going to walk?

CAROLINE: Hmmm not really, I'll probably just stop when I get tired.

HELPER: That sounds like a pretty good plan, but how would you feel about setting some more concrete times or distances for yourself?

CAROLINE: I guess that sounds like a good idea.

HELPER: Can you guess how long you would walk tomorrow?

CAROLINE: Oh, probably about an hour.

HELPER: That sounds like a pretty long walk. How do you think you would feel afterwards?

CAROLINE: I think I would feel better, but pretty tired. I haven't walked that long for at least the last 6 months.

HELPER: I'm wondering if it would make more sense to start out a little shorter and build up to an hour?

CAROLINE: Well if I only walked 30 minutes tomorrow, I would probably have more energy to walk other days this week.

HELPER: I'm really glad you said that! How many days this week do you think you could walk?

CAROLINE: I think every other day would be nice.

HELPER: Okay, that sounds like a great plan, but it also seems like a really big change to make in the course of a week. I'm wondering if you would be willing to commit to fewer days this week so you can build up to 4 days a week.

CAROLINE: Yeah, that probably makes more sense. In the past I've tried to start out doing a lot in the beginning and I get pretty tired of it soon.

HELPER: I think that's true for a lot of people Caroline. You're really excited about being more active and want to start immediately, but by taking on so much at once, you may get burned out quickly. Do you think you could walk 2 days this week and build up to 4 over the course of the next month?

CAROLINE: So does that mean I'll walk 2 days this week, 3 days next week, and four the following?

HELPER: Great question! I was actually thinking that maybe you could add 1 day per week every 2 weeks. So at the end of 4 weeks you would start walking 4 days per week. How does that plan sound to you Caroline?

CAROLINE: I think that makes sense. Hopefully this plan will keep me from getting burned out.

HELPER: I think it will help with that and also help you develop a routine instead of just feeling like you're adding a lot to your busy schedule. Also, if you really feel like you should be doing more, then feel free to go for it. Just remember how important it is to you to meet your weekly walking goals!

In this example, the helper assists the client in making her goal more concrete and realistic. It is much easier to feel a sense of accomplishment with a concrete goal in mind. Had the client walked until she was tired, she may have felt badly for not having as much stamina as she used to. By setting the goal of walking 30 min two times in the next week, the client knows exactly when she has accomplished her goal and might enhance her confidence in maintaining physical activity. Similarly, if successful in meeting her goals, the client can consider incrementally increasing her exercise goals. For example, Caroline may wish to walk 40 min four times a week, or increase her pace at 30 min. The helper also placed more emphasis on establishing a weekly walking schedule than on distance or length of time walking. This is because adherence rates in maintaining physical activity should increase as it becomes part of an established schedule. Now that a concrete goal (walking 30 min 2 days per week for the next 2 weeks, walking 30 min 3 days per week for the next 2 weeks, and walking 30 min 4 days per week for the last 2 weeks) has been established, the helper works to further schedule and structure the activity to increase the likelihood that it will be accomplished.

Implementing Behavioral Plans

BA uses scheduling structured activities to increase the likelihood that clients will follow through and translate intention into action. Scheduling refers to the exact description, frequency, and time of activities, while structuring refers to breaking down activities into smaller components.

Scheduling Activities

As mentioned above, clients will have a better chance of following through with exercise goals if their goals are concrete and specific. Once concrete, specific goals have been agreed upon, helpers can work with clients to schedule physical activities. Incomplete scheduling fails to specify times and locations for engaging in an activity and leaves room for ambiguity; thorough scheduling, on the other hand, identifies a specific time and place for an activity to occur. For instance, "So we're agreed. You are going to walk around your block for 20 min on Thursday morning before you go to work" is preferred over "So we're agreed you're going to walk for 20 min sometime this week." When activities are scheduled appropriately, there is no doubt as to when and where they should occur.

With predictable regularity, some clients will hesitate to commit to a specific time and place for engaging in physical activity. This is a normal and expectable response and is easier to work with when considered as resistance to change. When clients are noncommittal, helpers can implement skills from MI to remind clients of their reasons for increasing physical activity. Rolling with resistance, providing empathy and identifying discrepancies can aid the helper in scheduling regular activity. For example, a client may have to the goal of walking 4 days a week after work but can only go 3 days because their favorite TV program is on one of these days. The helper can gently empathize with the client, remain straightforward, and work to troubleshoot the situation. The helper may ask if the program can be recorded or if the client can walk before the program and reward themselves by watching it afterwards. The helper may also remind the client of their values related to increasing physical activity. Telling the clients that they need to give up something they enjoy will likely be ineffective and may also damage the therapeutic relationship. The helper may also benefit from assisting the client in setting up environmental and social contingencies to increase the likelihood that the client will follow through with their goals.

Ambiguity in scheduling may also reflect unrealistic goals, the client's personality style, or a less than optimal therapeutic relationship. If helpers believe that clients' goals are unrealistic, then helpers should work to break goals down into smaller pieces. For example, a client may have the goal of jogging 5 miles in 1 day, though they have not jogged in a year. The helper can ask how the client would feel about jogging 5 miles over the course of a week instead of in 1 day. Clients may possess personality styles that are not conducive to behavioral activation or do not mesh well with helpers' personalities. In these situations, helpers may benefit from being more empathic and as straightforward as possible.

Structuring

Structuring an activity refers to the process of breaking down an activity into smaller steps. The goal is to identify the core components, divide them into smaller steps, sequence each step, anticipate and troubleshoot potential obstacles, and introduce contingencies. To illustrate the process of activity structuring let us consider the example of a client, Jim, who wishes to join a recreational softball team. He and his helper determined that ensuring Jim had the proper equipment and finding a softball team to join were the primary components. They broke these components into smaller steps and sequenced them accordingly. First, Jim agreed to dig up an old mitt and buy a new pair of athletic shoes. Then, they brainstormed possible leads for joining a team. Jim knew a friend who played but was not sure if they needed extra players. The helper also suggested to look at classified ads in newspapers and on the internet for teams recruiting new players and to contact the community recreation offices. After finding a new team, Jim got cold feet and became anxious for not having played softball in sometime. The helper assisted Jim in developing a plan to practice before the first game whereby he made two visits to a local batting cage and asked a friend to play catch in a park. Finally, Jim embedded contingencies in his plan by contracting to call his helper if he deviated from his plan and to reward himself for each successfully completed step.

To conclude this discussion of activity scheduling and structuring, we highlight the importance of reviewing clients' experience with physical activity goals. As mentioned earlier, reviewing clients' activity goals reinforces clients to engage in future activities and gives helpers opportunities to assess what clients have learned, highlight improvements, and address barriers. When working with depressed clients on initial activation assignments, it is certain that not all clients will complete all components of every activity goal. Thus, it is essential for helpers to be comfortable addressing incomplete activity goals with a nonjudgmental, matter-of-fact attitude. Similarly, helpers will benefit from viewing partially completed activity goals as progress in the right direction and not as a failure or as a completed goal. Many helpers will find that much of BA involves troubleshooting problems with activity goals and that this process often sheds light on clients' patterns of avoidance or ambivalence about change. The task of the helper is to continually assign, review, troubleshoot, and reassign activities. It is important for helpers to maintain their own hope and optimism about change during this process and when clients have continual problems with completing activity goals, helpers are encouraged to consult with colleagues. Through such consultation, helpers may be aided in identifying specific barriers that can be targeted and develop ways to grade the tasks more effectively. Adopting this problem solving stance helps to counteract hopelessness about change, avoidance of reviewing activity goals, or adopting critical attitudes toward clients' challenges in completing activity goals.

In the next example, we consider David, a recovering alcoholic who plans to take up cycling to combat urges to drink.

HELPER: So David, I'm under the impression that you want to take up cycling.

DAVID: Yes I do. I have friends that are cyclists and I think it can help keep me out of the bars.

HELPER: Great idea! Do you have much experience cycling?

DAVID: Well I know how to ride a bike if that's what you mean. Also, one of my friends has an old road bike he said I could use if it helps me stay away from drinking.

HELPER: Those two things sound like a great start!
(Helper and client decide on the goal to ride 20 miles over the course of a week)

HELPER: How many miles do you think you can comfortably ride in 1 day David?

DAVID: I think 5 miles should be pretty easy. I'm in as good of shape as my friends and I know they ride further than that.

HELPER: That sounds like a great start! So if you think you can do 5 miles easily, how many days would you want to ride?

DAVID: Three, I guess. I can ride 5 miles 2 days and 10 miles 1 day.

HELPER: That sounds like a great plan. What days do you think you would want to go?

DAVID: The guys I've been talking about ride after work on Monday, Wednesday
            and Friday so maybe I could just go with them.
HELPER: Wow, sounds like you've already got this figured out! What days do you
            want to ride 5 miles and what day can you ride 10?
DAVID: Maybe I'll do 5 Monday and Wednesday and 10 on Friday when I have
            a little more time.
HELPER: Do your friends bring all of their cycling equipment with them to
            work?
DAVID: Yeah, they get ready to ride as soon as we get off work. They're usually
            on their bikes by 5:15.
HELPER: Do you have all the equipment you need and room in your car for
            everything?
DAVID: Yeah I do, everything I need is actually in my car now because I just
            picked up the bike and some equipment up from my friend's house last
            night.
HELPER: Oh okay, so are you planning on just leaving it there so you're always
            ready?
DAVID: Yeah, that's probably the best plan.
HELPER: I really like your plan David, but am wondering how it's going to keep
            you from drinking.
DAVID: Well I've only really ever had problems with drinking when I go straight
            to the bar for a 'few' drinks after work. I think if I can ride at the same
            time I'm used to drinking then that will help.
HELPER: I agree, it sounds like riding immediately after work is your best bet. We
            definitely want to interrupt those old patterns and replace them with
            healthy ones. I think you have great goals for this week, and now I am
            wondering how confident you are in accomplishing them.
DAVID: Hmmm, around 70% confident. Basically, I'll do it as long as I'm not
            too sore.

(The helper attends to David's ambivalence later.)

The helper started by structuring the client's goal of riding 20 miles into
smaller more reasonable goals. The helper also made sure the client has the necessary equipment and experience to take part in the activity. Next, the helper
worked on scheduling the activity so the client knows exactly when and where
he is going. In this case, the client has the benefit of joining friends who already
have an established routine. Opportunities like this should not be overlooked!
Another important feature of this scenario is that the helper worked to ensure
that cycling would interrupt David's drinking behavior. By scheduling his riding
time when he would be at the bars, David is giving himself the best chance at
overcoming his problematic alcohol use. After thorough structuring and scheduling, the client is ready to begin his goal of replacing drinking with a healthy
alternative.

Maintenance and Relapse Prevention

Self-Monitoring

Self-monitoring, the primary assessment tool used in BA, involves recording daily activities and assigning a corresponding mood rating. In the context of treating depression, information gathered from self-monitoring helps guide treatment by providing examples of pleasurable activities that can be increased and examples of activities that maintain depression that can be decreased (i.e., avoidance behaviors and ruminative thinking). Self-monitoring also permits clients and helpers to track progress with homework assignments, identify obstacles, and assess modifications to future assignments.

Self-monitoring does not end with the simple prescription to record and rate daily activities. Rather, the payoff depends on skillful reviews of monitoring assignments. Not only does a careful review reinforce clients' effort to self-monitor, it is often the only way to glean a nuanced understanding of the lives clients lead outside of treatment. By reviewing clients' activity, helpers may assist clients in understanding the relationship between physical activity and targeted outcomes.

The following example portrays an interaction between Caroline and her helper, who have been working together to increase Caroline's motivation and to set physical activity goals.

HELPER: Caroline, I want to show you an Activity Chart. I use this with all my clients to get a sense of how people's mood can impact their behavior and vice-versa. See here, there is a box for each hour of the day. You track in each box what you did and how you felt during that activity.

CAROLINE: Okay, that seems straightforward. But how do I track how I felt? Do I write something in there?

HELPER: Good question. You certainly can write in descriptions of how you felt. As we get started with the monitoring you can record a rating for your mood more globally. For instance, I often encourage people to rate their mood on a scale from 0 to 10 where 0 means your best mood ever and 10 means your worst mood ever. As you get more practice you can start to identify more specific emotions.

CAROLINE: That makes sense, but do I really have to fill this out for every hour of every day? That seems like a lot of work.

HELPER: Well, the more information we have the better, but to begin with I would just like you to start tracking some of your week—maybe 2 days during the week and 1 weekend day, but definitely on days you are exercising. Does that sound manageable?

By monitoring the client's mood throughout the day, and before and after engaging in physical activity, helpers and clients can get a clearer picture of how physical activity affects the client's mood. It will be crucial for helpers to remember that many, especially those who are sedentary, might not experience positive mood initially after exercising. In these situations it can be helpful to remind clients that they are acting in accordance with their goals and to ask how this affects their mood. Monitoring is also relevant outside the context of treating depression because people who feel better after engaging in an activity will be more likely to engage in it again. Clients can also reflect on how they feel about obtaining their goals, being active with others, or how they would have felt if they had not engaged in physical activity. These can be logged on the same monitoring sheet and help strengthen confidence and highlight the reward connection. Clients may also wish to monitor feelings such as cravings for alcohol or other substances or record objective data such as weight loss, heart rate, or steps taken.

Anticipating and Overcoming Obstacles

Clients will inevitably be faced with obstacles to maintaining regular physical activity. Common obstacles include weather, illness, injury, stress, and vacations or time away from home. While impossible to eliminate obstacles, helpers can work to limit the impact of obstacles on clients. The most important strategy when dealing with obstacles, especially ones that have already interfered with activity, is to not blame clients for not engaging in an activity. In these situations, helpers can adopt an empathic stance to let clients know that obstacles are expected and can be overcome. This is a normal part of the human experience and physical activity is not an exception. An insightful helper, however, can prepare for many obstacles and provide empathy when they are encountered. Overcoming obstacles is different than overcoming relapse. Obstacles are temporary setbacks while relapse involves falling back into old behavioral patterns. If helpers can assist clients in overcoming obstacles then they may be able to prevent relapse. For example, take the case of David explored above. David is confident that he can ride his road bike 3 days in the upcoming week despite his limited cycling experience.

HELPER: I'm by no means an expert in cycling, but am wondering if you could potentially feel very sore after your first day of cycling.

DAVID: That's an interesting point… I hadn't really thought about that. I do remember feeling really sore after riding in the past though.

HELPER: I'm wondering if there's anything else you could on the days you are planning to ride your bike, if in fact, you are too sore.

DAVID: I guess I could go for a jog or do some stretching.

HELPER: I think those are both really good ideas, but I'm worried jogging may
           prove to be overwhelming, if in fact, you are very sore.
DAVID: Well jogging would probably help me stretch as well as get some car-
           diovascular activity.
HELPER: I think you're right, but could also see how it may hurt just as much to
           jog as to ride your bike.
DAVID: That's definitely a possibility. Maybe I could just go for a walk instead.
HELPER: I think that's a much safer backup plan David! So if you're too sore to
           ride Wednesday or Friday you are going to go for a walk instead?
DAVID: Yeah, I can do that.

In the previous scenario, the helper identified a potential obstacle to David's physical activity goals. The helper also allowed David to come up with alternative activities and decide which one was the best fit for him. It will be important for the helper to schedule and structure the alternative activity, walking, just like they did with cycling so the client has a reasonable and achievable goal if they are unable to engage in their first chosen activity.

Plans for and Prevents Relapse

Anticipating obstacles is the first step to relapse prevention, but what can helpers do when clients who started an exercise program have completely stopped exercising? Similar to dealing with relapse in treating substance use, helpers must assist clients in viewing relapse as a temporary setback and not a failure. Earlier in the chapter we discussed how partial completion of a goal is still progress in the right direction. Relapse is just a step in the opposite direction and is not indicative of failure. Almost all forms of significant behavior change will involve periods of relapse and helpers will inevitably face this experience. Helpers can relate this perspective to their clients by handling relapse in an empathic straightforward manner and as a "normal" process in behavioral change. Helpers can work to motivate clients using skills learned in MI, set new goals, and schedule and structure the new activities. By repeating the initial process, clients learn how to recover from relapse and may become more self-sufficient in dealing with relapse. In the following example, the helper is working with Caroline to plan for and prevent relapse.

HELPER: Caroline, how long are you usually able to maintain your walking
           schedule on average?
CAROLINE: I think that 3 months is pretty average for me.
HELPER: What usually comes up after 3 months that makes it difficult to
           continue?

CAROLINE: Well sometimes a week of bad weather will set me back and I just stop going. Other times, my walking partner has got sick so I stopped going.

HELPER: I'm wondering what you could do to keep from getting sidetracked in the future. It seems like it may be really important to walk with other people.

CAROLINE: Maybe I could walk with more than one person so that if one person can't go then there are still others to walk with.

HELPER: It sounds like starting a walking club of sorts may really help hold everyone more accountable.

CAROLINE: I've overheard some of the other ladies in the office talking about going walking like I do with my friend. I could just invite them to come with us.

HELPER: Great idea Caroline! I'm still concerned about the weather holding your group up. Do you have any thoughts on another place you could walk or something else you could do?

CAROLINE: Hmmm, I guess we could go to an aerobics class or something, but that gets kind of expensive. I've heard of people going for walks in the mall though. That would be tough for me to do on my own, but I think if I were with friends it could actually be kind of fun.

HELPER: Alright, so it sounds like we have two plans. The first is to ask the other ladies at work if they would like to walk with you and your friend. The other is to plan on walking at the mall if the weather is too bad.

In this example, the helper identified obstacles that have kept the client from exercising regularly in the past. The helper then assisted the client in deciding the best way to overcome these obstacles, which could help prevent relapse. If the client has already relapsed, the helper can take the same action: Identify the obstacle and plan around it. Preventing and overcoming relapse is a difficult, but necessary, step in maintaining regular physical activity.

Brief-Supportive Follow-Up Contact

Providing supportive follow-up contact to clients is another important strategy in maintaining physical activity. Helpers may only have time to talk on the phone or over email, but limited contact provides far superior support than no contact. Ideally, clients would be able to talk to their helpers anytime they felt like they were having problems, but this is unrealistic. When helpers do have a chance to talk to clients, they can refer back to the principles of MI and BA discussed earlier in this chapter. Primary objectives in supportive follow-up contact include the following: praising the client for their successes, remaining empathic and straightforward when the client experiences a failure, identifying and overcoming obstacles, and reminding clients of their initial motivation to increase physical activity.

Summary

The strategies discussed in this chapter are proven means to change difficult behaviors and may also be effective in increasing physical activity. Fostering intrinsic motivation is a crucial and often overlooked step; merely telling a client they *need* to exercise is insufficient. The client must understand why they need to increase their physical activity and do so for their own reasons. After helpers assess clients' goals and capabilities, and clients are adequately motivated to realize them, they can use strategies from BA, such as setting physical activity goals and scheduling and structuring activities, to help clients increase physical activity. Struggles in following through with exercise plans may indicate that clients are not sufficiently motivated or that physical activity goals are not adequately structured. Intentional use of the strategies described in the implementing behavioral plans section may help clients succeed in sticking to and completing their physical activity goals. Planning for and preventing relapse will help keep clients on track despite obstacles they will encounter.

Increasing physical activity is an evolving field of behavior change. Helpers can stay on the lookout for new research concerning effective strategies to implement physical activity in the prevention and treatment of different disorders. Implementing individual-level behavioral change strategies is difficult. If it were easy, more people would be physically active and would not suffer from disorders caused or exacerbated by physical inactivity; however, increasing physical activity at an individual level is possible and necessary for many. As in the example with Caroline, incorporating social and environmental factors, such as starting a walking club at work or walking in the mall during bad weather, may be more effective and reach a wider audience than individual strategies.

The strategies described in this chapter may be applied to other areas of behavioral change and treatment providers can keep these strategies in mind when promoting other behaviors. In fact, the theories of behavior change described in this chapter apply to any area of behavior change and may be particularly helpful in changing behaviors associated with substance use and healthy eating behaviors. Finally, the field of behavior change would benefit greatly from large scale randomized controlled trials that can isolate the mechanisms of behavioral change responsible for increasing and maintaining regular physical activity. The strategies outlined in this chapter have been effectively used by many when establishing behavior change. Helpers can use these strategies to assist clients in increasing physical activity and leading healthier, more enjoyable lives.

Activity Chart

Instructions: Record your activity for each hour of the day (what were you doing, with whom, where, etc.). Record a mood rating associated with each activity. Mood is rated between 0 and 10, with "0" indicating "best mood ever" and "10" indicating "worst mood ever." Aim to record entries on your activity chart at least every 3–4 h each day.

	Monday	Tuesday	Wednesday	Thursday	Friday	Saturday	Sunday
7 a.m.							
8 a.m.							
9 a.m.							
10 a.m.							
11 a.m.							
12 p.m.							
1 p.m.							
2 p.m.							
3 p.m.							
4 p.m.							
5 p.m.							
6 p.m.							
7 p.m.							
8 p.m.							
9 p.m.							
10 p.m.							
11 p.m.							
12 a.m.							
1 a.m. –7 a.m.							

Adapted from: Dimidjian, S., Martell, C. R., Addis, M. E., Herman-Dunn, R. (2008). Behavioral activation for depression. In D. Barlow (Ed.) *Clinical handbook of psychological disorders: A step-by-step treatment manual* (4th ed., pp. 328–364). New York, NY: Guilford

References

Bandura, A. (1986). *Social foundations of thought and action: A social cognitive theory.* Englewood Cliffs, NJ: Prentice-Hall.

Behrman, A. (2006). Facilitating behavioral change in voice therapy: The relevance of motivational interviewing. *American Journal of Speech-Language Pathology, 15*(3), 215–225.

Bennett, J. A., Lyons, K. S., Winters-Stone, K., Nail, L. M., & Scherer, J. (2007). Motivational interviewing to increase physical activity in long-term cancer survivors—A randomized controlled trial. *Nursing Research, 56*(1), 18–27.

Brodie, D. A., & Inoue, A. (2005). Motivational interviewing to promote physical activity for people with chronic heart failure. *Journal of Advanced Nursing, 50*(5), 518–527.

Butterworth, S., Linden, A., McClay, W., & Leo, M. C. (2006). Effect of motivational interviewing-based health coaching on employees' physical and mental health status. *Journal of Occupational Health Psychology, 11*(4), 358–365.

Deci, E. L., & Ryan, R. M. (1985). *Intrinsic motivation and self-determination in human behavior*. New York: Plenum.

Dimidjian, S., Hollon, S. D., Dobson, K. S., Schmaling, K. B., Kohlenberg, R. J., Addis, M. E., et al. (2006). Randomized trial of behavioral activation, cognitive therapy, and antidepressant medication in the acute treatment of adults with major depression. *Journal of Consulting and Clinical Psychology, 74*(4), 658–670.

Dimidjian, S., Martell, C. R., Addis, M. E., & Herman-Dunn, R. (2008). Behavioral activation for depression. In D. Barlow (Ed.), *Clinical handbook of psychological disorders: A step-by-step treatment manual* (4th ed., pp. 328–364). New York, NY: Guilford.

Dishman, R. K. (1988). *Exercise adherence: Its impact on public health*. Champaign, IL: Human Kinetics Books.

Dunn, A. L., Trivedi, M. H., Kampert, J. B., Clark, C. G., & Chambliss, H. O. (2005). Exercise treatment for depression—Efficacy and dose response. *American Journal of Preventive Medicine, 28*(1), 1–8.

Elder, J. P., Lytle, L., Sallis, J. F., Young, D. R., Steckler, A., Simons-Morton, D., et al. (2007). A description of the social-ecological framework used in the trial of activity for adolescent girls (TAAG). *Health Education Research, 22*(2), 155–165.

Glanz, K., Rimer, B. K., & Viswanath, K. (2008). *Health behavior and health education: Theory, research and practice (Vol. 4)*. San Francisco, CA: Jossey-Bass.

Harland, J., White, M., Drinkwater, C., Chinn, D., Farr, L., & Howel, D. (1999). The Newcastle exercise project: A randomised controlled trial of methods, to promote physical activity in primary care. *British Medical Journal, 319*(7213), 828–832.

Haskell, W. L., Lee, I. M., Pate, R. R., Powell, K. E., Blair, S. N., Franklin, B. A., et al. (2007). Physical activity and public health—Updated recommendation for adults from the American college of sports medicine and the American heart association. *Circulation, 116*(9), 1081–1093.

Hillsdon, M., Thorogood, M., White, I., & Foster, C. (2002). Advising people to take more exercise is ineffective: A randomized controlled trial of physical activity promotion in primary care. *International Journal of Epidemiology, 31*(4), 808–815.

Hopko, D. R., Bell, J. L., Armento, M. E. A., Hunt, M. K., & Lejuez, C. W. (2005). Behavior therapy for depressed cancer patients in primary care. *Psychotherapy, 42*(2), 236–243.

Hopko, D. R., Sanchez, L., Hopko, S. D., Dvir, S., & Lejuez, C. W. (2003). Behavioral activation and the prevention of suicidal behaviors in patients with borderline personality disorder. *Journal of Personality Disorders, 17*(5), 460–478.

Jacobson, N. S., Martell, C. R., & Dimidjian, S. (2001). Behavioral activation treatment for depression: Returning to contextual roots. *Clinical Psychology: Science and Practice, 8*(3), 255–270.

Jakupcak, M., Roberts, L. J., Martell, C., Mulick, P., Michael, S., Reed, R., et al. (2006). A pilot study of behavioral activation for veterans with posttraumatic stress disorder. *Journal of Traumatic Stress, 19*(3), 387–391.

Marshall, S. J., & Biddle, S. J. H. (2001). The transtheoretical model of behavior change: A meta-analysis of applications to physical activity and exercise. *Annals of Behavioral Medicine, 23*(4), 229–246.

McMurran, M. (2009). Motivational interviewing with offenders: A systematic review. *Legal and Criminological Psychology, 14*(1), 83–100.

Miller, W. R., & Rollnick, S. (1991). *Motivational interviewing: Preparing people to change addictive behavior*. New York, NY: Guilford.

Pagoto, S., Bodenlos, J. S., Schneider, K. L., Olendzki, B., & Spates, C. R. (2008). Initial investigation of behavioral activation therapy for co-morbid major depressive disorder and obesity. *Psychotherapy, 45*(3), 410–415.

Physical Activity Guidelines Advisory Committee. (2008). *Physical activity guidelines advisory committee report, 2008*. Washington, DC: U.S. Department of Health and Human Services.

Prochaska, J. O., & Diclemente, C. C. (1983). Stages and processes of self-change of smoking—
    Toward an integrative model of change. *Journal of Consulting and Clinical Psychology, 51*(3),
    390–395.
Prochaska, J. O., Diclemente, C. C., & Norcross, J. C. (1992). In search of how people change—
    Applications to addictive behaviors. *American Psychologist, 47*(9), 1102–1114.
Rollnick, S., Miller, W. R., & Butler, C. C. (2008). *Motivational interviewing in health care.* New
    York: Guilford.
Ryan, R. M., & Deci, E. L. (2000). Self-determination theory and the facilitation of intrinsic motivation,
    social development, and well-being. *American Psychologist, 55*(1), 68–78.

Chapter 12
The Mandate for Movement: Schools as Agents of Change

John J. Ratey and Jacob Sattelmair

Introduction

We present a compelling evolutionary and scientific rationale for why movement (physical activity) must be viewed as essential in promoting students' physical and mental health, learning, and education. Because the human genome has encoded evolutionarily mandated cycling between periods of activity and rest, healthy gene expression and physiological function depend on regular movement. Yet our current culture, marked largely by sedentarism, has largely failed to heed the host of evidence that the mind and body require regular physical activity to function optimally. This disconcerting development has caused evolutionary cycles to stall, leading to metabolic derangement, epidemic chronic disease, and insidious patterns of mental disorders and addiction. Catalyzing change to combat this trend requires a global front in which every individual, community, and organization has a role. Schools, in particular, present a uniquely advantageous opportunity to acculturate future generations with the knowledge, skills, and behaviors needed for a lifetime of healthy activity.

Schools therefore have an imperative to change. Regular physical activity represents a critical component to improving physical fitness and preventing juvenile obesity, early-onset diabetes, and the like. Physical activity also offers equally compelling benefits to the brain, attention and focus, mood and self-efficacy, and thus to learning and memory. Movement is essential not just to the health of students but to the very goal of schools: *educating students*. Physical education (PE) in schools can be a big part of the solution, but historically PE has failed to engage students in

J.J. Ratey (✉)
Harvard Medical School, 328 Broadway, Cambridge, MA 02139, USA
e-mail: john_ratey@hms.harvard.edu

J. Sattelmair
Department of Epidemiology, Harvard School of Public Health,
677 Huntington Avenue, Boston, MA 02115, USA

A.L. Meyer and T.P. Gullotta (eds.), *Physical Activity Across the Lifespan*,
Issues in Children's and Families' Lives 12, DOI 10.1007/978-1-4614-3606-5_12,
© Springer Science+Business Media New York 2012

sufficient levels of activity to provide tangible benefits. A new model of PE has emerged that purposes to equip every student with the knowledge, skills, and behavioral patterns needed to pursue lifelong fitness and health, built on a foundation that stresses the importance of aerobic exercise and the pursuit of individual fitness goals. Moving well beyond weekly gym class, this new wave PE permeates the school culture and its surrounding communities. The desired result creates "moving schools" wherein movement and learning go hand-in-hand, encouraging student physical activity throughout the (school) day.

Achieving moving schools requires a dramatic ideological shift wherein teachers, administrators, students, parents, policy makers, and communities embrace a distinctly different paradigm for learning. Such a fundamental change that returns schools to a more evolutionarily sound and scientifically validated mode of educating that embraces movement often requires champions to advocate, educate, and inspire their communities to transcend the status quo. Numerous opportunities abound throughout the school day to engage students in physical activity; though, the logistical requirements to achieve this objective will differ for every school. Regardless of constraints on time, money, and other resources, committed schools find a way. Documented examples of successful transitions from sedentary schools to moving schools highlight the challenges and opportunities involved, provide evidence of dramatic benefits, and offer a road map to success.

The Evolutionary Mandate for Movement

Forces of natural selection, survival of the fittest, and adaptation have honed the human species throughout its evolutionary history. Achieving optimal physical and mental health and functioning thus requires working within an evolutionary mandate borne out of a fundamental understanding of human genome selection.

Hunter-Gatherers on the Move

An estimated 95 % of human biology and many human behaviors were naturally selected during the late Paleolithic era, when humans lived as hunter-gatherers, and the human genome has remained largely unchanged for the past 10,000 years. During this time humans engaged in daily physical activity such as foraging and hunting that was essential for existence and for procurement of food. Men typically hunted between 1 and 4 nonconsecutive days per week, and women gathered food every 2–3 days (Cordain, Gotshall, Eaton, & Eaton, 1998; Chakravarthy et al., 2004).

During this period of regular labor and physical movement, humans walked or ran an estimated 5–14 miles per day on average, alleviating any concern about exercising or "working out." Humans lived essentially in a constant "cross-training" mode; lifting, moving objects, stretching, and when relaxing, engaged in furious celebratory dances two to three nights per week. Skeletal remains show evidence of habitual physical activity and greater muscle mass and muscle strength than post-agricultural societies (Cordain, Gotshall, & Eaton, 1997).

Evolutionary Cycling and Thrifty Genes

Characterized by cycles of peak physical effort with alternate periods of rest, late Paleolithic existence corresponded to natural cycles between feast and famine. Inextricably linked to survival, physical activity and food procurement under these cycles of "physical activity/rest" and "feast/famine" together influenced gene selection (Chakravarthy & Booth, 2004). Some researchers believe that *thrifty genes* evolved to support the aforementioned cycles and endowed Paleolithic humans with the selective advantages of improved physical endurance and resilience during famine (Neel, 1962; Chakravarthy et al., 2004). Thrifty genes support oscillating metabolic pathways that include cycles of glycogen and triglyceride storage and oxidation essential in regulating insulin/sensitivity and metabolic regulatory proteins. Thus, the human "natural" or homeostatic metabolic state has evolved to rely on constant cycling of feast/famine and physical activity/rest (Chakravarthy et al., 2004).

Stalling Cycles and Metabolic Derangement

With the level of physical activity required for healthy gene expression and metabolic function contingent on the environmental-selective pressures of the late Paleolithic era, failing to achieve this threshold of physical activity now results in pathological gene expression, physiological dysfunction, and predisposes individuals over time to chronic health conditions such as type 2 diabetes, heart disease, and cancer. Over the past century, industrialized societies have advanced food production to such a degree that improved transportation and storage methods make food available 24 h a day and the average individual need only exert a minimal amount of physical work to obtain sustenance. As a result of the removal of periods of both famine and physical activity, feast/famine and physical activity/rest cycles have stalled in feast and rest. Consequently, cycling metabolic genes programmed to expect regular physical activity and famine have also stalled, resulting in metabolic malfunction or derangement—underlying the cellular and molecular mechanisms of many chronic diseases (Chakravarthy et al., 2004).

Because humans have an intrinsic biologic requirement for a threshold of physical activity, a sedentary lifestyle presents a disruption to the homeostatic mechanisms governing the proper metabolic cycling required to maintain health. Disrupting the balance of energy input and utilization in this way leads to chronic metabolic dysregulation that manifests as "syndromes of failed genetic homeostasis" such as metabolic syndrome (abdominal adiposity, high triglyceride, low HDL, atherosclerosis, hypertension, insulin resistance) and over 30 other chronic health conditions that affect hundreds of millions of Americans (Beaudet, Scriver, Sly, & Valle, 1995; Neel, 1999).

Chronic Inactivity and Chronic Disease

The Paleolithic mandate for robust and regular physical activity (with intermittent periods of rest) has been replaced with physical activity guidelines that call for 30 min a day of moderate-intensity physical activity (60 min for children and adolescents), a greatly attenuated level of activity nonetheless achieved by less than half of the US population (Centers for Disease Control and Prevention, 2007). The devastating ramifications of this sudden and dramatic decline in activity have appeared concurrent with similarly drastic deviations in dietary intake. For instance, the prevalence of type 2 diabetes (indicative of metabolic derangement and associated with numerous other chronic diseases) represents just 1 % or less in present-day hunter-gatherer societies (Diamond, 2003), whereas the CDC estimates that 33 % of those born in the US in the year 2000 will develop diabetes in their lifetime (CDC, 2009).

Because genes have not changed in the past 40 years (Diamond, 2003), the entirety of the epidemic rise in metabolic disorders and resultant chronic disease is due to the environmental modulation of existing genes (Chakravarthy et al., 2004). Though numerous environmental factors exert influence, physical activity deficiency plays a key role. Just 3 days of continuous bed rest (Lipman et al., 1972) places healthy humans into pre-diabetic conditions (decreased oral glucose tolerance with increased fasting plasma glucose and insulin concentration) and similar conditions ensue within only 10 days when trained individuals stop exercising (Heath et al., 1983). The dramatic impact of inactivity on the development of insulin resistance, a primary indicator of metabolic derangement, clearly demonstrates the principle that humans have a mandate to move regularly to realize optimal health and functioning.

Movement and Nutrition: In Perspective

Because of the mismatch between our genetically controlled biology and our current lifestyle (sedentary individuals with abundant access to food), the thrifty phenotype has now become disadvantageous. These individuals store excess energy as fat in anticipation of a famine that does not come. During prolonged states of continuous feeding with physical activity perpetually absent (now the norm in modern society), downregulation of the activity phenotype allows for the manifestation of metabolic dysfunctions that underlie chronic degenerative disorders that contribute to 75 % of deaths in the US (Booth, Chakravarthy, Gordon, & Spangenburg, 2002; Eaton, Konner, & Shostak, 1988; 2002).

Persuading a large proportion of the population to undertake significant caloric restriction has proven extremely difficult; yet even if hypothetically possible, from a public health perspective, excess caloric intake alone does not fully account for the current epidemic of metabolic disorders (Chakravarthy et al., 2004). Even severe caloric restriction concurrent with physical inactivity contributes to the induction of insulin resistance (Koffler & Kisch, 1996), indicating that dietary modulation alone is insufficient to break the stall in the cycling of metabolic processes (Pilegaard, Saltin, & Neufer, 2003) that lead to chronic diseases.

Compartmentalizing human behavior and physiology has lead to failures in our understanding of obesity and related metabolic disorders, hindering our success in addressing these afflictions. Conditional on energy expenditure as well as energy intake, energy balance involves basal metabolic rate and physical activity along with caloric consumption. Regular physical activity increases lean muscle mass and induces biochemical and hormonal changes that increase basal metabolic rate as well as activity-based expenditure. Moreover, metabolic activity affects energy consumed very differently contingent on the context of physical activity patterns; in the presence of increased physical activity, a shift from energy storage to immediate utilization leads to sustained metabolic homeostasis (De Vany, 2009). Dysfunctional gene expression and progression toward chronic disease (induced by an imbalance between expenditure and intake), however, can be prevented or delayed by re-introducing genes to habitual physical activity, thereby moving them away from a threshold at which symptoms of overt clinical disorders occur (Chakravarthy et al., 2004).

Frank Hu, Associate Professor of Nutrition and Epidemiology at the Harvard School of Public Health, who has spent years studying numerous nutritional and lifestyle health factors, has the following to say about exercise:

> Good nutrition is essential for health, but once promising discoveries have turned out not to be a magic health pill...the single thing that comes close to a magic bullet in terms of its strong and universal benefits is exercise...exercise can change virtually every tissue in the body, but because it works by many different pathways, metabolic, hormonal, neurological and mechanical, understanding it is not always easy—and it is often overlooked (Shaw, 2004).

Culture of Sedentarism

The problem extends beyond the lack of physical activity, as research reveals the independent hazards of excessive sitting. The extent of our sedentarism has become so extreme and rampant as to require the designation of a new term, Sedentary Death Syndrome (SeDS), to categorize the emerging array of sedentary-lifestyle-mediated disorders that ultimately result in increased mortality. SeDS is characterized by weak skeletal muscles, low bone density, hyperglycemia, glucosuria, low serum, HDL, obesity, low physical endurance, and resting tachycardia (Booth & Chakravarthy, 2002).

"There is no longer any need for physical activity for transportation, food seeking, or daily survival," says Joann Manson, M.D., Chief of Preventative Medicine at Brigham and Women's Hospital in Boston. Dr. Manson continues:

> Labor saving devices are everywhere, one can get through the day expending virtually no energy, doing virtually no physical activity, and they do. America loves to think of itself as

youthful nation focused on fitness, but in reality, we are inactive, unfit and increasingly overweight, as seventy-five percent of population fails to meet even minimum government recommendations (Shaw, 2004).

The abuse of, and addiction to "screen time" compounds the dramatic decline in physical activity (Ratey et al., 2008). American adults spend over 8 h a day, on average, in front of a screen (Council for Research Excellence, 2009), and American youth spend over seven and a half hours a day consuming media (Rideout, Foehrm, & Roberts, 2010). Excessive time spent watching television, using the computer, or playing video games exacerbates the already deleterious inactive lifestyle, independently leading to the viral spread of chronic diseases. The amount of time people spend sitting directly relates to blood pressure, cholesterol, and glucose levels, and increases the risk (by up to double) of obesity, type 2 diabetes, heart disease, and cancer, even when adjusting for time spent exercising (Owen, Bauman, & Brown, 2009).

The effects of sitting on the fat-metabolizing enzyme called lipase sheds light on the metabolic stalling that results from sedentarism. Whereas sitting shuts down the circulation of lipase, standing engages muscle and promotes the distribution of lipase, which prompts the body to process fat and cholesterol, independent of the amount of time spent exercising. Standing also metabolizes blood glucose, thus discouraging the development of diabetes. An "insidious hazard" and a main contributor to the fact that 47 million adults in the US have metabolic syndrome (Hamilton, Hamilton, & Zderic, 2007), "chair time" keeps the body's fat burning turned off. Sitting, independent of physical activity, can cause genetic and metabolic dysfunction that leads to increased risk of chronic disease. Leading researchers advocate that, "In the future, the focus in clinical practice and guidelines should not only be to promote and prescribe exercise, but also to encourage people to maintain their intermittent levels of daily activities" [that involve movement] (Bak, Hellenius, & Ekblom, 2010).

Among children, a relationship has been observed between media-related sedentary behavior (namely television viewing) and obesity, concerns about weight, high blood pressure (independent of weight), increased susceptibility to the temptation of smoking, and psychological distress—a precursor to substance abuse and other addictive behaviors (Leatherdale, Wong, Manske, & Colditz, 2008; Hamer, Stamatakis, & Mishra, 2009; Martinez-Gomez, Tucker, Heelan, Welk, & Eisenmann, 2009). This psychological distress can be viewed as part of a broader trend toward a societal lack of resilience that heightens susceptibility to addiction, for taking the path of least resistance to achieve stress relief makes one prone to addictive behaviors.

Despite some misguided claims that somehow suggest exaggeration or social construction behind the epidemic of childhood obesity, the evidence is indisputable: rates of childhood obesity have tripled in the last 25 years (CDC, 2010). Obesity can have a range of negative implications from impaired social interactions to accelerated mortality: overweight and obese children/adolescents report being subjected to social stigma (Puhl & Latner, 2007), are more likely to become obese as adults, and are twice as likely to die prematurely as their thinner counterparts (Franks et al., 2010).

Stress, Adaptation, Response

Owing to the evolutionary mandate for proper cycling of activity and rest, the body and brain experience physical activity as a stress that forces myriad physiologic adaptations that prepare the organism to meet future challenges. Vital to attaining and maintaining optimal health and performance, a recurring cycle of stress (physical activity), recovery (rest), and adaptation (physiologic advancement) promotes human health and resilience. Regular physical activity favorably affects numerous physiologic systems, including musculoskeletal (increased bone and muscle mass and strength), cardiovascular (improved cardiac function, vascular elasticity and endothelial function, blood content), metabolic (glucose, fat, insulin, mitochondria), and immune (reduced inflammation and oxidative stress) (Physical Activity Guidelines Advisory Committee, 2008). Conversely, avoidance of regular movement starves systems, tissues, and cells of a crucial stimulus, leading to derangement, loss of function, and eventual death.

Evolution, Movement, and the Brain

Throughout human evolution, physical activity and thrifty genes have been closely linked with brain function and development. The ability to acquire food and efficiently transform it into a usable energy source has been a major force in the evolution of humankind. This evolutionary process soldered together cooperative molecular mechanisms underlying activity, metabolism, and cognition. Individuals who could outrun and out-plan their peers could increase their likelihood of survival and reproduction:

> Rooted in even earlier evolutionary gains…the brain of early mobile organisms may have developed in complexity, incorporating perception and prediction as learning aspects, to maximize motor operations that increased the chances for obtaining food and survival (Vaynman & Gomez-Pinilla, 2006).

Some researchers view the concept of *motricity*—the need to generate physical movements to gain and compete for energy resources for survival—as the impetus for mental activity (Vaynman & Gomez-Pinilla, 2006). The moving brain evolved into our thinking brain, so much so that according to esteemed neuroscientist Rodolfo Llinas, "That which we call thinking is the evolutionary internalization of movement" (Llinas, 2001).

Our digitalized culture has us living almost exclusively in our heads, and we have lost the connection between movement and cognition. In other words, movement is as fundamental to the development of the brain as it is to the development of the body. The primary motor cortex and pre-motor cortex are both located in the frontal lobe, one of the most advanced parts of the brain responsible for higher executive functions such as thinking and planning. The executive brain receives a convergence of inputs from other areas of the brain and uses them to plan movements, whereas the primary motor cortex then controls those movements. Therefore, the parallel handling of motor and cognitive functions in the frontal lobe helps to facilitate cognitive functions. As life and the movements required become more complex, the interconnection between movement and cognitive processes increases in strength (Ratey et al., 2008).

Physical Activity and Neurophysiology

The physiological stress presented to the brain by physical activity balanced with recovery promotes adaptation and growth, preserves brain function, and enables the brain to respond to future challenges (Mattson, Maudsley, & Martin, 2004; Mattson, 2008). Physical activity requires that skeletal muscles do work, which increases the demand for energy. Activation of anaerobic and aerobic metabolic systems converts biological energy substrates such as carbohydrate and fat into ATP, the basic unit of energy that the body uses to fuel muscle contractions. Aerobic metabolism requires increased oxygen delivery, and this demand activates cardiovascular and pulmonary systems to deliver more oxygenated blood, as well as energy substrates, to the work-ing muscle and to clear carbon dioxide and metabolic waste products. Physical activity shunts blood away from internal organs and towards areas of increased oxygen and nutrient demand (i.e., muscles), altering blood flow dynamics to the brain in the process (Nybo & Secher, 2004), and thereby instigating a series of cas-cades in the brain that fundamentally changes the brain's activity, chemical milieu, and ultimately structure and function.

Physical activity-induced dynamic changes in blood flow to the brain are accom-panied by the flow of modulatory and growth factors from working muscle (e.g. IGF-1, VEGF, FGF-2, ANP) that together trigger myriad neurological responses. Physical activity enhances brain activity (neuronal firing); modulates major neu-rotransmitter systems (including dopamine, serotonin, epinephrine, and norepi-nephrine) essential to the regulation of attention, memory, emotions, and motivations; stimulates the release of neuronal growth factors (that help neurons survive and thrive) such as brain-derived neurotrophic factor (BDNF); promotes synaptic plas-ticity and long-term potentiation (LTP) (the physiologic basis of learning and mem-ory); and stimulates the growth of new neurons (neurogenesis) in the hippocampus (the area of the brain directly responsible for learning and memory) (Hillman, Erickson, & Kramer, 2008). Over time, these processes lead to gross structural and vascular plasticity (adaptive brain modifications).

A Global Crisis of Epic Proportion

Necessary for basic survival, movement has been mandatory throughout human life history; those unable to move faced the doom of extinction, with death often merci-fully quick. In contrast, the persistent inactivity of modern society robs humans of their potential by precipitating metabolic derangements that trigger the slow spiral of physical and mental degeneration that leads to lingering disease and eventual early or protracted death.

According to former US Surgeon General, Dr. Richard Carmona, "As we look to the future and where childhood obesity will be in 20 years…it is every bit as threatening to us as is the terrorist threat we face today. It is the terrorist threat from within" (Ornish, 2008). Heralding an equally dire warning, Dr. William J. Klish, Professor of Pediatrics at Baylor College of Medicine, asserts, "children today have a shorter life expectancy than their parents for the first time in one hundred years… that is scary…scary to think about." Dr. K.M. Venkat Narayan, CDC epidemiologist, projects that, "one in every three US children born after 2000 will become diabetic unless many more people start eating less and exercising more" (CDC, 2009).

Rather than cause alarm, the pervasive presence of chronic disease and its familiar avalanche of deleterious encroachment on quality and quantity of life have left many Americans seemingly indifferent, passively accepting disease as being inevitable. Still others find themselves overwhelmed and immobilized with fear, impotent to stand against such a behemoth of affliction.

However, empirical evidence consistently demonstrates that the vast majority of many chronic diseases can be entirely prevented through lifestyle modification, with physical activity as an integral component. Thus, we must face this profound threat to Americans of all ages head on by reinstating physical activity into our daily modern lifestyle, thereby taking great strides to reverse the trends of epidemic obesity, type 2 diabetes, metabolic syndrome, heart disease, and major mood disorders.

Strategy for Change: We Must Commit to Changes, Together as a Nation, So as to Foster and Promote Our National Health and Wellness

Changing such pervasive inactivity necessitates an extreme global front and requires re-engineering every major institution to incorporate a radical new paradigm for health promotion and education. Working together we can reclaim our heritage; everyone has a role. Individuals, families, and communities need to re-orient to embrace physically active lifestyles. The medical profession needs to adjust its thinking to recognize movement as vital for human survival and alter its prescribing habits to incorporate movement as a foundational component. Educators need to fundamentally revamp their approach to education by abandoning a sedentary school day for one characterized by movement. Politicians need to put aside ego and partisan politics and focus on the fundamentals required to promote movement at multiple levels. Built environments need modification to facilitate active lifestyles. This mammoth undertaking requires a concerted campaign to aggressively pursue all possible solutions; just as no one cause accounts for all of the recent decline in physical activity, no one solution, no silver bullet, will rectify all the consequent damage.

In her "Vision for a Healthy Nation," current US Surgeon General Regina Benjamin calls on one and all to join the cause:

> Every one of us has an important role to play in the prevention and control of obesity. Mothers, fathers, teachers, business executives, child care professionals, clinicians, politicians, and government and community leaders—we must all commit to changes that promote the health and wellness of our families and communities…I am calling on all Americans to join me in a national grassroots effort to reverse this trend…The real goal is not just a number on a scale, but optimal health for all Americans at every stage of life. To achieve this goal, we must all work together to share resources, educate our citizens, and partner with business and government leaders to find creative solutions in our neighborhoods, towns, and cities from coast to coast. Together, we can become a nation committed to become healthy and fit (USDHHS, 2010).

"Healthy People 2010," released by the US Department of Health and Human Services, echoes the importance of communities joining together to change the nation:

> Over the years, it has become clear that individual health is closely linked to community health—the health of the community and environment in which individuals live, work, and play. Likewise, community health is profoundly affected by the collective beliefs, attitudes, and behaviors of everyone who lives in the community…Indeed, the underlying premise of Healthy People 2010 is that the health of the individual is almost inseparable from the health of the larger community and that the health of every community in every State and territory determines the overall health status of the Nation. That is why the vision for Healthy People 2010 is "Healthy People in Healthy Communities" (USDHHS, 2000).

Schools: Agents of Change

The following sections highlight the *unique role of schools* in promoting movement and acculturating future generations to embrace healthy lifestyles and behaviors, a key strategy through which to combat the common enemy. Schools present a uniquely advantageous opportunity/setting through which to engage children and adolescents in regular physical activity, thereby improving health and physical fitness, enabling healthy cognitive development and overall mental well-being, enhancing academic performance, and reducing the risk of early-onset chronic conditions such as childhood obesity and juvenile-onset type 2 diabetes. Furthermore, the aforementioned physical and mental health benefits will go a long way in preventing the onset of addiction and substance abuse among students.

School Policy = Health Mandate

The mandate for schools to provide leadership to address crucial social issues that serve the next generations of Americans involves a concept that is neither radical nor new. The Texas Association of School Boards describes the fundamental role of public schools in the US as:

> …the backbone of our American way of life…[to] meet the changing needs of our evolving society through a commitment that every child can succeed and become a contributing

member of it…[with the purpose] first to care for and then to educate the offspring of every segment of society (Texas Association of School Boards, 2010).

In accord with the view that the public school system's responsibility is "first to care for and then educate," the National Association of State Boards of Education (NASBE) includes the following assertions in its model policy language:

- Schools have a duty to help prevent unnecessary injury, disease, and chronic health conditions that can lead to disability or early death.
- Health and success in school are interrelated. Schools cannot achieve their primary mission of education if students and staff are not healthy and fit physically, mentally, and socially.
- The nation's leading health authorities recommend that schools take an active role in preventing disabling chronic health conditions that create misery and consume a burdensome share of the nation's resources.
- Every school district and school shall develop, adopt, and implement a comprehensive plan for a thorough, well-coordinated school health program (National Association of State Boards of Education, 2010).

More specifically, the National Association of Sport and Physical Education underscores the importance of physical activity/education:

> Education policymakers are beginning to understand that physical education is as much an academic discipline as anything else taught in school—a discipline that gives students some of the most critical skills they need to be productive citizens of the 21st century. Like other academic courses of study, physical education should be based upon rigorous national standards that define what students should know and be able to do as a result of participation (Wechsler, McKenna, Lee, & Dietz, 2004; National Association of Sport and Physical Education, 2004).

The Child Nutrition and WIC Reauthorization Act of 2004, in recognition of the declining health status of American students, mandates that schools promote health and wellness. The National School Lunch program requires every participating school district to adopt a local school wellness policy that addresses healthy eating and physical activity. These policies must include nutrition education, nutrition standards, physical education and physical activity opportunities, other school-based activities designed to promote student wellness, and implementation and measurement. The policy goals include engaging parents and the community in policy development, implementation, and review; giving students opportunities for physical activity on a daily basis and access to affordable, nutritious, and appealing foods; and providing all students with nutrition education and physical education to foster lifelong healthy habits (Child Nutrition and WIC Reauthorization Act, 2004).

Evidence

The overwhelming evidence for the beneficial effects of physical activity on students' health, physiology, cognition, psychosocial well-being, and academic performance speaks to the enormous impact on students' well-being and education that schools can have by implementing the aforementioned policies, as well as the tragic outcomes that result when schools remain sedentary. We will look at some of the key scientific data that support the claim that a "fit body optimizes brain function."

Exercise and Health

By fulfilling the evolutionary mandate for movement, school-based physical activity programs that combine daily physical education (PE), activity breaks, and physically active homework have been shown to lower students' body fat, improve aerobic fitness, and lower cardiovascular risk (Kriemler et al., 2010). One daily in-school physical activity program among students of low socioeconomic status, notable by its ease of implementation, reduced the prevalence of childhood obesity by 4 %, and improved cardiorespiratory fitness by 14 % and fat-free mass by 2.6 (Walther, Machalica, Muller, & Schuler, 2009). A moderate aerobic exercise program improved insulin sensitivity (an essential component to the prevention of type 2 diabetes) among both lean and obese sedentary adolescents, irrespective of weight loss (van der Heijden, Toffolo, Manesso, Sauer, & Sunehag, 2009).

The Perils of Sitting

The science of sitting warns of the hazards of a sedentary school day. Many educators ascribe to the traditional belief that concentration requires quiet, disciplined sitting, prompting an ideal in which the student remains physically inert while passively and attentively receiving information. Primary school children spend up to 10 h per day sitting, yet our elementary schools often give no consideration whatsoever to the impact that this inactivity has on kids' health, psychosocial well-being, and learning. This amount of static, passive sitting has devastating effects on the postural and locomotive systems that leads to functional degeneration (i.e., chronic back pain) (Breithecker, 2010). Addictive technologies ranging from video games to text messaging further contribute to sedentarism, effectively turning many members of younger generations into "cyber slaves."

In order to stay focused and alert, children have to be able to move when seated. Forcing children to sit passively and inertly for prolonged periods is abusive. Children who undergo prolonged periods of academic instruction become more fidgety or restless and experience reduced concentration (Mahar, Murphy, & Rowe, 2006). "A continual rhythmic exchange between being passivity and activity, strain and relief, tension and relaxation," represents an anthropological need; this basic behavior by children and adolescents serves to ensure a "balanced physical, mental, and emotional state (Breithecker, 2010)." Temporary fidgeting or restlessness expresses a physiological need; a strategy for survival that today leads children to detentions and being labeled ADHD (Breithecker, 2010).

Prolonged passive sitting can be avoided by substituting active-dynamic sitting that allows leg movement, rocking, standing at desk, and frequent postural shifts, together with intermittent breaks for standing or movement. Dynamic sitting can be facilitated by ergonomic chairs, stability balls, customized desks, etc. Active or intermittent sitting facilitates chronic low-level physical exertion and activates motor and vestibular cortices that influence pre-frontal executive centers to enable students to better focus (Breithecker, 2010).

Schools can adopt numerous strategies to achieve "activity-permissive" class-rooms. The use of stability balls in classrooms allows students to move constantly throughout lessons without being disruptive. Stability balls help students struggling with attention problems to focus better (Pytel, 2007), and students overwhelmingly prefer them (Kilbourne, 2009). Similarly, adjustable-height school desks promote attentiveness among students by allowing easy switching between sitting and standing, while liberating legs to swing at will (Saulny, 2009).

Exercise, Fitness, and Cognitive Ability

The short- and long-term benefits of exercise on cognitive abilities (such as learning and memory and executive function) have been exhaustively demonstrated in animal models (Vaynman, Zhe, & Fernando, 2004) as well as among aging humans, where physical activity has been shown to delay or prevent cognitive decline and dementia (including Alzheimer's-type dementia) (Kramer, Stanley, Colcombe, Dong, & Greenough, 2004). Among children and adolescents, research broadly supports a positive relation among physical activity and physical fitness and cognitive ability. A meta-analysis of studies among school-aged children found a positive correlation with physical activity and numerous facets of cognitive performance, including: per-ceptual skills, intelligence quotient, achievement, verbal tests, mathematical tests, and developmental level/academic readiness (Sibley & Etnier, 2003). A randomized trial of aerobic exercise among overweight children demonstrated improvements in aspects of executive functioning (planning) among those exercising compared to control groups (Davis et al., 2007). Another trial among adolescents associated improved attentional performance with acute coordinative exercises as compared to normal sport lessons (Budde, Voelcker-Rehage, Pietrabyk-Kendziorra, Ribeiro, & Tidow, 2008). Among young adults, improvement in executive functions that rely on working memory resulted only from aerobic exercise, and not resistance exercise (Pontifex, Hillman, Fernhall, Thompson, & Valentini, 2009).

Among pre-adolescent students, an acute bout (20 min) of moderate aerobic activity (treadmill walking) improved both academic achievement tests and behav-ioral as well as neuroelectric indexes of the cognitive control of attention (Hillman et al., 2009). Among children and adolescents, research has similarly found a posi-tive relation between measures of cognition and physical fitness. Among pre-adolescents, researchers have associated physical fitness with improved attention, working memory, response speed, and interference control (Hillman,

Castelli, & Buck, 2005; Buck, Hillman, &. Castelli, 2008). Improved cognitive performance on executive control tasks among higher-fit (aerobic capacity) children, compared with their lower-fit peers, shows a relation to increased cognitive control, greater allocation of attentional resources during stimulus coding, and reduced conflict during response selection; evidence that suggests a general rather than selective relationship between aerobic fitness and cognition (Hillman, Buck, Themanson, Pontifex, & Castelli, 2009). Scientists have shown that an "enriched environment" which entails physical, social and intellectual stimulation enhances cognition, stimulates neuroplasticity, and prevents cognitive decline with aging (Lewis, 2004; Bruel-Jungerman, Laroche, & Rampon, 2005; Mora, Segovia, & del Arco, 2007).

Recently, Maria Aberg and her group (2009) completed a large study of 1.2 million Swedish men looking at the effect of physical activity on cognition as well as assessing the effect of familial and genetic influences. They compared their physical and cognitive scores when they completed high school at the age of 15 and again at 18 when they entered military service. Those that had improved their cardiovascular fitness improved their cognitive scores. Moreover, the researchers found the cognitive and achievement benefits conferred by cardiovascular fitness predictive even for 1,600 sets of monozygotic twin pairs, thereby becoming the first study to rule out genetic predisposition as one of many potential alternative explanations for the consistently observed association between physical fitness and cognitive and academic outcomes. Based on their interpretation of the implications of these findings, the authors were compelled to make these policy recommendations:

> We believe the present results provide scientific support for educational policies to maintain or increase physical education in school curricula as a means to stem the growing trend toward a sedentary lifestyle, which is accompanied by an increased risk for diseases and perhaps intellectual and academic underachievement (Aberg et al., 2009).

Obesity and the Brain

In contrast to Sweden, in the US one-third of children and adolescents (and nearly one-fifth of 4-year-olds) are overweight or obese, with many forced to remain sedentary throughout the school day. Over the past 40 years, childhood obesity rates have quadrupled among children ages 6–11 and more than tripled among youth ages 12–19 (Anderson & Whitaker, 2009; CDC, 2010). One of the most pressing health issues affecting our nation's students, obesity not only represents a precursor to chronic diseases but also leads to loss of cognitive functioning and detrimental effects on academic performance. The brains of obese adults show severe signs of brain damage or deterioration and have 8 % less tissue than their lean adult counterparts, deficiencies that appear in areas including the frontal and temporal lobes as well as the anterior cingulate gyrus (areas involved in planning, memory, and executive functions) (Raji, Ho, & Parikshak, 2010). Researchers associate childhood obesity among students with lower cognitive ability, lower academic achievement, increased incidence of behavioral problems, and occurrence of white matter lesions in the brain similar to those seen in Alzheimer's patients (Miller et al., 2006; Li, Dai, Jackson, & Zhang, 2008). Regarding the latter, these researchers attribute the cause of these white matter lesions to abnormal hormonal levels caused by excessive adipose tissue that causes accumulation of metabolic byproducts that interfere with neuronal myelination (Miller et al., 2006). Others have associated higher body mass index (BMI) with lower verbal, social, and motor skills (Vaynman & Gomez-Pinilla, 2006).

Exercise, Fitness and Psychosocial Well-Being

A student's mental well-being influences their capacity for learning and memory through factors such as mood, anxiety, stress, and attention control. The positive effects of exercise on components of mental well-being suggest indirect pathways mediating improved academic performance. Attaining the right "frame of mind" greatly facilitates the learning process for students.

Students obtain numerous behavioral and psychosocial benefits from physical activity, including improvements to relationships (Field, Diego, & Sanders, 2001); self-esteem (Ekeland, Heian, Hagen, & Coren, 2005); psychological well-being (Parfitt & Eston, 2005); attention, motivation, and concentration anger expression (Tkacz, Young-Hyman, & Boyle, 2008); and classroom behavior (Barros, Silver, & Stein, 2009); as well as prevention/mitigation of chronic stress, impulsivity, and learned helplessness (Greenwood, Foley, Burhans, Maier, & Fleshner, 2005) and depression and anxiety (Strong et al., 2005). Physical activity helps put students in the right frame of mind to learn by modulating dopamine and serotonin, neurotransmitters essential for mood, attention, and motivation; the author has previously described physical activity as "like taking a little bit of Ritalin and a little bit of Prozac" (Ratey et al., 2008). "Play," a popular outlet for physical activity among children and adolescents, similarly promotes healthy cognitive development by stimulating frontal lobe maturation, alleviating impulsiveness, and promoting pro-social minds through the maturation of behavioral inhibition (Panksepp, Burgdorf, Turner, & Gordon, 2003; Panksepp, 2007; 2008).

Exercise and Addiction: Reclaiming the Biology of Self Control

As described in detail elsewhere in this book, exercise represents a potent factor in both the prevention and treatment substance abuse (drugs, alcohol, and tobacco), as well as other potential addicting behaviors such as texting, video games, and television. Exercise may re-set an addicted individual's out-of-control reward system. Regular physical activity, as part of a holistic approach to wellness, stimulates neurobiological modifications that quell addictive urges, while providing structure and motivation. Exercise provides life experience, challenge, feelings of pleasure and pain, and goal setting and accomplishment that serve as an inoculation against addictive behaviors. PA also influences major neurotransmitter systems, including dopamine and serotonin, as well as endorphins and endocannabinoids, leading to lower levels of tension, anxiety, and depression; blunted cravings; and improved mood, satisfaction, inhibitory control, self-regulation, and hopefulness (Dietrich & McDaniel, 2004; Ratey et al., 2008).

Physical Activity, Physical Fitness, and Academic Performance

Numerous studies have found a similar positive relationship between physical activity/physical fitness and measures of academic performance (such as grades and test scores) and of concentration, memory, and classroom behavior (Strong et al., 2005). A cross-sectional study involving 8,000 schoolchildren found that academic ratings have a significant correlation with exercise levels and performance on physical fitness tests (Dwyer, Sallis, Blizzard, Lazarus, & Dean, 2001). Another cross-sectional study of school-aged children in Iceland revealed that the combination of BMI and physical activity explain up to 24 % of variance in academic achievement (Sigfusdottir, Kristjansson, & Allegrante, 2007). A large cross-sectional study conducted in 2002 by the California Department of Education demonstrated a strong association between physical fitness and academic performance (California Department of Education, 2005). Based on an evaluation of nearly one million students in grades five, seven, and nine using the Fitnessgram (a six-faceted measure of overall fitness) and students' state standardized test grades (SAT-9), investigators consistently found that those students with higher levels of fitness scored higher. The research clearly ascribes a positive linear relationship to the number of fitness standards achieved and standardized test scores; this result held for boys and girls in both math and reading, being most pronounced in math. Smaller follow-up studies have replicated this finding (Castelli, Hillman, Buck, & Erwin, 2007; Chomitz, Slining, & McGowan, 2009), wherein aerobic capacity in particular related positively to test scores in mathematics and reading, while BMI related inversely to scores (Castellie et al., 2007). Because of the cross-sectional nature of their designs, these studies do not allow us to infer per se that physical activity or fitness causes enhanced academic performance (despite consistently showing a strong association between activity and fitness and academic performance).

Physical Education and Academic Performance

Several studies have assessed the relation between physical education and academic performance. In a 16-month Canadian, in-school physical activity intervention, researchers found neither increased nor decreased standardized test scores compared to control schools (Ahamed et al., 2007). Other reviewers have asserted that, at the very least, time spent in physical education does not hinder academic performance and may even lead to an improvement (Hillman et al., 2008; Trudeau & Shephard, 2008). Many researchers have previously correlated the addition of physical education to school curricula with modest improvements in academic performance (Dwyer, Coonan, Leitch, Hetzel, & Baghurst, 1983; Sallis et al., 1999; Dishman, Renner, White-Welkley, Burke, & Bunnell, 2000). Other researchers found that a reduction of 4 h per week of academic class time replaced with physical education led to higher scores on standardized math examinations (Shephard, 1997).

A longitudinal analysis conducted by the US Centers for Disease Control and Prevention (Carlson et al., 2008) found that teacher-reported estimates of the time students spent in physical education correlated with higher academic performance among girls but not among boys. In a review of physical activity and academic outcomes among school-aged children, one author concluded that "there is evidence to suggest that short-term cognitive benefits of physical activity during the school day adequately compensate for time spent away from other academic areas" (Taras, 2005). Another author highlighted that:

1. The addition of PE to curriculum results in small positive gains in academic performance
2. Allocating more curricular time to programs of PA does not negatively affect academic performance, even when time allocated to other subjects is reduced
3. Evidence exists for a relative increase in academic performance per unit time of PE (Strong et al., 2005)

On the other hand, a recent middle-school intervention study found that adding physical education to school curricula did not improve grades or standardized test scores. Instead, only vigorous exercise performed outside of school positively predicted grades. Interestingly, the physical education classes under investigation included, on average, only 19 min of adequately vigorous physical activity in a 55-min class (Coe, Pivarnik, Womack, Reeves, & Malina, 2006). The authors suggest that failing to achieve activity levels in physical education class high enough to meet recommended activity standards for children, such as those reported in this study, provides students little benefit; whereas students able to achieve the higher PA levels (outside of school activities) positively affect academics.

Clearly, the quality of physical education is vitally important to cognitive and academic outcomes. Physical activity predicts higher academic performance, but physical education with insufficient levels of activity does not. This suggests that the quality of the programs under investigation has limited the available evidence relating physical education to academic outcomes, thus likely producing data that underestimates the potential academic benefit of daily, quality physical education. Animal and human research primarily supports the importance of aerobic activity to enhance cognitive function. Physical education classes that fail to encourage aerobic activity of sufficient duration and intensity will likely also fail to produce notable improvements in student fitness, health, weight control, or academic achievement.

Achieving Moving Schools: A Change in Paradigm

In the face of this preponderance of evidence demonstrating the benefits of physical activity among students, many US schools over the last several decades have become increasingly sedentary, cutting back on physical education, recess, and other PA opportunities for students. Schools have simultaneously increased classroom time, wherein students often must remain sedentary. This crisis of passivity requires a fundamental paradigm shift wherein every school culture embraces an evolutionarily sound, empirically proven, and scientifically justified principle that recognizes regular movement as essential to human health and performance, as well as learning and education.

A sedentary school culture is catastrophic for students' health and education. In juxtaposition, a moving school culture, wherein moving and learning are embraced as co-reinforcing, holds the potential to favorably affect all of a school's most fundamental objectives: improved attendance, reduced violence and disciplinary incidences, improved classroom behavior, higher grades and test scores, as well as lower prevalence of physical and mental health conditions. Ideally, this paradigm shift toward moving schools arises within a broader metamorphosis that considers wellness as a crucial component of the pursuit of happiness and success. Schools need to equip all students with the necessary knowledge, skills, tools, and behavioral patterns to instill each individual with the self-motivated pursuit of a healthy lifestyle throughout the life course. And though physical activity represents a critical component, updated programs must also stress the importance of healthful diet, anti-smoking, alcohol and substance abuse prevention, sexual health education, communicable disease prevention, environmental health, and education regarding healthcare. Schools similarly need to embrace environmental changes that benefit human physiological and cognitive performance, such as lighting (natural light and broad spectrum lighting vs. fluorescent lighting), temperature, seating and posture, biological rhythms, breathing, intelligent class length, kinesthetic learning, and educating by engaging multiple senses (Jensen, 1994).

Redefining Physical Education

A new conceptual framework at the core of this paradigm shift elevates PE from "step child" to a bona fide science of the body–brain connection:

> Early man needed to live by his wits to exploit a hostile environment of fugitive and random food source. Consequently, the human mind had to become clever, and man the strategic "adaptive opportunist." The mind, body, metabolic connection, a unique three in one interface, is the basis for optimum mental and physical health and human performance (De Vany, 2009).

The predominant view of physical education today misses the point. To fully know and appreciate the human condition requires a holistic understanding that humans are physical beings. Faculties of the brain and functions of body operate in concert; mind, body, and metabolism inextricably connect and intertwine.

Attempts at compartmentalization of the human body by systems can lead to incomplete and misleading observations. For instance, the leg muscles serve essential functions for multiple sub-systems of the body: movement in the musculoskeletal system, venous pumps in the cardiovascular system, and major metabolic centers in the metabolic system. To understand and address obesity, we must go beyond inadequate concepts of "dieting" to properly understanding the combined effects of nutritional intake in concert with physical activity, while assessing factors as varied as muscle mass, metabolic activity, hormonal messaging, and energy balance. The science of physical activity needs to incorporate the science of the body–brain connection; the primary goals of physical education must be educating, inspiring, and training students to embody and actualize a global view of the human organism working in concert.

We must stop relegating physical education to the gym; rather, all education must be physical, recognizing movement as essential to physical health and learning. We must stop viewing biology, physics, mathematics, health, and PE as disparate subjects; instead, material in each of these subjects should be used to support the others, taught in an integrated manner so as to educate students regarding brain–body paradigms. Incorporating human health and brain–body science into standardized testing would provide additional incentives for schools to educate students in this way.

Putting Physical Activity Back into Physical Education

Following from this conceptual paradigm, the New PE integrates educational (i.e., learning brain–body science) and behavioral (i.e., physical activity) components into most every subject interspersed throughout the school day. However, time set aside for daily PE as traditionally conceived remains an essential component and a prime driver of moving schools; yet the authors in no way argue for a return to traditional PE class. Instead, we strongly advocate for physical education that emphasizes cognitively, socially, and aerobically demanding physical activity. This New PE provides students with the knowledge, skills, and behavioral patterns necessary to pursue a lifetime of active, healthy living.

The New PE focuses on personal progress and lifelong fitness activities by encouraging enjoyable, engaging, and challenging modes of physically strenuous play. For younger students (grades K–4), PE should consist largely of recess-like supervised play (active recess; play with a little push), encouraging students to pursue physically strenuous, creative, social play with their peers. For older students (grades 5+), we recommend a more structured approach that encourages students to pursue more formal exercises, albeit with choice for preferred activities and a continued emphasis on enjoyment and play. PE should encourage students to pursue their personal fitness goals, with personal progress made the main criteria for grading (as opposed to rigid objective measures of skill or fitness). The competitive sport model that characterizes many PE programs today generally fails to provide a sufficient level of PA to offer tangible benefits and tends to marginalize the very students who would benefit the most from PA. The final result sought by the New PE thus involves a dramatic divergence from traditional PE programs.

Technology represents one way to provide critical accountability to students and educators alike to ensure that their New PE program engages participants in a sufficiently beneficial level of physical activity. For instance, using heart rate monitors to track intensity of activity provides students with a window into their own physiology and a tool with which to ensure appropriate intensity of activity, while also allowing educators to monitor and reward student activity. Other helpful tools include pedometers, accelerometers, fitness equipment feedback, etc. Monitoring and evaluating PE outcomes (including physical fitness, obesity, academic performance, behavioral outcomes, disciplinary incidents, etc.) will support accountability and inform progress towards optimally advantageous programs.

As stated above, the New PE incorporates a strong educational component, wherein PE teachers provide students with the scientific rationale for movement and other health behaviors to reinforce behavioral patterns. Ideally, PE should take place daily. However, in many instances daily PE may not be immediately feasible, in which case numerous alternative solutions abound. In either case, schools should educate and inspire their entire school community, including faculty and students, through a quality PE program to engage in physical activity throughout the school day.

Providing comprehensive and integrated physical education to students will advance schools' academic objectives, while acculturating the next generation with an appreciation for the mandate for physical activity and a new paradigm and behavioral pattern geared toward holistic health. However, switching to a New PE program represents just the beginning. In a genuinely moving school, movement transforms into a pervasive part of the school culture, community, grounds, and schedule. Success requires wholesale adoption and involvement by students, teachers, staff, administrators, families/parents, and other community members.

Daily fitness-based PE for EVERY student has never been more necessary. Whereas previous generations of children often engaged in physical activity during their commute to and from school and in after-school and outdoor activities, many children today have a sedentary commute and engage in sedentary after-school and at-home activities. This trend has been particularly marked among those students from lower socioeconomic status families and neighborhood environments. As optional after-school physical activities often do not reach those students most in need of daily activity, these programs should therefore supplement, rather than replace, daily PE.

Movement Throughout the Day

Logistic considerations and available resources vary greatly between schools. However, any school can avail itself of numerous opportunities, many low cost and readily accessible, available throughout the school day through which to engage students in physical activity. Committed schools find a way to become moving schools, regardless of constraints on time, money, and other resources. Schools need to capitalize on any and all opportunities to get their students active throughout the day; the following list cites several that have worked in practice:

- Active Transport—Provide students with safe opportunities to walk or cycle to school. This program can include working with town/community officials to ensure safe routes to school, enlisting teachers or parents as chaperones, or even having the bus drop students off a mile from school and having everyone walk together.
- Zero Hour PA—Make exercise the first thing students do upon arrival at school, before they start in on courses. Some schools invite students to arrive early or carve out time at the beginning of the official school day. In other cases, schools take advantage of time when many students loiter while waiting for school to begin.
- Morning Exercise—Replace morning assembly with morning workout (or incorporate exercises into assembly) as a great way to reach all students at once, start the day on the right foot, and engender a culture of activity and wellness.

Recess—Recess provides a valuable opportunity to allow students, particularly younger students, to engage in creative, undirected, physically active play. Provide students with simple equipment and encourage active recess to promote exercise, play, creativity, and improved health and learning. While recess is traditionally phased out after 5th and 6th grade, recess opportunities may be beneficial throughout early adolescence as well.

- Lunch—Depending on the school schedule, lunch can sometimes provide a substantial amount of optional extra time during which students should be allowed and encouraged to move and play.
- Downtime—Open the gym/playground to students who wish to get active during periods of downtime that may be interspersed throughout the day.
- After School—As budget allows, provide students with structured or unstructured opportunities to engage in physical activities and sports after school.
- Active Homework—To encourage activity in the home and community, assign students activity homework. This practice raises awareness among parents/families and enables students with sedentary home environments to change their family dynamic.
- Active Learning—Perhaps the most important opportunity to promote movement in schools, incorporating movement into the classroom can take many forms, including dynamic sitting, learning while standing and moving, or taking short activity breaks during the course of a class period. Such breaks (i.e., dancing, yoga, plyometrics, or stretching) can last less than 10 min, integrate grade appropriate learning materials, involve no equipment, and require little teacher preparation.
- Micro Exercise—The principle underlying many of the opportunities described above incorporates short, classroom-based exercise breaks throughout the school

day to rejuvenate the body and mind, improving mood, classroom behavior, concentration, and productivity (i.e., on-task behavior during academic instruction) (Mahar et al., 2006).

School Strategy

At present, many schools operate far afield from the movement culture that we advocate, characterized rather by diminished or largely ineffective PE programs and a sedentary culture that offers students a dearth of opportunities for movement during or between classes. Such schools require radical change; however, many cite administrative or faculty recalcitrance, logistical or political barriers, financial limitations, and general inertia as barriers to achieving reform. Many other schools simply do not want to put in the effort required to engage students and provide them with opportunities to move. Several consistent strategies emerge from successful schools:

- School Champion—A single person, or small group of people, who truly believes in the necessity of movement in schools and passionately and adamantly advocates for reform can be extremely effective in overcoming barriers. Champions convert colleagues and students to the cause and lead the way toward a moving school. Champions can come from among the PE teachers, other teachers, students, administrators, school board members, parents, politicians, business leaders, and other community members.
- Physical Activity Committee—Tasked with identifying and executing strategies to promote physical activity throughout the school day, this committee often but not necessarily draws its chair from within the PE department.
- Wellness Policy—Among the requirements for schools receiving federal money for subsidized lunches, adopting a formal wellness policy provides nutritional guidelines for foods served, as well as goals for nutritional education, physical activity, and other school-based activities. Schools can use this policy to advance programs and attitudes that provide all students with opportunities for regular movement throughout the school day.
- Community Engagement—Partner with community organizations to support or develop wellness programs and integrate school activities with community, business, and healthcare initiatives, including programs and activities during or after the school day, as well as summer programs, etc.

Case Study: The Naperville Model for the New PE

Fifteen years ago, Madison Junior High PE teacher Phil Lawler spearheaded what they refer to as the "New PE" in Naperville, Illinois, District 203. The CDC has since identified his new PE program as a national model for physical education, repeatedly highlighted in US national media, that serves as an international proto-type and training center for school systems seeking to change to moving schools.

In 2007 testimony to the Congressional House Subcommittee on Education, Phil Lawler explained that the "old school" PE met the needs of just 30 % of students, leaving the majority of students with a lifetime of bad memories and demeaning experiences. Today's PE, he explained, seeks to develop a healthy lifestyle among all students, thereby serving as a vehicle in the national crusade to improve physical fitness and combat obesity (Lawler, 2007).

The New PE championed by Lawler in Naperville focuses on aerobic exercise and lifelong fitness, while taking an individual approach that encourages each student to progress toward their own personal fitness goals. The program aims to get students hooked on moving by promoting fun activities, while providing the tools and skills to monitor and maintain their own health and activity. The program exposes students to a broad menu of activities—from kayaking to dancing to rock climbing and typical team sports like volleyball, basketball, and swimming—so that every student feels comfortable and can excel at fitness activities. Done properly, the intent is for students to become positively inclined to pursue similar activities for a lifetime. Students are expected to participate in PE every day; maybe spend 1 day working out in a state-of-the-art fitness center, the next doing a cardiovascular run/walk, with the remaining 3 days each week allotted to participation in individual and team sports of their choosing (Furger, 2001; Naperville, 2008; Viadero, 2008,).

A visionary junior high physical education teacher, Lawler, started this revolutionary movement with equal parts of idealism and self preservation. Lawler frequently relates his dramatic conversion to heart rate monitors. During weekly mile runs, he tested a heart rate monitor on a sixth grade girl, thin and not the least bit athletic. Jogging very slowly, an observer might easily have thought the student was not "giving it her all." Yet when he downloaded her stats, he placed her average heart rate at 187, and she crossed the finish line at 207. As an 11-year-old, a heart rate of 209 represents her maximum. This "ah-ha" moment would cause dramatic changes and serve as the springboard and impetus for a revolutionary movement (Furger, 2001; Ratey et al., 2008).

Lawler believes in the necessity of both students and teachers using these tools. "It's like driving a car without a speedometer," he says. "Without the heart-rate monitor, we just can't know how hard kids are really working. Not only is it unfair to some students, it can also be dangerous." Heart rate monitors provide students and their instructors with a clear picture of the intensity of workouts, as well as information about their "target zone," thereby helping to teach physiology in PE (Furger, 2001).

Naperville has since extended its technological reach beyond heart rate monitors to include state-of-the-art tools to support the physical health and education of its adolescent students. Students exercise at a complete fitness center, dubbed the "Madison Health Club," complete with a rock climbing wall and a series of computer-enabled fitness test stations (where students create a total health portfolio that will eventually follow them from sixth grade through high school graduation). Integral to Madison's commitment to emphasizing fitness over raw athletic ability, the fitness-testing system measures flexibility, blood pressure, body composition, upper-body strength, and cardiovascular health. Students exercise on treadmills, elliptical machines, rock-climbing walls, Dance-Dance Revolutions (DDRs), and video-game-like interactive stationary bikes, all the while wearing heart rate monitors to make sure exercise remains within their optimal aerobic zones (Furger, 2001; Naperville Central Physical Education Program, 2008).

Lawler's New PE in Naperville has had a dramatic impact—the district yearly ranks at the top in Illinois academically, despite lower expenditure per student (spending at the state-wide median amount) compared with similarly ranked districts. In 1999, Naperville students took the Trends in International Mathematics and Science Study (TIMSS) test and finished first in science (ahead of Singapore) and sixth in math world-wide—compared to the overall US ranking of 18th in science and 19th in math. Measured as low as 3 %, the prevalence of being overweight among Naperville sophomores compares favorably to the national average of 30 % (Pascopella, 2001; Ratey & Hagerman, 2008).

In 2005, Lawler and partner Paul Zientarski expanded the scope of Naperville's PE program by implementing Learning Readiness Physical Education (LRPE) class. Based on a philosophy that recognizes physical activity as critical to cognitive abilities and academic performance, Naperville enrolled students in a special reading program into a vigorous exercise session (achieving 80–90 % of maximum heart rate) preceding literacy class. After one semester, students participating in LRPE immediately before literacy class increased their reading and comprehension scores by 1.4 on a grade level equivalency scale—nearly twice as much as comparable students who had a significantly longer time frame between LRPE and literacy class. The school encountered similar results for LRPE and math scores; students enrolled in a PE class immediately before math increased their algebra readiness by an average of 20 % compared to only 4 % for the students who took PE several hours after math class (Ratey et al., 2008).

Naperville's success did not occur overnight; changes happened because of the multi-level commitment of staff, school and district administrators, coupled with ongoing professional development and an ironclad commitment to incorporating knowledge for the emerging science of exercise and the brain. In addition to his job at Madison, Lawler's responsibilities eventually expanded to coordinating the PE programs for the entire Naperville school district, advocating what might be called an enlightened approach to physical fitness (Ratey et al., 2008). Lawler points to two seminal reports—"Healthy People 2000" (now Healthy People 2010) and "The Surgeon General's Report on Youth Fitness"—as the impetus for his department's switch from an old-style PE curriculum narrowly focused on raw speed and ability to a New PE program that emphasizes fitness and well-being over athleticism (Furger, 2001).

As the Naperville program blossomed and became a prominent model of the New PE, a partnership was established with PE4Life, a non-profit organization with a kindred mission that engages in government advocacy, PEP grant assistance, and community/business coalition building. PE4Life has aimed to replicate the Naperville model by indoctrinating administrators and teachers from around the country with Lawler's vision. The PE4Life vision seeks to have physical education offered to every child every day; available to all students, not just the athletically inclined; to provide a wide variety of sports and fitness activities to promote an active and healthy lifestyle; to assess students on their personal progress toward fitness and physical activity goals; to incorporate technology on a regular basis; and to extend beyond the walls of the gymnasium (Ratey et al., 2008).

Thanks to federal funding and forward-thinking school leaders, PE4Life has set up "PE4life Academies" in schools around the country, setting a new standard for PE in the process. So far, PE4Life Academies have trained about 1,000 educators at over 350 schools to emulate their program and join the new wave of PE, with Naperville serving as a hub for training and recruiting in the new PE revolution (PE4Life, 2007; Ratey et al., 2008). Results from PE4Life schools track those from Naperville, generally demonstrating increased fitness levels, lower absenteeism, and improved classroom behavior and academic performance. Many have found the impact of PE on school discipline of paramount importance.

Woodland Elementary School, a K-5 school in the urban core of Kansas City, Missouri, integrated PE4life's Core Principles into their program in the 2005–2006 school year. After just 1 year, the number of out-of-school suspensions dropped by 67 % (from 1,177 to 392), and the number of disciplinary incidents dropped 59 % (from 228 to 94). Woodland has also documented a sustained, significantly lower decrease in disciplinary incidents over the 4 years since the integration of PE4life's Core Principles, as the average number of out-of-school suspensions has decreased 51 % (PE4Life, 2007).

Few schools have the resources to develop a Naperville-like program overnight. However, Naperville provides empirical evidence for the dramatic effect that the New PE can have on student health and education and stands as a beacon emblazing the realm of possibility open to others to emulate. Schools that draw from the Naperville model to implement simple, low-cost solutions find similar benefits. Charleston Progress Academy, a public magnet school including grades 4–8 whose students are all on school lunch/breakfast programs, implemented 40 min of exercise in the morning before school beginning in 2006. Held in the gym and staffed by volunteer teachers, the session followed a "station" format that included basketball, DDR, double-Dutch jump-roping and pogo stick jumping. This before-school program had dramatic results on disciplinary referrals and suspensions, with referrals dropping 47 % (from 661 to 353) in just 1 year and suspensions dropping 66 % (from 71 to 24) over the same period of time (Charleston Progressive Academy, 2008).

Inspired by a visit to Naperville, the Johannes Skolen in Copenhagen, Denmark, increased PE from once a week to five times per week. Daily activities offered consisted of ball play, running, hip hop dance, aerobics, spinning, indoor rowing, and military boot camp training, as well as after-school activities. Concurrently, the school removed all "junk food," instead offering only healthy "super foods." After only 3 months, the school observed a 38 % drop in absenteeism, a 33 % improvement in concentration abilities, improved teacher-reported classroom behavior, and an average 1.5 grade level improvement among students (Johannes, 2009).

Conclusions

Forged over the course of human evolution, the requirement for regular movement and physical activity remains integral to proper gene expression, physiological adaptation, and physical and mental health and performance. We must come to perceive the modern sedentary environment and culture as pathological, acting as major contributors to epidemic levels of metabolic disorders, chronic disease, mental disorders, and addiction. Science and the state of our health dictate a return to evolutionarily sound lifestyles; schools present a unique opportunity to lead this societal transformation and to acculturate future generations with the knowledge, skills, and behaviors necessary for a lifetime of healthy living. However, our schools require a paradigm shift to realize this opportunity by replacing the outdated concept of a sedentary school culture with that of the "moving school," with students encouraged and required to move regularly and remain active throughout the day. Doing so will enable students to comply with evolutionary, physiological, and psychological demands that help realize physical and mental health and academic potential. Schools that have adopted the New PE and embraced a culture of movement provide us glimpses of the future. Leading the charge toward a healthier future, today's PE reformers can be found brewing a social revolution in our schools.

References

Aberg, M. A., Pedersenn, N. L., Tore'n, K., Svartengren, M., Backstrand, B., Johnsson, T., et al. (2009). Cardiovascular fitness is associated with cognition in young adulthood. *Proceedings of the National Academy of Sciences of the United States of America, 106*(49), 20906–20911.

Ahamed, Y., MacDonald, H., Reed, K., Naylor, P. J., Liu-Ambrose, T., & McKay, H. (2007). School-based physical activity does not compromise children's academic performance. *Medicine and Science in Sports and Exercise, 39*(2), 371–376.

Anderson, S. E., & Whitaker, R. C. (2009). Prevalence of obesity among US preschool children in different racial and ethnic groups. *Archives of Pediatric & Adolescent Medicine, 163*(4), 344–348.

Bak, E. E., Hellenius, M. L., & Ekblom, B. (2010). Are we facing a new paradigm of inactivity physiology? *British Journal of Sports Medicine, 44*(12), 834–835.

Barros, R. M., Silver, E. J., & Stein, R. E. K. (2009). School recess and group classroom behavior. *Pediatrics, 123*, 431–436.

Beaudet, A. L., Scriver, C. R., Sly, W. S., & Valle, D. (1995). Genetics, biochemistry, and molecular basis of variant human phenotypes. In C. R. Scriver, A. L. Beaudet, W. S. Sly, D. Valle, J. B. Stanbury, J. B. Wyngaarden, & D. S. Fredrickson (Eds.), *The metabolic and molecular bases of inherited disease* (7th ed., Vol. 1, p. 79). New York: McGraw-Hill.

Booth, F. W., & Chakravarthy, M. V. (2002). Cost and consequences of sedentary living: New battleground for an old enemy. *President's Council on Physical Fitness and Sports: Research Digest, 3*(16), 1–8.

Booth, F. W., Chakravarthy, M. V., Gordon, S. E., & Spangenburg, E. E. (2002). Waging war on physical inactivity: using modern molecular ammunition against an ancient enemy. *Journal of Applied Physiology, 93*, 3–30.

Breithecker, D. (2010). *Beware the sitting trap in learning and schooling. "Ergo-dynamic" concepts are decisive.* Retrieved June 12, 2010, from http://www.designshare.com/index.php/articles/sitting-trap/.

Bruel-Jungerman, E., Laroche, S., & Rampon, C. (2005). New neurons in the dentate gyrus are involved in the expression of enhanced long-term memory following environmental enrichment. *European Journal of Neuroscience, 21*, 513–521.

Buck, S. M., Hillman, C. H., & Castelli, D. M. (2008). The relation of aerobic fitness to Stroop Task performance in preadolescent children. *Medicine and Science in Sports and Exercise, 40*, 166–172.

Budde, H., Voelcker-Rehage, C., Pietrabyk-Kendziorra, S., Ribeiro, P., & Tidow, G. (2008). Acute coordinative exercise improves attentional performance in adolescents. *Neuroscience Letters, 441*(2), 219–223.

California Department of Education (CDE). (2005, April). *California physical fitness test: A study of the relationship between physical fitness and academic achievement in California using 2004 test results*. Sacramento, CA: California Department of Education. Retrieved August 29, 2010, from www.cde.ca.gov/ta/tg/pf/documents/2004pftresults.doc.

Carlson, S. A., Fulton, J. E., Lee, S. M., Maynard, M., Brown, D. R., Kohl, H. W., III, et al. (2008). Physical education and academic achievement in elementary school: Data from the early childhood longitudinal study. *American Journal of Public Health, 98*, 721–727.

Castelli, D. M., Hillman, C. H., Buck, S. M., & Erwin, H. E. (2007). Physical fitness and academic achievement in third- and fifth-grade students. *Journal of Sport & Exercise Psychology, 29*, 239–252.

Centers for Disease Control and Prevention (CDC). (2007). *US physical activity statistics*. Retrieved June 12, 2010, from http://apps.nccd.cdc.gov/PASurveillance/StateSumResultV.asp?CI=&Year=2007&State=0#data.

Centers for Disease Control and Prevention (CDC). (2009). *Diabetes—Successes and opportunities for population-based prevention and control: At a glance*. Retrieved June 12, 2010, from http://www.cdc.gov/chronicdisease/resources/publications/AAG/ddt.htm.

Centers for Disease Control and Prevention (CDC). (2010). *Healthy youth. Childhood obesity*. Retrieved June 12, 2010, from http://www.cdc.gov/HealthyYouth/obesity/.

Chakravarthy, M. V., & Booth, F. W. (2004). Eating, exercise, and "thrifty" genotypes: connecting the dots toward an evolutionary understanding of modern chronic diseases. *J. App. Physiol. 96*, 3–10.

Charleston Progressive Academy. (2008). Direct Correspondence.

Child Nutrition and WIC Reauthorization Act. (2004, June 30). *Local wellness policy* (Section 204 of Public Law 108-265). Retrieved August 29, 2010, from http://www.fns.usda.gov/tn/healthy/108-265.pdf.

Chomitz, V. R., Slining, M. M., & McGowan, R. J. (2009). Is there a relationship between physical fitness and academic achievement? Positive results from public school children in the northeastern United States. *Journal of School Health, 79*(1), 30–37.

Coe, D. P., Pivarnik, J. M., Womack, C. J., Reeves, M. J., & Malina, R. M. (2006). Effect of physical education and activity levels on academic achievement in children. *Medicine and Science in Sports and Exercise, 38*, 1515–1519.

Cordain, L. O., Gotshall, R. W., & Eaton, S. B. (1997). Evolutionary aspects of exercise. *World Review of Nutrition and Dietetics, 81*, 49–60.

Cordain, L. O., Gotshall, R. W., Eaton, S. B., & Eaton, S. B. I. I. I. (1998). Physical activity, energy expenditure and fitness: an evolutionary perspective. *International Journal of Sports Medicine, 19*, 328–335.

Council for Research Excellence (CRE). (2009). *Video consumer mapping study*. Muncie: Ball State University, Center for Media Design, Sequent Partners. Retrieved August 29, 2010 from http://www.researchexcellence.com/VCMFINALREPORT_4_28_09.pdf.

Davis, C. L., Tomporowski, P. D., Boyle, C. A., Waller, J. L., Miller, P. H., & Naglieri, J. A. (2007, December). Effects of aerobic exercise on overweight children's cognitive functioning: a randomized controlled trial. *Research Quarterly for Exercise and Sport, 78*(5), 510–519.

De Vany, A. (2009). *Essay on evolutionary fitness*. Retrieved June 12, 2010, from http://www.arthurdevany.com/categories/20091026.

Diamond, J. (2003). The double puzzle of diabetes. *Nature, 423*, 599–602.

Dietrich, A., & McDaniel, W. F. (2004). Endocannabinoids and exercise. *British Journal of Sports Medicine, 38*, 536–541.

Dishman, R. K., Renner, K. J., White-Welkley, J. E., Burke, K. A., & Bunnell, B. N. (2000). Treadmill exercise training augments brain norepinephrine response to familiar and novel stress. *Brain Research Bulletin, 52*, 337–342.

Dwyer, T., Coonan, W. E., Leitch, D. R., Hetzel, B. S., & Baghurst, P. A. (1983). An investigation of the effects of daily physical activity on the health of primary school students in South Australia. *International Journal of Epidemiology, 12*, 308–313.

Dwyer, T., Sallis, J. F., Blizzard, L., Lazarus, R., & Dean, K. (2001). Relation of academic performance to PA and fitness in children. *Pediatric Exercise Science, 13*, 225–237.

Eaton, S. B., Konner, M., & Shostak, M. (1988). Stone agers in the fast lane, chronic degenerative disease in evolutionary perspective. *American Journal of Medicine, 84*, 736–749.

Eaton, S. B., Konner, M., & Shostak, M. (2002). Evolutionary health promotion, consideration of common counterarguments. *Preventive Medicine, 34*, 119–123.

Ekeland, E., Heian, F., Hagen, K. B., & Coren, E. (2005). Can exercise improve self esteem in children and young people? A systematic review of randomised controlled trials * Commentary. *British Journal of Sports Medicine, 39*(11), 792–798.

Field, Y., Diego, M., & Sanders, C. E. (2001). Exercise is positively related to adolescents' relationships and academics. *Adolescence, 36*, 105–110.

Franks, P. W., Hanson, R. L., Knowler, W. C., Sievers, M. L., Bennett, P. H., & Looker, H. C. (2010). Childhood obesity, other cardiovascular risk factors, and premature death. *The New England Journal of Medicine, 362*(6), 485–493.

Furger, R. (2001). The new PE curriculum: An innovative approach to teaching physical fitness. *Edutopia*. Retrieved June 12, 2010, from http://www.edutopia.org/new-p-e-curriculum.

Greenwood, B. N., Foley, T. E., Burhans, D., Maier, S. F., & Fleshner, M. (2005). The consequences of uncontrollable stress are sensitive to duration of prior wheel running. *Brain Research, 1033*, 164–178.

Hamer, M., Stamatakis, E., & Mishra, G. (2009). Psychological distress, TV viewing, and physical activity in children aged 4-12 years. *Pediatrics, 123*(5), 1263–1268.

Hamilton, M. T., Hamilton, D. G., & Zderic, T. W. (2007). Role of low energy expenditure and sitting in obesity, metabolic syndrome, type 2 diabetes, and cardiovascular disease. *Diabetes, November, 56*(11), 2655–2667.

Heath, G. W., Gavin, J. R., III, Hinderliter, J. M., Hagberg, J. M., Bloomfield, S. A., & Holloszy, J. O. (1983). Effects of exercise and lack of exercise on glucose tolerance and insulin sensitivity. *Journal of Applied Physiology, 55*, 512–517.

Hillman, C. H., Buck, S. M., Themanson, J. R., Pontifex, M. B., & Castelli, D. M. (2009). Aerobic fitness and cognitive development: Event-related brain potential and task performance indices of executive control in preadolescent children. *Developmental Psychology, 45*(1), 114–129.

Hillman, C. H., Castelli, D., & Buck, S. M. (2005). Aerobic fitness and neurocognitive function in healthy preadolescent children. *Medicine and Science in Sports and Exercise, 37*, 1967–1974.

Hillman, C. H., Erickson, K. I., & Kramer, A. F. (2008). Be smart, exercise your heart: Exercise effects on brain and cognition. *Nature Reviews. Neuroscience, 9*, 58–64.

Hillman, C. H., Pontifex, M. B., Raine, L. B., Castelli, D. M., Hall, E. E., & Kramer, A. F. (2009). The effect of acute treadmill walking on cognitive control and academic achievement in preadolescent children. *Neuroscience, 159*, 1044–1054.

Jensen, E. (1994). *The learning brain*. Del Mar: Turning Point Publishing.

Johannes, S. (2009). Copenhagen Denmark. Direct Correspondence.

Kilbourne, J. (2009). Sharpening the mind through movement: Using exercise balls in a university lecture class. *The Chronicle of Kinesiology and Physical Education in Higher Education, 20*(1), 10–15. Retrieved August 29, 2010, from http://www.balldynamics.com/research/a1237990661.pdf.

Koffler, M., & Kisch, E. S. (1996). Starvation diet and very-low-calorie diets may induce insulin resistance and overt diabetes mellitus. *Journal of Diabetes and its Complications, 10*, 109–112.

Kramer, A. F., Stanley, J., Colcombe, L. B., Dong, W., & Greenough, W. T. (2004). Environmental influences on cognitive and brain plasticity during aging. *Journal of Gerontology Medical Sciences, 59A*, 940–957.

Kriemler, S., Zahner, L., Schindler, C., Meyer, U., Hartmann, T., Hebestreit, H., et al. (2010). Effect of school based physical activity programme (KISS) on fitness and adiposity in primary schoolchildren: cluster randomized controlled trial. *British Medical Journal, 340*, c785.

Lawler, P. (2007, May 10). *Using school wellness plans to help fight childhood obesity.* Testimony before House Sub-Committee on Healthy Families and Community (p. 1). Washington, D.C.: Department of Health and Human Services. Retrieved August 29, 2010, from http://edlabor. house.gov/testimony/051007PhilLawlertestimony.pdf.

Leatherdale, S. T., Wong, S. L., Manske, S. R., & Colditz, G. A. (2008). Susceptibility to smoking and its association with physical activity, BMI, and weight concerns among youth. *Nicotine & Tobacco Research, 10*(3), 499–505.

Lewis, M. H. (2004). Environmental complexity and central nervous system development and function. *Mental Retardation and Developmental Disabilities Research Reviews, 10*, 91–95.

Li, Y., Dai, Q., Jackson, J. C., & Zhang, J. (2008). Overweight is associated with decreased cognitive functioning among school-age children and adolescents. *Obesity, 16*(8), 1809–1815.

Lipman, R. L., Raskin, P., Love, T., Triebwasser, J., Lecocq, F. R., & Schnure, J. J. (1972). Glucose intolerance during decreased physical activity in man. *Diabetes, 21*, 101–107.

Llinas, R. (2001). *I of the vortex: From neurons to self* (p. 302). Cambridge: MIT Press.

Mahar, M. T., Murphy, S. K., & Rowe, D. A. (2006). Effects of a classroom-based program on physical activity and on-task behavior. *Medicine and Science in Sports and Exercise, 38*(12), 2086–2094.

Martinez-Gomez, D., Tucker, J., Heelan, K. A., Welk, G. J., & Eisenmann, J. C. (2009). Associations between sedentary behavior and blood pressure in young children. *Archives of Pediatrics and Adolescent Medicine, 163*(8), 724–730.

Mattson, M. P. (2008). Hormesis defined. *Ageing Research Reviews, 7*(1), 1–7.

Mattson, M., Maudsley, S., & Martin, B. (2004). BDNF and 5HT: a dynamic duo in age-related neuronal plasticity and neurodegenerative disorders. *Trends in Neurosciences, 27*(10), 589–594.

Miller, J., Kranzler, J., Liu, Y., Schmalfuss, I., Theriaque, D. W., Shuster, J. J., et al. (2006). Neurocognitive findings in Prader-Willi syndrome and early-onset morbid obesity. *The Journal of Pediatrics, 149*(2), 192.

Mora, F., Segovia, G., & del Arco, A. (2007). Aging, plasticity, and environmental enrichment: Structural changes and neurotransmitter dynamics in several areas of the brain. *Brain Research Reviews, 55*, 78–88.

Naperville Central Physical Education Program. (2008). Naperville Central Physical Education Department. Retrieved August 29, 2010, from http://www.ncusd203.org/central/html/what/physed/.

National Association for Sport and Physical Education (NASPE). (2004). *Moving into the future: National standards for physical education* (2nd ed.). Reston: McGraw Hill.

National Association of State Boards of Education (NASBE). (2010). *General school health policies.* Retrieved June 12, 2010, from http://nasbe.org/index.php/component/content/article/78-model-policies/118-general-school-health-policies.

Neel, J. V. (1962). Diabetes mellitus: a "thrifty" genotype rendered detrimental by "progress"? *American Journal of Human Genetics, 4*, 353–362.

Neel, J. V. (1999). The "thrifty genotype" in 1998. *Nutrition Review, 57*, S2–S9.

Nybo, L., & Secher, N. H. (2004). Cerebral perturbations provoked by prolonged exercise. *Progress in Neurobiology, 72*(4), 223–261.

Ornish, D. (2008, May 27). A plan for overweight kids. *Newsweek, 1.* Retrieved August 29, 2010, from http://www.newsweek.com/2008/05/26/a-plan-for-overweight-kids.html.

Owen, N., Bauman, A., & Brown, W. (2009). Too much sitting: a novel and important predictor of chronic disease risk? *British Journal of Sports Medicine, 43*, 81–83.

Panksepp, J. (2007). Can PLAY diminish ADHD and facilitate the construction of the social brain? *Journal of the Canadian Academy of Child and Adolescent Psychiatry, 16*, 57–66.

Panksepp, J. (2008). Play, ADHD, and the construction of the social brain: Should the first class each day be recess? *American Journal of Play, 1*, 55–79.

Panksepp, J., Burgdorf, J., Turner, C., & Gordon, N. (2003). Modeling ADHD-type arousal with unilateral frontal cortex damage in rats and beneficial effects of play therapy. *Brain and Cognition, 52*, 97–105.

Parfitt, G., & Eston, R. G. (2005). The relationship between children's habitual activity level and psychological well-being. *Acta Paediatrica, 94*, 1791–1797.

Pascopella, A. (2001, October 1). *TIMMS: Tired of criticism about your schools' math and science test scores? Find out how these U.S. schools are boosting their results.* The free library, District Administration (p. 1). Retrieved June 12, 2010, from http://www.thefreelibrary.com/TIMMS:+tired+of+criticism+about+your+schools%27+math+and+science+test...-a097117368.

PE4life. (2007). *Results.* Retrieved June 12, 2010, from http://www.pe4life.org/sub/Results/index.cfm.

Physical Activity Guidelines Advisory Committee. (2008). *Physical activity guidelines advisory committee report.* Washington, DC: U.S. Department of Health and Human Services.

Pilegaard, H., Saltin, B., & Neufer, P. D. (2003). Effect of short-term fasting and refeeding on transcriptional regulation of metabolic genes in human skeletal muscle. *Diabetes, 52*, 657–662.

Pontifex, M. B., Hillman, C. H., Fernhall, B., Thompson, K. M., & Valentini, T. A. (2009). The effect of acute aerobic and resistance exercise on working memory. *Medicine and Science in Sports and Exercise, 41*(4), 927–934.

Puhl, R. M., & Latner, J. D. (2007). Stigma, obesity, and the health of the nation's children. *Psychological Bulletin, 133*(4), 557–580.

Pytel, B. (2007, November 21). No more classroom chairs: Students are sitting on exercise balls. *Student Health Issues,* 1. Retrieved August 29, 2010, from http://student-health-issues.suite101.com/article.cfm/no_more_classroom_chairs.

Raji, C. A., Ho, A. J., & Parikshak, N. N. (2010). Brain structure and obesity. *Human Brain Mapping, 31*, 353–364.

Ratey, J., & Hagerman, E. *Spark: The Revolutionary New Science of Exercise and the Brain* Little Brown, January 2008.

Rideout, V.J., Foehrm, U.G., & Roberts, D.F. (2010, January). *Generation M2: Media in the lives of 8- to 18-year olds.* Washington, D.C.: Kaiser Family Foundation Study (p. 1). Retrieved August 29, 2010, from http://www.kff.org/entmedia/entmedia012010nr.cfm.

Sallis, J., McKensie, T. L., Kolody, B., Lewis, M., Marshall, S., Rosengard, P., et al. (1999). Effects of health related physical education on academic achievement: Project SPARK. *Research Quarterly for Exercise and Sport, 70*, 127–134.

Saulny, S. (2009). Students stand when called upon, and when not. *New York Times,* A1. Retrieved February 25, 2009.

Shaw, J. (2004, March–April). The deadliest sin. *Harvard Magazine,* 36–44.

Shephard, R. J. (1997). Curricular physical activity and academic performance. *Pediatric Exercise Science, 9*, 113–126.

Sibley, B. A., & Etnier, J. L. (2003). The relationship between physical activity and cognition in children: A meta-analysis. *Pediatric Exercise Science, 15*, 243–256.

Sigfusdottir, I. D., Kristjansson, A., & Allegrante, J. P. (2007). Health behaviour and academic achievement in Icelandic school children. *Health Education Research, 22*, 70–80.

Strong, W. B., Malina, R. M., Blimkie, C. J. R., Daniels, S. R., Dishman, R. K., Gutin, B., et al. (2005). Evidence based physical activity for school-age youth. *Journal of Pediatrics, 146*, 732–737.

Taras, H. (2005). Physical activity and student performance at school. *Journal of School Health, 75*, 214–218.

Texas Association of School Boards (TASB). (2010). *The fundamental role of public schools.* Retrieved June 12, 2010, from http://www.tasb.org/about/schools/role.aspx.

Tkacz, J., Young-Hyman, D. Y., & Boyle, C. A. (2008, November). Aerobic exercise program reduces anger expression among overweight children. *Pediatric Exercise Science, 20*(4), 390–401.

Trudeau, F., & Shephard, R. J. (2008). Physical education, school physical activity, school sports and academic performance. *International Journal of Behavioral Nutrition and Physical Activity, 5*(10), 1–12.

U.S. Department of Health and Human Services (USDHHS). (January. (2010). *The Surgeon General's vision for a healthy and fit nation*. Rockville: U.S. Department of Health and Human Services, Office of the Surgeon General.

U.S. Department of Health and Human Services (USDHHS). (November. (2000). *Healthy people 2010: With understanding and improving health and objectives for improving health* (2nd ed.). Washington: U.S. Government Printing Office.

van der Heijden, G. J., Toffolo, G., Manesso, E., Sauer, P. J. J., & Sunehag, A. L. (2009). Aerobic exercise increases peripheral and hepatic insulin sensitivity in sedentary adolescents. *The Journal of Clinical Endocrinology and Metabolism, 94*(11), 4292–4299.

Vaynman, S., & Gomez-Pinilla, F. (2006). Revenge of the "sit": how lifestyle impacts neuronal and cognitive health through molecular systems that interface energy metabolism with neuronal plasticity. *Journal of Neuroscience Research, 84*(4), 699–715.

Vaynman, S., Zhe, Y., & Fernando, G. P. (2004). Hippocampal BDNF mediates the efficacy of exercise on synaptic plasticity and cognition. *European Journal of Neuroscience, 20*, 2580–2590.

Viadero, D. (2008). Exercise seen as priming the pump for students' academic success. *Education Week, 27*, 14–15.

Walther, C., Machalica, K., Muller, U., & Schuler, G. (2009, November 17). Students with a lower socioeconomic background benefit from daily school physical activity. *American Heart Association, Abstract*. Retrieved August 29, 2010, from http://www.newsroom.heart.org/index.php?item=859&s=43.

Wechsler, H., McKenna, M.L., Lee, S.M., & Dietz, W.H. (2004, December 1–9). The role of schools in preventing childhood obesity. *The State Education Standard*. Retrieved August 8 29, 2010, from http://www.cdc.gov/HealthyYouth/physicalactivity/pdf/roleofschools_obesity.pdf.

Epilogue

Across a dozen chapters and several hundred manuscript pages, with what impressions are we left? Unquestionably, active living is essential to the human body and soul. In childhood it appears to serve both cognitive and social purposes. Childhood active living equates to play. Running, jumping, tumbling, and joyous unstructured activity seems crucial to the formation of neural pathways to promote intelligence and to nurture behaviors that will morph into the personality characteristics of empathy, cooperation, and understanding in later life.

Indeed, there is correlational evidence that young people's academic performance increases with physical activity. There is even the interesting suggestion that physical exercise might aid in development of frontal areas of the brain whose impoverishment appears linked to ADHD—a hypothesis worth examining. Despite this information and a disturbing rise in obesity and diabetes as the result of poor dietary choices and inactivity, the time devoted to physical exercise of any type among school children is declining. Moreover, a growing evidence base indicates that the sedentary lifestyle our children and youth experience each day (e.g., sitting at a desk, playing video games, staying inside) may be more harmful to them than a lack of rigorous physical exercise. Indeed, this generation of youth may be the first to experience a shorter life expectancy than their parents for reasons of poor health that are completely preventable.

The importance of active living does not diminish with age. In fact, the evidence grows more robust with time. Physical exercise seems to maintain an adult's cognitive executive control functions. It is a critical factor that can delay or even prevent diabetes and some types of heart disease. The connection between maintaining a healthy weight and exercise are well established, but less well known is that being overweight results in chemical changes in the brain that result in obese people having 8 % less brain tissue than lean adults.

Interestingly, this book documents that not all physical activity should be valued equally. For example, organized sports activity that places an emphasis on winning at all costs, putting the best team on the field at the expense of encouraging all to play, skill development of the few over the many, and cheating is counterproductive

A.L. Meyer and T.P. Gullotta (eds.), *Physical Activity Across the Lifespan*,
Issues in Children's and Families' Lives 12, DOI 10.1007/978-1-4614-3606-5,
© Springer Science+Business Media New York 2012

to the development of healthy contributing young members of our society. Teams with coaches that practice these behaviors are likely to cause distress and/or disengagement from activity within their members, reducing the number of youth who continue to be active in sports. Such experience can lead vulnerable youth to experience physical activity as aversive.

Only recently has attention been redirected to the neighborhoods in which we live and play. The great progressive parks movement at the beginning of the last century that established areas in cities to enable tenant dwellers to escape their stifling apartments fell into gradual disuse after the World War II exodus to the suburbs. In these new towns, community playgrounds were either the backyard swing set or the schoolyard and walking paths were the sides of the road. Wisely, town planners and local governments are demanding sidewalks in new developments and installing them in areas close to schools thus enabling children to walk rather than be bused to their education. The federal government has played an important role in encouraging these actions by using transportation funding to have curb cuts installed in sidewalks thus enabling those using wheelchairs increased freedom of mobility, bike paths and walking paths have also benefited from this enlightened decision. More attention needs to be paid to our older communities whose well-established park grounds suffer from inattention to care which in turn discourages their use by children and families.

Evidence supporting the use of physical activity for the treatment and prevention of obesity is positive. This is encouraging, given the data that 17 % of young people presently are considered obese and, if this trend remains unaltered, are expected to grow to 30 % by the year 2030. Evidence also suggests that developing the "habit" of active living needs to be encouraged early in life if sporadic episodes of gym membership (or use of the thigh master) are to be avoided.

Nearly as impressive is the use of active living in the prevention and management of depression. We know that for nearly everyone there are increases in brain chemicals like serotonin, norepinephrine, and dopamine connected to mood after exercising. As a preventive intervention, the importance of active living for adolescents should not be brushed aside. With a reoccurrence rate of 70 % after the first clinical depression, adolescents are at risk for this potentially crippling disorder. Further, preliminary evidence hints that ongoing physical activity encourages neurogenesis in the hippocampus area of the brain that is damaged by reoccurring depressions.

Finally, what do we know about active living and substance abuse? The short answer is not as much as we wished we did. While we have many more questions than answers, particularly as it relates to drug abuse prevention, we can offer some tantalizing tidbits of research for rumination. Physical exercise is helpful in enabling cigarette smokers to kick the habit. There is preliminary evidence that physical exercise is a useful adjunct to helping alcoholics become and stay sober. In these instances the new habit physical activity helps adults develop is that of intentional self-regulation, more commonly known as self-discipline. The ability to intentionally self-regulate one's urges enables the individual to calm oneself when tempted, ignore and tolerate desires to return to old behaviors, and choose to engage in healthy behaviors. While we know less about how physical activity can help children learn to self-regulate, the promise of that possibility is substantial.

We are excited about the application of active living to the problems of obesity, depression, and substance abuse. Rather than a new pill, the use of experiential interventions that utilize physically active approaches and promote the health of our children and the general public demands serious public and research attention. Given the existing evidence about the benefits of physical activity across multiple health behaviors and the ways that both work and play are becoming less and less active in recent times, we should strive to make our homes, schools, workplaces, and communities as settings where active living can be practiced daily.

Index